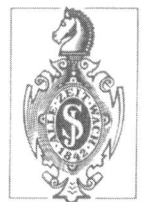

Receptor-Mediated Uptake in the Liver

Edited by
H. Greten E. Windler and U. Beisiegel

With 149 Figures and 18 Tables

Springer-Verlag Berlin Heidelberg GmbH

Prof. Dr. med. Heiner Greten
Priv.-Doz. Dr. med. Eberhard Windler
Dr. rer. physiol. Ulrike Beisiegel

Med. Kernklinik und Poliklinik
Universitätskrankenhaus Eppendorf
Martinistraße 52
D-2000 Hamburg 20

Intern. Symposion on Receptor-Mediated Uptake in the Liver
Hamburger Gastroenterologisches Symposium II
Hamburg, 8th — 10th May 1985
Chairmen: H. Greten and H.W. Schreiber

This symposium was part of the research programm "Function and defects of receptor systems" (Deutsche Forschungsgemeinschaft, Sonderforschungsbereich 232)

ISBN 978-3-540-16181-3   ISBN 978-3-642-70956-2 (eBook)
DOI 10.1007/978-3-642-70956-2

Originally published by Springer-Verlag Berlin Heidelberg New York Tokyo in 1986
Softcover reprint of the hardcover 1st edition 1986

2127/3140-543210

Preface

Cell surface receptors are multifunctional proteins with binding sites towards the external environment and effector sites which mediate intracellular events. The purpose of this symposium was to bring together investigators who have a common interest in those receptors which are located in the liver, and who have studied endocytic mechanisms for various macromolecules like insulin, lipoproteins, epidermal growth factor and others. Experiments in this particular field of research date back to the early 60-ies but have only recently led to new and important insight in the molecular basis of receptor mediated uptake in the liver. The structural features which control these mechanisms are currently under intense investigation in many laboratories. Though this symposium largely emphasizes lipoprotein uptake and catabolism by the liver, it was the particular intention of the organizers to discuss methodology and results with investigators who are also interested in hepatic uptake of macromolecules. This might then eventually lead to new and common concepts for both receptor-ligand interaction and internalization processes in the liver. Biochemists, pathologists and gastroenterologists met for two and a half days and discussed their latest data in this so rapidly developing field of basic research. This conference is part of a series on current topics in gastroenterology and hepatology arranged regularly by the Departments of Medicine and Surgery at the University Hospital Eppendorf. If is our hope, that such exchange of information between the different disciplines in medicine will continue.

H.W. Schreiber
Director,
Department of Surgery

H. Greten
Director,
Department of Medicine

Contents

Mechanisms of Uptake and Processing of Macromolecules by the Liver

R. J. HAVEL

Cardiovascular Research Institute and the Department of Medicine, University of California, San Francisco

The author's research was supported by the National Institutes of Health Grant HL 14237 Arteriosclerosis SCOR

This conference on receptor-mediated uptake in the liver brings together investigators who have studied endocytic mechanisms for a variety of macromolecules. A large emphasis has been placed on the plasma lipoproteins, which in mass terms probably contribute the most to these processes.

Some of the earliest evidence of receptor-mediated endocytosis in any system came from studies of the transport of lipids to the developing ovum. In a 1964 paper, Roth and Porter reported an elegant electron microscopic investigation of the uptake of vitellogenin (a lipoprotein) into the oocyte of the mosquito, Aedes aegypti [1]. They demonstrated clearly the role of coated pits in the endocytic event as well as the loss of the coat material from the endosome and the further processing of the contents to form yolk granules. Subsequent studies have shown that similar events occur in higher species (i. e., Perry and Gilbert's morphologic investigation of lipoprotein-endocytosis in hen oocytes [2] and the description by Paavola et al. of somewhat different lipoprotein processing in cultured granulosa cells of the rat [3]. The current biochemical era of investigation of receptor-mediated endocytosis was initiated by Brown and Goldstein's discovery of the low density lipoprotein (LDL) receptor in cultured human fibroblasts and their elucidation of the pathway within these cells which leads to degradation of LDL in lysosomes [4].

Although it has been appreciated for many years that the terminal catabolism of some mammalian plasma lipoproteins occurs predominantly in the liver, most detailed investigations of receptor-mediated processing of macromolecules in this organ until recently have been concerned with other plasma proteins and polypeptides. The most intensely studied have been the asialoglycoproteins, which are taken up with high efficiency into hepatic parenchymal cells via a specific receptor [5]. In addition, research on the processing of hormones of the endocrine and autocrine systems (i. e., insulin and epidermal growth factor) and of proteins that are secreted into the bile (immunoglobulin A) has intensified the interest in hepatic endocytic mechanisms [6]. During the past year, the structure of six receptors, all of which are active in the liver, has been determined by isolating and sequencing their complementary DNAs [7-12]. These achievements should make it possible soon to understand the molecular basis for ligand-binding, the localization of receptors or receptor-ligand complexes in coated pits, and some of the subsequent events, such as ligand receptor-dissociation and receptor-recycling.

The first detailed studies of receptor-mediated endocytosis of lipoproteins in the liver were facilitated by the discovery that administration of pharmacological

Receptor-Mediated Uptake
in the Liver
Edited by H. Greten, E. Windler, U. Beisiegel
© Springer-Verlag Berlin Heidelberg 1986

amounts of 17-α-ethinyl estradiol to rats induces a manyfold increase in the number of LDL receptors on the surface of hepatocytes and increases in comparable degree the uptake and catabolism of LDL by the liver *in vivo* [13-15]. From combined biochemical and morphological approaches, it was possible to show that the various steps of lipoprotein binding, internalization, movement to the Golgi-lysosomal region and lysosomal processing resemble closely those described for asialoglycoproteins in hepatic parenchymal cells [15, 16]. Recently, the same pathway has been demonstrated for remnants of chylomicrons and very low density lipoproteins (VLDL) which, in the rat, comprise the bulk of the lipoproteins that are endocytosed into hepatocytes [17]. Because of the large and continuous uptake of remnant lipoproteins, some of the steps of the endocytic pathway can be visualized directly: these particles (diameter 30-100 nm) can be stained and identified by transmission electron microsopy. Their presence in endosomes imparts a characteristic appearance to these structures that differs from that of most other cells in which few lipoproteins are taken up normally or in cultured cells in which no lipoproteins are present.

Before describing some of the steps of the pathway for lipoproteins in hepatocytes, I would like to point out that more than one receptor seems to participate in lipoprotein catabolism in the liver, and that processes other than receptor-mediated endocytosis may also participate in hepatic lipoprotein catabolism.

Experiments in a mutant rabbit that lacks LDL receptors (Watanabe heriditary hyperlipidemic [WHHL] rabbit) have provided persuasive evidence that LDL receptors are not necessary for efficient uptake of chylomicron remnants [18]. Uptake of chylomicrons into hepatic parenchymal cells in these animals seems to occur via endocytic vesicles, just as it does in normal rats [19]. Thus, a distinct chylomicron remnant receptor evidently participates in a classical receptor-mediated endocytic pathway through which these particles are catabolized in lysosomes. A third lipoprotein receptor, present mainly in sinusoidal endothelial cells and also in Kupffer cells, efficiently removes certain chemically modified lipoproteins, such as acetyl-LDL, from the blood [20-22]. The importance of this "scavenger" receptor for lipoprotein catabolism is uncertain because the extent to which lipoproteins are modified *in vivo* so as to permit them to be recognized are unknown. LDL and, presumably, VLDL remnants are also taken up into hepatic parenchymal cells of WHHL rabbits, albeit inefficiently [23]. Therefore, other processes, which remain to be defined, may normally participate in the hepatic catabolism of these particles. Binding sites for high density lipoprotein (HDL) have been found on isolated hepatocytes and membrane preparations from liver [24], and HDL components, particularly the major core lipids of HDL (cholesteryl esters) are taken up into the liver of normal rats [25]. This process may not involve endocytosis, however, because the rate of uptake of the cholesteryl esters substantially exceeds that of the major protein of HDL, apolipoprotein A-I [24, 26, 27].

Chylomicron remnants and VLDL remnants contain apolipoprotein E as well as apolipoprotein B and the former protein seems to be responsible for remnant binding to lipoprotein receptors [28]. As described elsewhere in this volume by Schneider, the LDL receptor, which is responsible for the uptake of VLDL remnants, has seven domains in its cysteine-rich NH$_2$-terminal region that could bind apolipoprotein E. It is known that particles containing several molecules of this protein can bind to multiple LDL receptor sites. It is possible, therefore, that remnant particles containing more than one molecule of apolipoprotein E can bind polyvalently to a single LDL receptor [29]. By contrast, LDL presumably bind to the receptor via a single site on apolipoprotein B. These differences are associated with large differences in binding affinity of the two particles. The affinity of VLDL remnants is much higher than that of LDL, presumably because these remnants bind polyvalently [30]. This difference in affinity seems to have major consequences for lipoprotein catabolism because VLDL remnants are removed from the blood within minutes, whereas LDL circulate for many hours. Presumably, the rapid removal of chylomicron remnants by the chylomicron remnant receptor also reflects the binding of multiple apolipoprotein E molecules on the remnant particles to binding sites on this receptor. The rapid catabolism of asialoglycoproteins also seems to be a function of polyvalent binding [5] to galactose residues, which comprise the recognition sites for the asialoglycoprotein receptor. A triantennary structure of the carbohydrate side chain, in which galactose residues are present at the termini, is required for high affinity binding.

In estradiol-treated rats, the initial binding of LDL to the surface of hepatocytes seems to occur mainly on the sinusoidal plasma membrane microvilli, rather than coated pits. This localization has been visualized with LDL-gold complexes by Handley and associates [31] and by Renaud, Hamilton, and me [32]. We found that these complexes are rapidly taken up into Kupffer cells in estradiol-treated rats. However, most of the uptake could be directed into parenchymal cells by blocking the Kupffer cell activity by prior injection of gadolinium chloride. Under these conditions, intravenously injected LDL-gold complexes were rapidly distributed along the microvilli and flat portions of the sinusoidal plasma membrane of parenchymal cells. This localization is consistent with that reported for the early association of asialoglycoproteins with parenchymal cells. This ligand is present initially over the sinusoidal cell surface, but is concentrated in coated pits [33].

These observations suggest that the ligand-receptor complexes move to coated pits after the binding event. The subsequent localization of LDL-gold complexes in endocytic organelles is consistent with that deduced from autoradiographic observations of radioiodinated LDL injected into estradiol-treated rats [15]. In particular, the LDL-gold complexes seem to be associated initially with the inner side of the membrane of endosomes lying near the cell surface; later they are dispersed within the contents of larger endosomal structures, including multivesicular bodies (MVBs), together with particles the size of VLDL and chylomicron remnants. MVBs contain most of the LDL-gold complexes 15 to 30 minutes after injection and are located near the Golgi apparatus in the bile canalicular pole of the cell. Subsequently, the gold particles are seen predominantly within secondary lysosomes in the same region. In experiments in which radioactive gold was used to prepare the LDL-gold complexes, we have observed a steady excretion of gold in the feces of the animal, beginning about three days after injection. By one month after injection, most of the gold taken up into the liver of these animals was excreted in this manner. This observation suggests that lysosomes may gradually deliver some of their contents into biliary canaliculi, but the mechanism of this process remains to be defined.

Additional aspects of the lipoprotein processing mechanism have been elucidated by examining certain properties of MVBs isolated from the liver of estradiol-treated rats [34]. The isolation procedure is described by Hamilton elsewhere in this volume, together with our evidence that MVBs contain endocytosed remnant lipoproteins whereas morphologically similar secretory vesicles of the Golgi apparatus contain nascent lipoproteins.

Remnant lipoproteins appear to fill the MVB compartments both within hepatocytes and in isolated MVBs, suggesting that the lipoproteins are not bound to membrane-associated receptors. However, at least some of them could be bound to the internal bilayer vesicles of the MVBs, several of which are present in each organelle. We have found LDL receptors in MVB fractions by ligand and immunoblotting procedures, and quantitative binding studies with radioiodinated LDL show that LDL receptors are concentrated in MVBs with respect to the homogenate from which they were derived [35]. MVBs contain two morphologically distinct appendages [34], at least one of which could contain uncoupled receptors, as described by Geuze and associates for asialoglycoprotein receptors in hepatocytes [36].

LDL dissociate from the LDL receptor under acidic conditions. MVB fractions contain an active proton pump, whose characteristics are indistinguishable from those of the proton pump of coated vesicles from rat liver [37]. Dissociation of the lipoprotein contents of MVBs from the LDL receptor should have occurred in the acidic environment of the organelle. Consistent with this observation, most of the lipoprotein contents of MVBs can be separated by ultracentrifugal flotation after simple rupture of the limiting membranes [34]. However, suramin, a polyanion that prevents binding of LDL to its receptor, dissociates virtually all of the lipoprotein contents of ruptured MVBs from the membrane of the organelle [35].

As described by Hamilton elsewhere in this volume, most MVBs in the liver and in purified subcellular fractions contain only trace amounts of lysosomal enzyme activity. However, in cytochemical studies we have obtained evidence for fusion of primary lysosomes with MVBs. From this and other evidence, we have concluded that MVBs constitute the immediate prelysosomal compartment of the endocytic pathway in hepatocytes. The ability to isolate MVBs in highly purified form should facilitate the investigation of a number of aspects of the processing of endocytosed macromolecules. Some of the proteins associated with MVB membranes undoubtedly have specific functions related to the acquisition of lysosomal enzymes. Some may serve as useful markers of the endosomal pathway, which could be used to develop reagents for isolation of other endosomal structures. It may be possible to isolate from MVBs their characteristic internal vesicles, the function of which remains unclear.

References

1. Roth TF, Porter KR (1964) J Cell Biol 20: 313-332
2. Perry MM, Gilbert AB (1984) J Cell Sci 39: 257-272
3. Paavola, LG Strauss, JF Boyd, CO Nestler, JE (1984) J Cell Biol 100: 125-1247
4. Brown MS, Anderson RGW, Goldstein JL (1983) Cell 32: 663-667

5. Schwartz AL (1984) CRC Critical Rev Biochem 16: 207-232
6. Jones AL, Renston RH, Burwen SJ (1982) In: Progress in Liver Diseases, Vol. VII (Popper H and Schaffner F eds.) Grune & Stratton, Inc., pp. 51-69
7. Yamamoto T, Davis CG, Brown MS, Schneider WJ, Casey ML et al. (1984) Cell 39: 27-38
8. Chiacchia KB, Drickamer K (1984) J Biol Chem 259: 15440-15446
9. Mostov KE, Friedlander M, Blobel G (1984) Nature 308: 37-43
10. Ullrich A, Coussent L, Hayflick JS, Dull TJ, Gray A et al. (1984) Nature 309: 418-425
11. Schneider C, Owen MJ, Banville D, Williams JG (1984) Nature 311: 675-678
12. Ullrich A, Bell JR, Chen EY, Herrera R, Petruzzelli LM et al. (1985) Nature 313: 756-761
13. Chao Y-s, Windler E, Chen CG, Havel RJ (1979) J Biol Chem 254: 11360-11366
14. Kovanen PT, Brown MS Goldstein JL (1979) J Biol Chem 245: 11367-11373
15. Chao, Y-s, Jones AL, Hradek GT, Windler EET, Havel RJ (1981) Proc Natl Acad Sci USA 78: 597-601
16. Hornick CA, Jones, AL Renaud G, Hradek G, Havel RJ (1984) Am J Physiol 256: G187-194
17. Jones AL, Hradek GT, Hornick CA, Renaud G, Windler EET, Havel RJ (1984) J Lipid Res 25: 1151-1158
18. Kita T, Goldstein JL, Brown MS, Watanabe Y, Hornick CA, Havel RJ (1982) Proc Natl Acad Sci USA 79: 3623-3627
19. Hamilton RL, Yamada N, Havel RJ Unpublished data
20. Blomhoff R, Helgerud P, Rasmussen M, Berg T, Norum DR (1982) Proc Natl Acad Sci USA 79: 7326-7330
21. Nagelkerke JF, Barto KS, van Berkel TJC (1983) J Biol Chem 258: 12221-12227
22. Pitas RE, Boyles J, Mahley RW, Bissell M (1985) J Cell Biol 100: 103-117
23. Pittman RC, Carrew TE, Attie AD, Witztum JL, Watanabe Y, Steinberg D (1982) J Biol Chem 257: 7994-8000
24. Havel RJ (1985) Methods in Enzymology. New York, NY: Academic Press, in press
25. van't Hooft FM, van Gent T, van Tol A (1981) Biochem J 196: 877-885
26. Glass CR, Pittman RC, Weinstein DB, Steinberg D (1983) Proc Natl Acad Sci USA 80: 5435-5439
27. Stein Y, Dabach Y, Hollander G, Halperin G, Stein O (1983) Biochim Biophys Acta 752: 98-105
28. Havel RJ (1985) Annu. Rev. Physiol. Palo Alto, CA: Annual Reviews, Inc., in press
29. Pitas RE, Innerarity TL, Mahley RW (1980) J Biol Chem 255: 5454-5460
30. Windler EET, Kovanen PT, Chao Y-s, Brown MS, Havel RJ, Goldstein JL (1980) J Biol Chem 255: 10464-10471
31. Handley DA, Arbeeny CM, Eder HA, Chien S (1981) J Cell Biol 90: 778-787
32. Renaud G, Hamilton RL, Havel RJ, Unpublished data
33. Wall DA, Hubbard AC (1981) J Cell Biol 90: 687
34. Hornick CA, Hamilton RL, Spaziani E, Enders GH, Havel RJ (1985) J Cell Biol 100: 1558-1569
35. Belcher J, Havel RJ Unpublished data
36. Geuze HJ, Slot JW, Strous JAM, Lodish HF, Schwartz AL (1983) Cell 32: 277-287
37. Van Dyke RW, Hornick CA, Belcher J, Scharschmidt BT, Havel RJ (1985) J Biol Chem 260: 11021-11026

The LDL Receptor — Structural Insights

W. J. SCHNEIDER

The University of Alberta, Edmonton, Canada

Introduction

Low density lipoprotein (LDL), the major cholesterol-carrying class of lipoproteins in human plasma, is taken up by hepatic and extrahepatic cells via receptor-mediated endocytosis. In this process, LDL particles bind to cell-surface receptors, the LDL receptors, which are localized in specialized regions of the plasma membrane called coated pits. Coated pits make up 2% of the surface area of a normal human fibroblast and are characteristic indentations displaying an electron-dense coat on their cytoplasmic side consisting mainly of a polypeptide called clathrin. After LDL has bound to LDL receptors, it is rapidly taken up into the cell through invagination and pinching-off of the coated pits to form coated vesicles containing the receptor-LDL complex. Along its intracellular route, in the endosome compartment, the complex dissociates; LDL is delivered to lysosomes where the particles are degraded, and unoccupied LDL receptors recycle back to the cell surface, ready to bind and internalize new LDL particles. Normal functions of the LDL receptor pathway is of great importance for cellular cholesterol homeostasis; the LDL-derived cholesterol exerts feedback-control on the level of the enzyme catalyzing the rate-limiting step in cellular cholesterol synthesis, 3-hydroxymethyl-glutaryl-CoA reductase, as well as on the number of LDL receptors, thereby protecting the cell from overaccumulation of cholesterol. In addition, the cholesterol derived from LDL is rapidly converted to cholesterylesters for storage in droplets via stimulation of acyl-CoA: cholesterol acyltransferase.

The LDL Receptor and Familial Hypercholesterolemia

The importance of this regulatory pathway at the physiological level is underscored by the dramatic consequences of mutations at the LDL receptor locus found in patients with the clinical phenotype of familial hypercholesterolemia (FH). FH is the most common single-gene mutation disease known occurring in the heterozygous state in about 0.2% of the general population. The frequency of patients that have inherited two mutant LDL receptor genes is 1 in 1 million. In these so-called homozygous FH patients, the complete absence of normal LDL receptors leads to accumulation of LDL cholesterol in the bloodstream to levels as high as 600% of normal; atherosclerosis and myocardial infarctions typically occur in childhood.

Receptor-Mediated Uptake
in the Liver
Edited by H. Greten, E. Windler, U. Beisiegel
© Springer-Verlag Berlin Heidelberg 1986

In an effort to understand the detailed molecular defects in the LDL receptor leading to FH, we have purified the receptor, obtained partial amino acid sequence of receptor fragments, and have used this information to clone a full-length cDNA for the human LDL receptor. The complete sequence of the 839 residue glycoprotein revealed 5 domains: First, an aminoterminal cysteine-rich domain of 292 residues containing the LDL binding site; second, a region of about 400 residues that shares 35% sequence homology with the precursor to mouse epidermal growth factor; third, a small domain of 42 residues, 18 of which are either Ser or Thr residues and containing a high number of carbohydrate chains in 0-linkage; fourth, 22 amino acids constituting the only membrane-spanning region of the LDL receptor; and fifth, the carboxyterminal cytosolic domain consisting of 50 residues.

Biosynthetic studies have revealed that the LDL receptor is first synthesized as a precursor molecule of apparent relative molecular mass (M_r) of 120,000 which undergoes rapid posttranslational processing of its N- and O-linked carbohydrate chains. About 60 minutes after initiation of synthesis, mature receptors with an apparent M_r of 160,000 appear on the cell surface. The characteristic increase in apparent M_r upon maturation of the receptor is due to the addition of galactose and sialic acid units to 18 N-acetylgalactosaminyl residues which are linked to the hydroxylgroups of Ser and Thr residues clustered in the third domain of the receptor.

Five Groups of LDL Receptor Mutations

When biosynthesis and posttranslational processing of LDL receptors expressed in fibroblasts from patients with homozygous FH were investigated, several groups of mutations could be distinguished. The first group is characterized by the absence of detectable (i. e., immunoprecipitable) receptor protein; the second group synthesizes receptor precursors of normal or abnormal M_r which fail to undergo posttranslational processing; in the third group, precursors of normal or abnormal M_r apparently contain normal signals for posttranslational processing and hence for transport to the cell surface; in the fourth group, such processing occurs, but at a greatly diminished rate; this kind of abnormality was found in the Watanabe heritable hyperlipidemic (WHHL) rabbit, an animal model for the human disease FH; the fifth group of mutant LDL receptors is functionally defined: cells from patients of this group are able to bind small amounts of LDL, but cannot internalize the lipoprotein. In this so-called internalization-defective form of FH, LDL receptors fail to cluster in coated pits due to mutations that alter or abolish the cytosolic receptor domain.

Internalization-Defective Familial Hypercholesterolemia: LDL Receptors Truncated at the Carboxyterminus

Through genomic cloning of the segments of DNA encoding the COOH-terminal regions of the LDL receptor derived from 4 individuals with the internalization-defective phenotype of FH, we were able to define the molecular defects in these mutant LDL receptors. In one patient, a point mutation has converted a Tyr to a Cys residue at a position 18 amino acids inside the plasma membrane. At least two other mutations have occurred causing drastic changes in the cytosolic domain of the LDL receptor: a frameshift mutation (insert of AGAA) at the codon for the sixth residue from the membrane, such that the new cytosolic tail of the receptor consists of 14 amino acids, 6 of which are normal and 8 new ones; and a nonsense mutation changing the codon for a Trp residue (at the position of the third amino acid on the cytoplasmic side of the plasma membrane) into a termination signal. In all of these mutant receptors, a membrane spanning region is maintained but the cytosolic domain is altered. Thus, these receptors are anchored in the plasma membrane but due to their altered cytoplasmic structure lack the ability to cluster in coated pits and cannot internalize LDL.

In one case of internalization-defective FH, there is a 5 kb deletion mutation in the DNA, and as a consequence, not only is the cytosolic portion of the receptor missing altogether, but the deletion has also obliterated the membrane spanning region as well as a small part of the region just outside the plasma membrane. The truncated receptors specified by this mutant allele are secreted into the extracellular environment. A small portion of these receptors for reasons yet unknown, however, adhere to the outside of the cell where they apparently are able to bind small amounts of LDL, thus leading to the internalization-defective phenotype.

Conclusion and Outlook

Molecular analysis of LDL receptor mutations occurring in FH has provided us with substantial insights into structure-function relationships of the normal LDL receptor molecule. It is clear from these studies that even a small change in the cytoplasmic domain of the receptor (consisting of only 50 amino acids) can destroy the receptor's important function to cluster in coated pits and bring about FH. By analysis in the fashion outlined here of mutant receptors in any of the four remaining groups of mutant LDL receptors, we hope to learn about the importance of other receptor regions for normal function.

Partial Purification and Characterization of Hepatic Low Density Lipoprotein (LDL) Receptor from Rabbit Liver

E. GHERARDI and D. E. BOWYER

Department of Pathology, University of Cambridge, Tennis Court Road, CB2 1QP Cambridge, U.K.

Introduction

The presence in liver cells of a membrane receptor for LDL similar to the one described in extrahepatic cells has been originally demonstrated by binding experiments to liver membranes [1-5] and isolated hepatocytes [6]. Further evidence indicating the presence of LDL receptors in liver cells has come from *in vivo* experiments in which the uptake of LDL [7-10] or anti-receptor antibodies [11] has been studied. These experiments indicated that liver plays the major role in receptor-mediated clearance of LDL from plasma.

Purification of the LDL receptor has been obtained by W. Schneider and co-workes from bovine adrenal glands, the tissue which exhibits the highest receptor specific activity. The receptor has been found to be an acidic glycoprotein of 164 kdaltons containing approximately 10 kdaltons of carbohydrates per mole of protein [12].

We report here a 500-570 fold purification of hepatic LDL receptor from rabbit liver and its preliminary characterization. Hepatic LDL receptor copurifies with a membrane fraction enriched in sinusoidal plasma membranes and Golgi membranes. It has a Mr of 120-125 kdaltons and a pI < 5.0. The protein appears to be indistinguishable by all criteria used from the LDL receptor of plasma membrane of cultured rabbit fibroblasts [13].

Materials and methods

Animals and Treatment

Male adult (2.0-2.5 kg) New Zealand Rabbits were used in this study. Rabbits were fed a standard diet and received 7 subcutaneous injections of 17-alpha-ethynyl estradiol (5 mg/kg). Blood samples were obtained before and after treatment after overnight fasting.

Receptor-Mediated Uptake
in the Liver
Edited by H. Greten, E. Windler, U. Beisiegel
© Springer-Verlag Berlin Heidelberg 1986

Liver Fractionation

Liver was obtained after rabbits were killed by intravenous injection of sodium pentabarbitone (150 mg/kg), washed in ice-cold 0.05 M Tris-maleate, 0.15 M NaCl, 0.002 M $CaCl_2$, 0.001 M PMSF and homogenized in the same buffer using a Polytron homogenizer (maximum setting, 15 + 15 seconds) at a concentration of 175 g of wet tissue/litre. Homogenate was centrifuged at 4 °C in a Sorvall SS34 rotor at 1,000 g for 10 minutes and supernatant centrifuged at 14,000 g for 10 minutes. The 14,000 g supernatant was centrifuged at 104,000 g for 60 minutes. For sucrose density centrifugation of 14,000-104,000 g membranes, 20-25 mg of membrane protein were resuspended in 1.5 ml of 2.1 M sucrose in 0.01 Tris-maleate, 0.002 M $CaCl_2$, 0.001 M PMSF, pH 7.0. Membrane proteins were overlayered with 2.0 ml of 1.15 M sucrose and 1.5 ml of 0.25 M sucrose and centrifuged at 75,000 g for 4 hours at 4 hours. 0.25 ml fractions were collected and assayed for protein and receptor activity (see below).

Assays of LDL Receptor

LDL receptor activity of membrane fractions was assayed according to Kovanen et al. [1]. Soluble LDL receptor was assayed as in Schneider et al. [14]. In both assays LDL receptor activity was measured as the difference between binding of LDL to membrane proteins in the presence of 0.002 M $CaCl_2$ and in the presence of 0.01 M EDTA. Ligand blotting of the LDL receptor was performed following separation of membrane proteins by polyacrylamide gel electrophoresis in the presence of sodium dodecyl sulphate [15] and electrophoretic transfer to nitrocellulose. Nitrocellulose strips were incubated of with human LDL (5 ug/ml) in phosphate buffered saline containing 0.002 M $CaCl_2$ followed by incubation with anti-human LDL rabbit Ig G (5 ug/ml) and peroxidase — conjugated anti — rabbit Ig G. Peroxidase was detected by incubation with 0.003 M alpha-chloro naphthol and 0.005 M H_2O_2.

DEAE-Sephacel and LDL-Sepharose Chromatography of Soluble 14,000-104,000 g Proteins

14,000-104,000 g membrane proteins (4-6 mg/ml) were solubilised in 0.05 M Tris-maleate, 0.05 M NaCl, 0.002 M $CaCl_2$, 0.001 M PMSF, pH 6.5 containing 10 g/l Triton X-100 for 30 minutes at 4° C. Insoluble material was removed by centrifugation (104,000 g for 60 minutes) and supernatant applied to a DEAE-Sephacel column equilibrated in the same buffer. Bound proteins were eluted with a gradient of NaCl (0.05-0.35 M) in 0.03 M octyl-D-glucoside, dialysed against 500 volumes of detergent — free buffer (4 buffer changes) and applied to an LDL — Sepharose column equilibrated with 0.05 M Tris-Cl, 0.05 M NaCl, 0.002 M $CaCl_2$, pH 8.0. Bound proteins were eluted with 0.0035 M sodium suramin in 0.05 M Tris-maleate, pH 6.0 [12].

Other Assays

Protein on membrane fractions and total liver homogenate was measured according to [16]. LDL apolipoprotein B in serum was measured by rocket immunoelec-
trophoresis using a sheep anti — rabbit apolipoprotein B antiserum following separation of LDL from triacylglycerol — rich lipoproteins on a Sepharose 6B column (1.5 x 50 cm).

Results

Induction of Hepatic LDL Receptor

Since the specific activity of LDL receptor in liver membranes is substantially lower than in adrenal membranes we attempted to increase it by administration of
17-alpha-ethynyl estradiol, which has been found very effective in increasing hepatic LDL receptor activity in rats [17]. The hormone induced a 1.5 to 2.0 fold increase in receptor binding of ^{125}I-LDL to liver membranes and a 50% drop in the
concentration of serum LDL apolipoprotein B.

*Fractionation of Liver Homogenate and Distribution of LDL Receptor Activity
among Subcellular Fractions*

Liver homogenate was fractionated as indicated in Materials and Methods and LDL
receptor activity in the three major membrane fraction ($<$ 1,000 g; 1,000-14,000 g
and 14,000-104,000 g) measured by binding of ^{125}I-LDL to membranes as well by
receptor blotting. LDL receptor was present in all three membrane fractions the
highest specific activity being associated with the 14,000-104,000 g fraction. No receptor activity was found in the 104,000 g supernatant by receptor blotting experiments. The 14,000-104,000 g fraction was then used for further studies and sub-
fractionated by sucrose gradient centrifugation into a "heavy" (rich in endoplasmic reticulum membranes) and "light" (rich in sinusoidal plasma membranes and
Golgi membranes) fractions (Fig. 1a). LDL receptor was associated with both fractions although receptor specific activity in the sinusoidal plasma membranes was
markedly higher than in the endoplasmic reticulum membranes (Fig. 1b).

Partial Purification of LDL Receptor from 14,000-104,000 g Membranes

A partial purification of the LDL receptor from the 14,000-104,000 g membrane
pellet was achieved using a combination of DEAE and LDL-Sepharose column
chromatography [12]. When 14,000-104,000 g membrane proteins were solubilised
in Triton X-100 and applied to DEAE-Sephacel at pH 6.5 10 to 15% of the protein
was retained by the column and eluted with a linear gradient of NaCl (Fig. 2a, lane c).
The bulk of the LDL receptor eluted in the bound fractions as shown by binding
assay and receptor blotting (Fig. 2b). Following removal of the detergent proteins

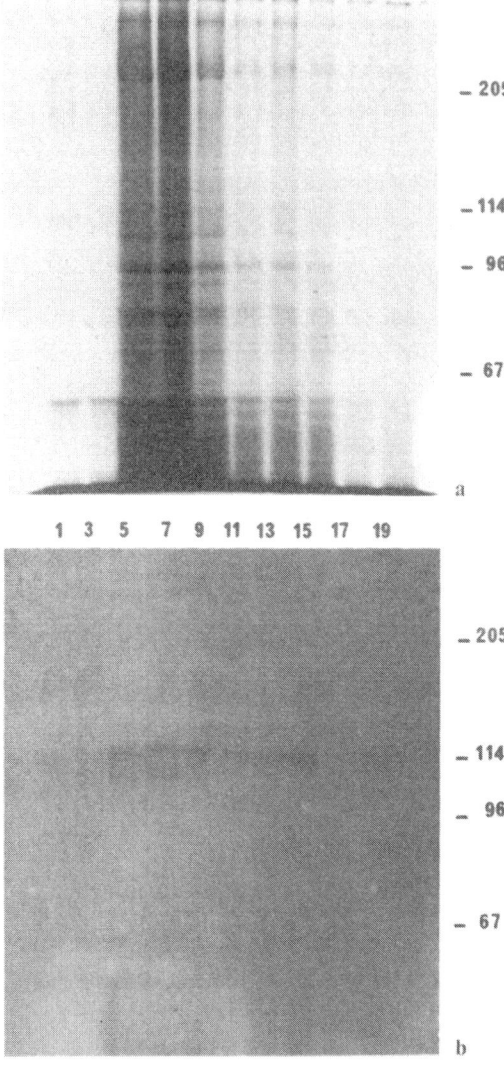

Fig. 1. Sucrose density gradient centrifugation of 14,000-104,000 g membranes. 25 mg of 14,000-104,000 g membrane protein were separated on a discontinuous sucrose gradient into "heavy" (endoplasmic reticulum membranes, fractions 4-11) and "light" (sinusoidal plasma membranes and Golgi membranes, fractions 13-15) fractions in a SW 50.1 rotor. 50 ul aliquots of each fraction were used for polyacrylamide gel electrophoresis (Fig. 1a) and for receptor blotting (Fig. 1b). Numbers at the top of the figures indicate the fraction number. Molecular weight markers are indicated

bound to DEAE were applied to an LDL-Sepharose column and bound proteins eluted with 0.0035 M sodium suramin, pH 6.0. LDL receptor was recovered in the bound fraction (Fig. 2b) at 15-20% purity (Fig. 2a).

Discussion

We have reported here a partial purification of hepatic LDL receptor from rabbit liver. The purification achieved after DEAE-Sephacel and LDL-Sepharose column

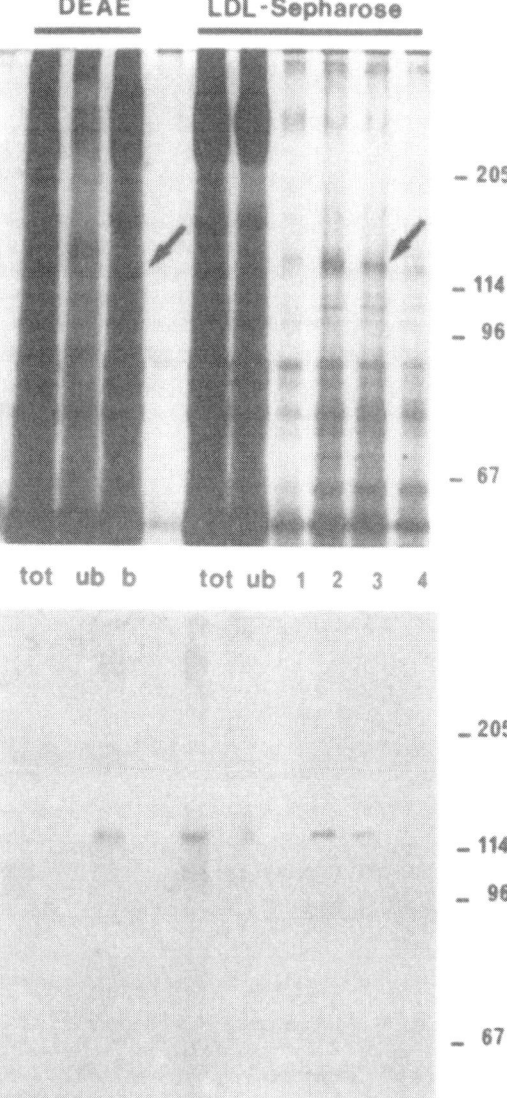

Fig. 2. Partial Purification of LDL Receptor from 14,000-104,000 g Membranes. 14,000-104,000 g membrane proteins were solubilised in the presence of 10 g/l Triton X-100 and applied to a DEAE-Sephacel column at pH 6.5 (Fig. 2a, tot). The unbound fraction was collected as a single pool Fig. 2a, ub). Bound proteins were eluted with a NaCl gradient in 0.03 M octyl-D-glucoside (Fig. 2a, b). LDL receptor was eluted in the bound fraction which was pooled, dialysed for 36 hours against detergent-free buffer and applied to a 3 ml LDL-Sepharose column (5.5 mg LDL protein/ml of gel). Bound proteins (Fig. 2a, lanes 1-4) were eluted at pH 6.0 in the presence of 0.0035 M sodium suramin. Fig. 2b is a receptor blotting of the same fractions shown in Fig. 2a. Molecular weight markers are indicated as for Fig. 1

chromatography has been in the order of 500-750 fold compared to liver homogenate and yielded a preparation containing approximately 15-20% receptor as judged by densitometric scanning of the gel. This indicates the purification to homogeneity of LDL receptor from the liver of rabbits treated with 17-alpha-ethynyl estradiol requires a purification factor of 3,000-4,000. This figure is much greater than required for the purification of LDL receptor from bovine adrenal glands [12] and closely agrees with previous estimates of LDL receptor specific activity in the two tissues [5, 11, 18, 19]. As a result the two step purification procedure used in this study, which is quite similar to the one used by Schneider and coworkers for the purification of the receptor from adrenal glands, has provided a partial purification of the protein. Purification to homogeneity will probably require an additional step such as an anti — receptor antibody column or a lectin column. Work on these lines is now in progress.

The molecular weight and isoelectric point of hepatic LDL receptor are identical with those of the receptor of rabbit fibroblasts in culture. The latter can be labelled on the cell surface by lactoperoxidase — catalysed iodination and immunoprecipitated with anti — LDL antibodies following binding of the receptor to LDL [13]. Furthermore, binding of hepatic receptor to LDL is dependent upon the presence of $CaCl_2$ in the medium and is abolished by reductive methylation of LDL as shown for the LDL receptor of peripheral cells.

Hepatic LDL receptor is responsible for the uptake and catabolism of the vast majority of plasma LDL in several animal species [7-10] and probably in man and thus regulates LDL levels in plasma. It may also be important for the clearance of IDL although the apo E receptor [20] may be involved in this process as well. The latter receptor has now been partially purified and characterized by Mahley and coworkers and it will soon be possible to study the mechanisms which regulate the expression of the two lipoprotein receptors in liver cells. This would certainly contribute to understand the way in which the concentration of plasma lipoproteins (especially those which are atherogenic) is ultimately controlled.

Acknowledgements. This work has been supported by a Grant of British Heart Foundation and by a Grant in Aid of Science Research Council of Italy.

References

1. Kovanen PT, Brown MS, Goldstein JL (1979) J Biol Chem 254: 11367
2. Bachorik, PS, Kwitevorich PO, Cooke JC (1978) Biochemistry 17: 5287
3. Kovanen PT, Bilheimer DW, Goldstein JL, Jaramillo JJ, Brown MS (1981) Proc Natl Acad Sci 78: 1194
4. Kovanen PT, Brown MS, Basu SK, Bilheimer DW, Goldstein JL (1981) Proc Natl Acad Sci 78: 1396
5. Kita T, Brown MS, Watanabe Y, Goldstein JL (1981) Proc Natl Acad Sci 78: 2268
6. Soltys PA, Portman OW (1979) Biochim Biophys Acta 574: 505
7. Slater HR, Packard CJ, Bicker S, Sheperd J (1982) J Biol Chem 255: 10210
8. Pittman RC, Attie AD, Carew TE, Steinberg D (1982) Biochim Biophys Acta 710: 7
9. Spady DK, Bilheimer DW, Dietschy JM (1983) Proc Natl Acad Sci 80: 3499
10. Pittman RC, Attie AD, Carew TE, Steinberg D (1979) Proc Natl Acad Sci 76: 5345
11. Huettinger M, Schneider WJ, Ho YK, Goldstein JL, Brown MS (1984) J Clin Invest 74: 1017
12. Schneider WJ, Beisiegel U, Goldstein JL, Brown MS (1982) J Biol Chem 257: 2664
13. Gherardi E, Bowyer DE (1985) manuscript in preparation
14. Schneider WJ, Goldstein JL, Brown MS (1980) J Biol Chem 255: 11442
15. Laemmli UK (1970) Nature 2276: 680
16. Markwell MAK, Haas SM, Bieber LL, Tolbert NE (1978) Anal Biochem 87: 206
17. Windler ET, Kovanen PT, Chao Ys, Brown MS, Havel RJ, Goldstein JL (1980) J Biol Chem 255: 10464
18. Brown MS, Kovanen PT, Goldstein JL (1979) Recent Prog Horm Res 35: 215
19. Russell DW, Yamamoto T, Schneider WJ, Slaughter CJ, Brown MS, Goldstein JL (1983) Proc Natl Acad Sci 80: 7501
20. Mahley RW, Hui DY, Innerarity TL, Weisgraber KH (1981) J Clin Invest 68: 1197

DNA Polymorphisms of the Low Density Lipoprotein (LDL) Receptor Gene

B. HORSTHEMKE, ANNA M. KESSLING, R. WILLIAMSON, and ST. E. HUMPHRIES

Department of Biochemistry, St. Mary's Hospital Medical School, Norfolk Place, London W2 1PG, UK

Summary

We have used a cloned cDNA probe for the human LDL receptor to look for gross alterations in the LDL receptor gene of patients with Familial Hypercholesterolaemia (FH). Among the genes of 60 UK patients analysed to date, we have identified one defective allele which seems to result from a 2 kb deletion in the 3' part of the gene. Presymptomatic diagnosis based on DNA analysis will thus be possible in this particular family. The cDNA probe also detects a common restriction fragment length polymorphism (RFLP) with the enzyme PvuII. The variable PvuII site appears to be within an intervening sequence in the 3' part of the gene. The rare allele frequency of this polymorphism in both the normolipidaemic population (n = 63) and for patients with heterozygous Familial Hypercholesterolaemia (FH) (n = 36) is 0.2. 30% of individuals are heterozygous for the polymorphism and potentially informative for familiy studies and early diagnosis of FH based on genetic linkage analysis.

Introduction

Over the last years it has been shown by Brown, Goldstein and coworkers that mutations in the low density lipoprotein (LDL) receptor gene have a causal role in Familial Hypercholesterolaemia (FH) [1, 2]. This disaese is characterised in the heterozygote by high levels of serum and LDL cholesterol, tendon xanthomata in some cases, and increased risk of myocardial infarction after the age of thirty-five years [3, 4]. The rare homozygotes seldom survive for more than twenty-five years. With an allele frequency of about 0.002 [5], FH contributes significantly to the number of individuals suffering from coronary arterial disease. If individuals with FH could be identified before they developed elevated cholesterol levels, they could be treated prophylactically to reduce their future risk of myocardial infarction. To date, however, the disease cannot always be diagnosed unequivocally in early childhood.

The cloning of human LDL receptor cDNA [6] has now made it possible to analyse the defects at the DNA level. The present communication describes the identification of a deletion in the LDL receptor gene from a FH patient and a neutral restriction fragment length polymorphism (RFLP), which can be used for presymptomatic diagnosis.

Receptor-Mediated Uptake
in the Liver
Edited by H. Greten, E. Windler, U. Beisiegel
© Springer-Verlag Berlin Heidelberg 1986

DNA rearrangements

In order to identify gross alterations in the LDL receptor gene we have digested DNA samples from 55 unrelated heterozygous and 5 homozygous FH patients (= 65 defective genes) with XbaI and probed with the LDL receptor cDNA. The probe hybridises to fragments of 23 kb, 10 kb, 6.6 kb and 1.7 kb from the normal gene and thus covers about four fifths of the 50 kb gene [7]. Only one sample showed an abnormal pattern (see Fig. 1). Preliminary mapping experiments indicate that the abnormal 8.0 kb band in patient T.D. is derived from the 10 kb fragment by a deletion of 2 kb. The deletion cosegregates with the FH phenotype in the family of this patient (Fig. 2). This finding is compatible with the deletion being the

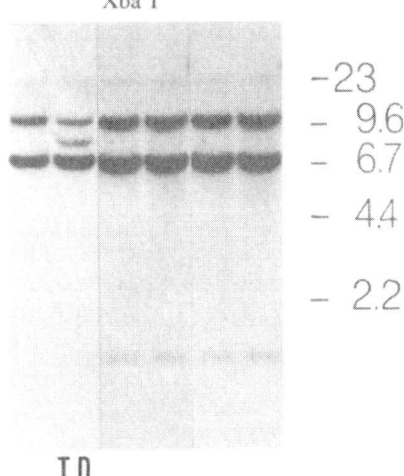

Fig. 1. Genomic Southern blot analysis of the LDL receptor gene in FH patients. Six samples are shown. 5 µg of DNA was digested with XbaI, size fractionated on an agarose gel, transferred to filter membranes and hybridised with the radioactively labelled LDL receptor probe as described [9]. The probe was a kind gift of Dr. D.W. Russel and consists of a 1.9 kb fragment (base pairs 1573-3486) of the 3' part of the LDL receptor cDNA. The size markers were derived from a HindIII digest of λ DNA

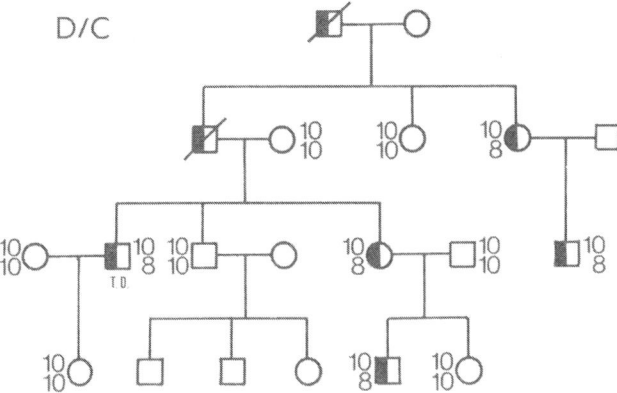

Fig. 2. Segregation of deletion and FH phenotype in the D/C familiy. Symbols used are: normal male and female □ ○
FH male and female (heterozygous) ◨ ◑
individual deceased ⊠ ⊘
"10" denotes the normal 10 kb XbaI fragment and "8" the abnormal 8 kb fragment

underlying defect of the disease in this case. Presymptomatic diagnosis based on DNA analysis will thus be possible in this particular family. A deletion of 5 kb in the LDL receptor gene of another FH patient has recently been reported by Lehrman et al. [7]. Although our screening method would not identify small deletions or insertions, the results suggest that the majority of defects in the LDL receptor gene are due to point mutations. Presymptomatic diagnosis in these cases could be based on genetic linkage analysis using restriction fragment length polymorphisms.

Neutral DNA polymorphisms

In order to find RFLPs in or adjacent to the LDL receptor gene, DNA samples from 9 unrelated normolipidaemic individuals were digested with ten different restriction enzymes and analysed by Southern blot hybridisation with a cDNA probe for the human LDL receptor gene. A variation in the patterns of bands among the individuals was observed only in digests using the restriction enzyme PvuII (see Fig. 3a). We interpret these patterns as being the products of two alleles, which we designate V1 (19 kb + 4.8 kb fragments) and V2 (16 kb + 4.8 kb + 2.6 kb). Individuals showing all four fragments are heterozygous for the polymorphism

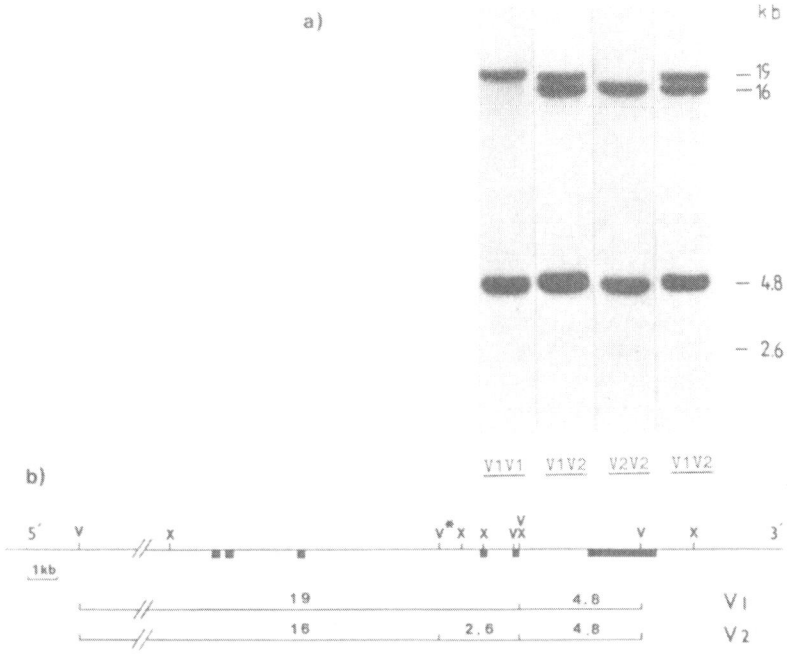

Fig. 3. The DNA polymorphism detected with the LDL receptor probe. A) 5 μg of DNA were digested with PvuII and analysed as described in [10]; B) Map of the LDL receptor gene showing the variable PvuII-Site marked as V* and the DNA fragments detected in Southern blot hybridisations of PvuII digests. The map was derived from [7] and the double digests mentioned in the text. The shaded boxes represent exons

S
―

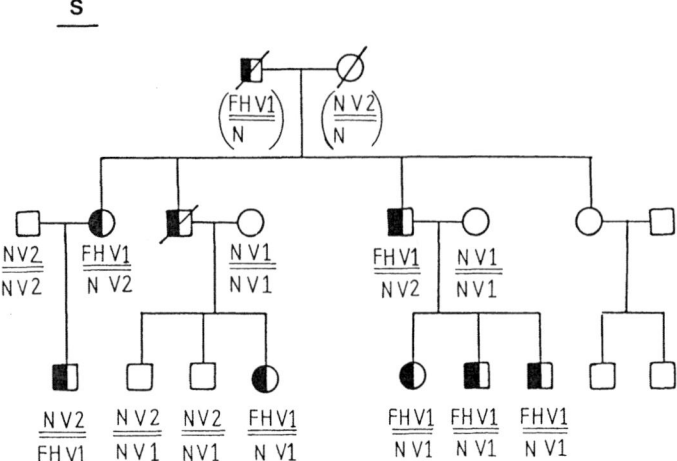

Fig. 4. Segregation of FH-phenotype and the PvuII-RFLP in a FH family. Symbols are explained in the legend to Fig. 2. N, normal

and designated *V1V2*. Double digests of DNA samples from a *V1V1*, a *V1V2* and a *V2V2* individual with PvuII and other enzymes indicate that the polymohrpism is due to the absence *(V1)* or presence *(V2)* of a PvuII site within an intervening sequence of the 3' end of the gene (Figure 3b). The rare allele frequency of this RFLP in both the normolipidaemic population (n = 63) and for patients with heterozygous FH (n = 36) is 0.2. The distribution of genotypes is close to the expected value if the population is in Hardy-Weinberg-equilibrium, and there is no apparent strong linkage disequilibrium of either allele with the LDL receptor mutations in our FH population. Approximately 30% of individuals are heterozygous for the polymorphism and potentially informative for family studies and presymptomatic diagnosis of FH. Figure 4 shows one FH family, in which the FH phenotype cosegregates with the *V1* allele.

To detect more RFLPs we have used the cDNA probe to screen a genomic library which was constructed by cloning 15-20 kb genomic DNA fragments from a partial Sau3AI digest into the BamHI site of λL47.1 (Horsthemke et al., in preparation). Several recombinants containing genomic DNA downstream of the LDL receptor gene have been isolated. Single copy sequences in these recombinants have been subcloned and are being used as probes to detect RFLPs downstream of the LDL receptor gene. 5' cDNA and single copy sequences upstream of the gene will be used in a similar way for the RFLP search. We hope that this approach will provide us with the 3-4 common RFLPs necessary to have informative genetic markers for early diagnosis in virtually all FH families.

Conclusions

We have identified a deletion and a neutral DNA polymorphism in the LDL receptor gene. Within the near future more RFLPs will be available allowing presymptomatic diagnosis in virtually all FH families. Affected children could then be treated prophylactically and encouraged from an early age to live on a low saturated fat diet, take physical exercise and not start smoking. The recent results of the Primary Coronary Prevention Study offer the hope that early therapeutic intervention will effectively lower the risk of developing premature atherosclerosis [8].

Acknowledgements. This work was supported by grants of the British Heart Foundation (RG5) and the MRC. B. Horsthemke is in receipt of an EMBO long term fellowship.

The authors would like to thank Drs. D. W. Russel, M. Brown and J. Goldstein for supplying the LDL receptor probe and Joy Dexter and Pauline McAree for help in preparing the manuscript.

References

1. Brown MS, Goldstein JL (1974) Expression of the familial hypercholesterolaemia gene in heterozygotes — Mechanism for a dominant disorder in man. Science 185: 61-63
2. Brown MS, Goldstein JL (1974) Familial hypercholesterolaemia — Defective binding of lipoproteins to cultured fibroblasts associated with impaired regulation of 3-hydroxy-3-methyglutaryl Coenzyme A reductase activity. Proc Natl Acad Sci USA 71: 788-792
3. Harlan WR, Graham JB, Estes EH (1966) Familial hypercholesterolaemia, a genetic and metabolic study, Medicine (Baltimore); 45: 77-110
4. Goldstein JL, Schrott HG, Hazzard WR, Bierman EL and Motulsky AG (1973) Hyperlipidaemia in coronary heart disease, Part 2, (Genetic analysis of lipid levels in 176 families and delineation of a new inherited disorder, combined hyperlipidaemia). J Clin Invest 52: 1544-1568
5. Fredrickson DS, Goldstein JL, Brown MS (1978) The familial hyperlipoproteinanaemias. In: Stanbury JB, Wyngaarden JB, Fredrickson DS (eds) The Metabolic Basis of Inherited Disease, McGraw-Hill, New York, p. 604-655
6. Yamamoto T, Davis LG, Brown MS, Schneider WJ, Casey ML, Goldstein JL, Russell DW (1984) The human LDL receptor: a cysteine-rich protein with multiple Alu sequences in its mRNA. Cell 39: 27-38
7. Lehrman MA, Schneider WJ, Sudhof TC, Brown MS, Goldstein JL, Russell DW (1985) Mutations in LDL receptor: Alu-Alu recombination deletes exons encoding transmembrane and cytoplasmic domains. Science 227: 140-146
8. Lipid Research Clinics Program. The Lipid Research Clinics Coronary Primary Prevention Trial Results. II The Relationship of Reduction in Incidence of Coronary Heart Disease to Cholesterol Lowering. JAMA 1984; 251: 356-374
9. Horsthemke B, Kessling AM, Seed M, Wynn V, Williamson R, Humphries SE. Indentification of a Deletion in the Low Density Lipoprotein (LDL) Receptor Gene in a Patient with Familial Hypercholesterolaemia. Human Genet.; *in press*
10. Humphries SE, Kessling AM, Horsthemke B, Donald JA, Seed M, Jowett N, Holm M, Galton DJ, Wynn V, Williamson R (1985) A Common DNA Polymorphism of the Low Density Lipoprotein (LDL) Receptor Gene and its Use in Diagnosis. Lancet; *in press*.

LDL-Binding to Human Liver Plasma Membranes

G. RENAUD, JACQUELINE MARAIS, and R. INFANTE

INSERM U.9, Hôpital Saint-Antoine, 184, rue du Fg Saint-Antoine 75571 Paris F

Introduction

Among the circulating lipoproteins, low density lipoproteins (LDL) have been shown to be the most atherogenic. In peripheral cells (fibroblasts, endothelial cells, monocytes) LDL binding followed by their uptake and degradation plays and important role in the regulation of cholesterol homeostasis. Since the pioneering work of Goldstein and Brown demonstrating the existence of a specific receptor for LDL on the surface of human fibroblasts [1] and its partial or total defect in familial hypercholesterolemia, a variety of cell types have been shown to possess LDL receptors.

In swine, rat and rabbit, the liver is the most active organ involved in LDL catabolism and second to the adrenals when this activity is expressed per unit weight [2]. In these species, studies performed with hepatocytes in primary culture revealed the existence of specific receptors for LDL on the cell surface [3-5]. Recently, the LDL receptor has been purified from bovine adrenals [6] and its cDNA has been cloned [7].

In the human, however, the existence of such receptors at the surface of the hepatocytes is not firmly established. Human hepatoma cell line Hep G2 possess LDL receptors which are subject to down regulation when the cells are exposed to high LDL concentrations [8-11]. Studies lead with normal human liver biopsies are sometimes controversial: Mahley et al. could not find any LDL binding on hepatic membranes isolated from human liver as they observed in immature dog and swine [12]. On the contrary, Harders-Spengel et al. found that LDL binding to human hepatic membranes is EDTA sensitive and decreases in familial hypercholesterolemic patients [13]. Hoeg et al. observed an EDTA sensitive and saturable LDL binding on liver human liver membranes at 37° C but not at 0° C [14]. This binding was sharply decreased when membranes from hypercholesterolemic patients were used. Chylomicron remnants and intermediate density lipoproteins (IDL) bind to human liver membranes through a calcium dependent mechanism, but no saturable component could be demonstrated for IDL [15].

Finally, specific apoprotein-B binding to hepatic membranes is increased in abetalipoproteinemia and increases after portocaval shunt in familial hypercholesterolemic patients [16].

In this study, we show some characteristics of LDL binding to hepatic membranes isolated from normocholesterolemic adults.

Receptor-Mediated Uptake
in the Liver
Edited by H. Greten, E. Windler, U. Beisiegel
© Springer-Verlag Berlin Heidelberg 1986

Materials and Methods

Patients

Human livers were obtained from normocholesterolemic (69-155 mg/dl), organ donors during renal transplantation.

Isolation, modification and labeling of lipoproteins

Human blood was obtained from human donors. After addition of EDTA (0.02%), sodium azide (0.02%) and gentamicin sulfate (5 mg/dl) to the serum, VLDL (d < 1.006), LDL (1.025 < d < 1.050) and HDL (d < 1.21) were isolated by differential ultracentrifugation [17]. Each lipoprotein class was purified by a second centrifugation at its own density. After isolation, each lipoprotein class was dialyzed against 0.155 M NaCl containing 0.02% EDTA, 0.02% sodium azide and 0.01% gentamicin sulfate, pH 7.4. LDL were labeled by the iodine monochloride method [18] modified for lipoproteins [19]. ^{125}I-LDL were separated from unbound iodine by Sephadex G-50 column chromatography and dialyzed against 5 mM Tris-HCl, 50 mM NaCl, 0.04% EDTA, 0.01% NaN$_3$, 0.05% gentamicin sulfate, pH 7.4 (dialysis buffer). Lipoprotein fractions were sterilized by filtration on 0.45 μm Minisart filters (Sartorius). ^{125}I-LDL specific activity ranged from 150 to 350 cpm/ng protein. Lipoprotein protein concentration was determined by a modification of the method of Lowry using bovine serum albumin (fatty acid poor Sigma A-6003) as a standard [20]. Modification of the arginine residues of the LDL was obtained by treatment of the LDL with 1,2-cyclohexanedione (CHD-LDL) as described by Shepherd et al. [21].

Liver membrane preparation

Immediately after surgery, liver samples (usually 10 g) were rinsed in sterile cold saline and immediately frozen in liquid nitrogen. The membranes were prepared within 24 hours of surgery. After thawing, the liver was homogenized in 20 mM Tris-HCl, 150 mM NaCl, 1 mM CaCl$_2$ (pH 7.5) with two ten second pulses (setting 6) in a Polytron homogenizer (Kinematica, Switzerland) and membranes were prepared as described by Kovanen et al. [22]. Membrane pellets were kept in liquid nitrogen unless specified otherwise.

^{125}I-LDL binding to human liver membranes

On the day of the experiment, the membrane pellets were thawed and resuspended in 1 ml of 20 mM Tris-HCl, 50 mM NaCl, 1 mM CaCl$_2$, pH 7.5 (buffer B) by flushing five times through a 22 gauge needle and then five times through a 25 gauge needle. The membrane suspension was then sonicated twice for 20 seconds each at 0° C with a 200 Watts NSU 157 generator (Ultrasonic, Annemasse, France).

The binding assay mixture consisted of 20 μl of the membrane suspension (80-120 μg of membrane protein), 40 μl of 50 mM Tris-HCl, 0.63 mM $CaCl_2$, 20 mM NaCl and 20 mg/ml of fatty acid poor bovine serum albumin (Sigma A-6003) pH 7.5, containing the ^{125}I-LDL and 20 μl of dialysis buffer. The different concentrations of ^{125}I-LDL and of the different lipoproteins added to the assay system are indicated in the figures. Incubations were carried out at different temperatures for 120 minutes.

At the end of the incubation period, 70 μl of the incubation mixture were layered onto 125 μl of 0.25% sucrose in dialysis buffer. The bound ^{125}I-LDL were separated from the unbound ^{125}I-LDL by centrifugation in a Beckman 42.2 rotor at 100,000 g for 30 minutes. The membrane pellets were washed twice without resuspension with 175 μl of dialysis buffer and recentrifuged at 100,000 g for 10 minutes. After slicing the tubes with a razor blade, the radioactivity associated with the membrane pellet was determined in a gamma counter (Compugamma 1282, LKB, Sweden). For each experiment, a series of tubes containing the different concentrations of ^{125}I-LDL were incubated in the same conditions in the absence of membranes. The radioactivity found in those tubes was subtracted from the corresponding experimental values. All experiments were done in triplicate. Blank values did not exceed 6% of the ^{125}I-LDL bound in the presence of membranes. The amount of membrane protein present in the tubes at the end of the experiment was determined after solubilization of the pellets in 5% sodium deoxycholate.

Results and Discussion

As observed in other binding assay systems, the amount of ^{125}I-LDL in our experiments is proportional to the amount present in the assay. The equilibrium between the bound and unbound LDL in the assay system is reached within 45 minutes after the addition of the ^{125}I-LDL.

The total amount of ^{125}I-LDL bound is proportional to the ^{125}I-LDL present in the assay within the range of LDL concentrations used in our assays (50-500 μg/ml) (Fig. 1). When an excess of unlabeled-LDL (20-50 times) was added to the incubation medium, a fraction of ^{125}I-LDL still bound to the plasma membrane. This fraction represents the non specific binding. The difference between the total binding and the non specific binding is classically called the "specific" binding of the ligand. Within the range of the LDL concentrations used in our experiments, this "specific" component of the LDL binding did not show any saturation and represented between 45 and 65% of the total LDL binding.

Increasing the temperature of the incubation medium lead to a doubling of the total amount of ^{125}I-LDL bound between 21 and 37° C. No significant change could be observed between 4 and 21° C (Fig. 2). The non specific component of the binding seems to be independent of the temperature. As a consequence, the "specific" component of the binding increased in parallel with the total binding. This phenomenon could result from changes in the tertiary structure of the lipoprotein which is determined in part by the interaction between the protein and the lipid components of the lipoprotein. Membrane fluidity may be affected by the

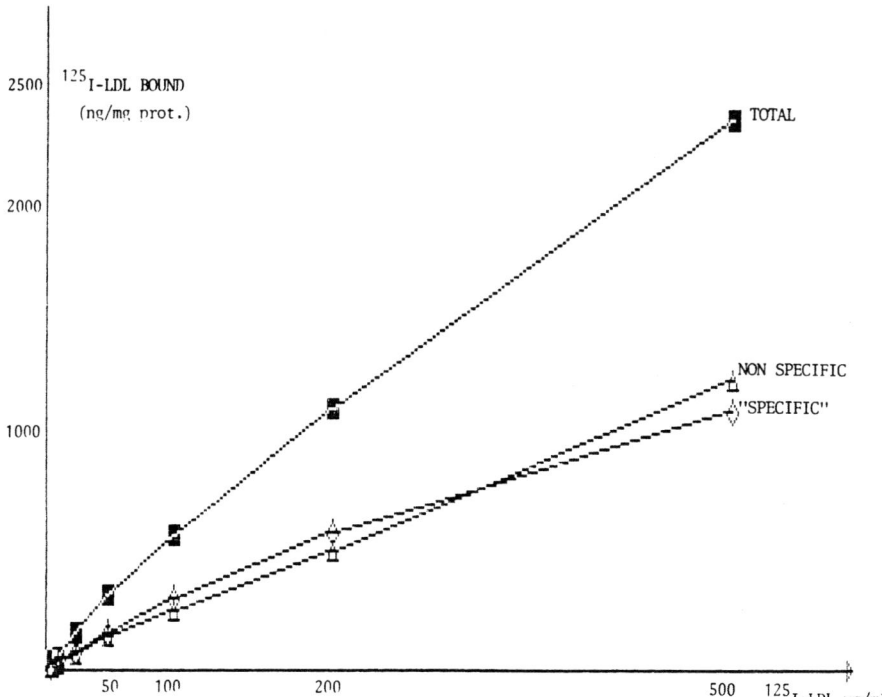

Fig. 1. ^{125}I-LDL binding to human liver plasma membranes

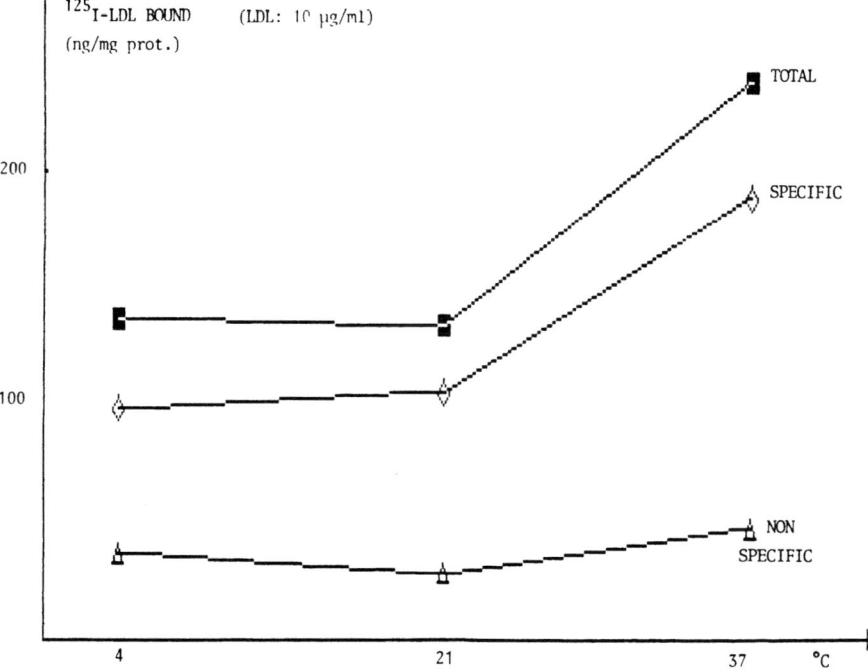

Fig. 2. Effect of temperature on LDL binding

temperature and this could also influence the interaction between LDL and the membranes.

In order to test the stability of the membrane binding activity, we kept several aliquots of the same membrane preparation in incubation buffer at -80° C for various periods of time before the binding assay. As shown in Fig. 3, the "specific" binding of the LDL decreases sharply with time and is almost negligible after 26 days. This loss of binding activity with time supports the view of a role played by an interaction between the lipoprotein and a protein of the plasma membrane, since it is very unlikely that an interaction involving only lipids would be affected by storage at -80° C. In our subsequent experiments, we kept the membrane pellets in liquid nitrogen as described in Materials and Methods.

The B/E receptor has been shown to be EDTA sensitive (i. e. calcium dependent [1]. We measured the ^{125}I-LDL binding (10 and 50 μg/ml) to liver membranes in the presence of increasing concentrations of EDTA (0-10 mM). Within this range of EDTA concentrations and for the two LDL concentrations studied, no effect of EDTA could be shown (Fig. 4). The concentration of EDTA used in our experiments was high enough to complex all the calcium ions present in the assay above 2 mM. Furthermore, the addition of calcium to an assay medium devoid of calcium did not modify the LDL binding to the liver membranes (Fig. 5). This confirms that in our experimental conditions and contrasting to the apo-B/E receptor, LDL binding to normal human liver membranes does not require the presence of calcium ions.

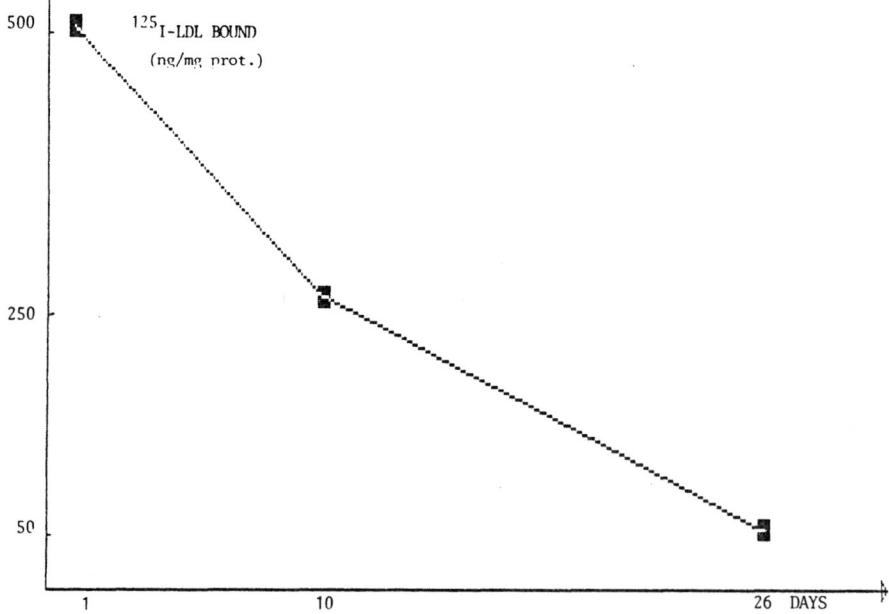

Fig. 3. Effect of time on ^{125}I-LDL binding to plasma membrane stored at -80° C

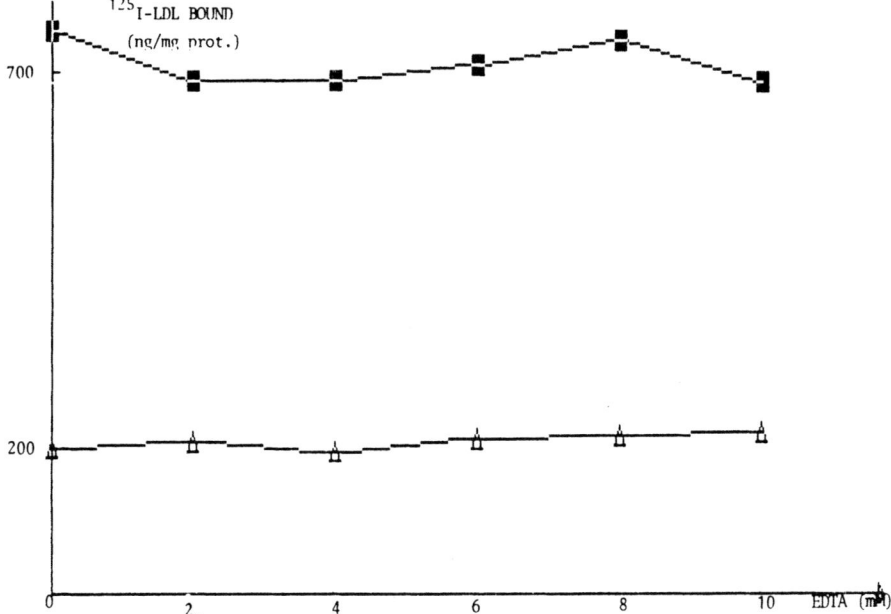

Fig. 4. Effect of EDTA on LDL binding to liver plasma membranes

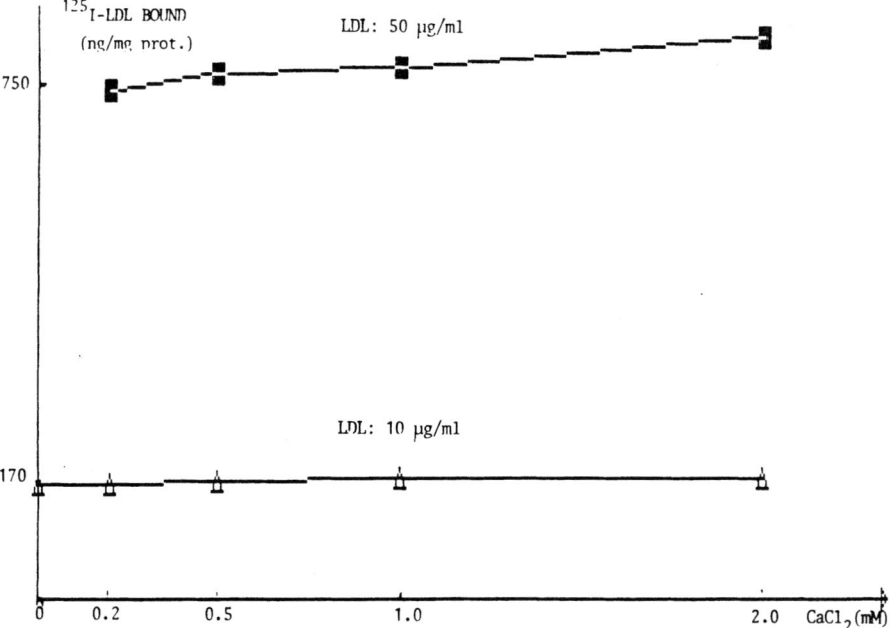

Fig. 5. Effect of CaCl$_2$ on LDL binding to plasma membrane

In order to study the specificity of this binding, we measured the binding of ^{125}I-LDL (10 μg/ml) in presence of increasing amounts (10-200 μg/ml) of unlabeled human albumin or lipoproteins isolated from normal plasma (Fig. 6). All the lipoproteins studied, including modified LDL (CHD-LDL) which are not recognized by the B/E receptor, competed with ^{125}I-LDL for membrane binding. Albumin, however, had very little effect on LDL binding. Thus, it is very unlikely that the albumin which is present in the incubation buffer at 20 mg/ml could block a specific LDL receptor.

Among the competitors, VLDL and HDL compete much more than LDL for the lipoprotein binding site. CHD-LDL competed as well as LDL. This data do not support the existence of a high affinity receptor for LDL on the surface of normal adult liver.

In addition, the possibility of an exchange between the fraction of label present in the LDL-lipid (usually less than 10%) and the membrane lipids should be considered. This exchange is expected to be negligible when the binding assays are performed at 0° C.

Acknowledgements. We thank Mrs Marie-Elisabeth Bouma for her help in providing the human liver and Dr Arie Van Tol for interesting discussion.

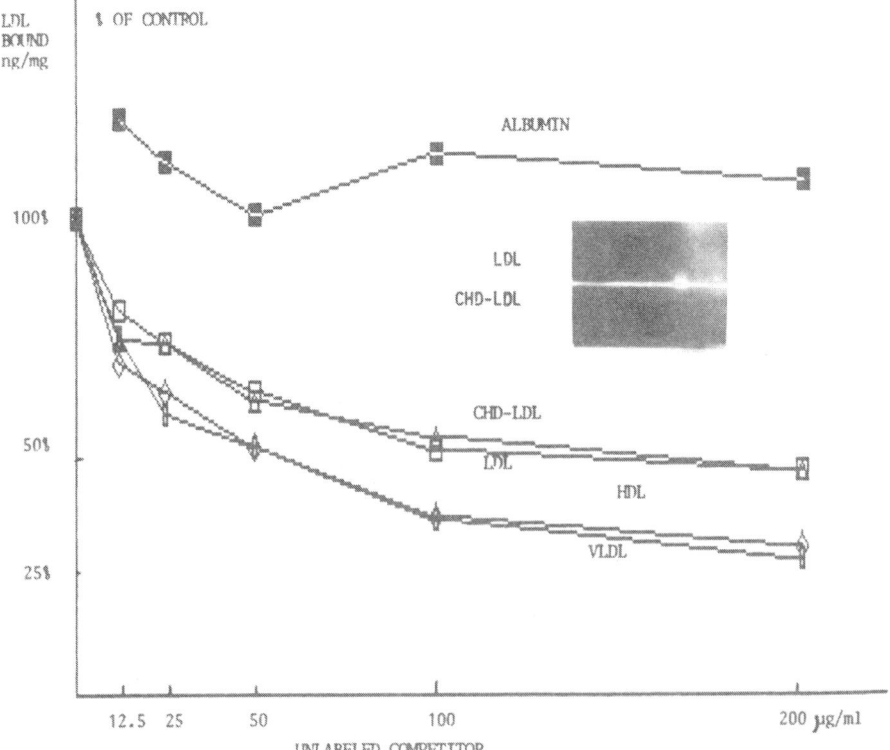

Fig. 6. Displacement of ^{125}I-LDL (10 μg/ml) by lipoproteins and albumin

References

1. Brown MS, Dana SE, Goldstein JL (1973) Proc Natl Acad Sci 70: 2162-2166
2. Pittman RC, Steinberg D (1984) J Lipid Res 25: 1577-1585
3. Bachorik PS, Franklin FA, Virgil DG, Kwiterovich PO (1982) Biochemistry 21: 5675-5684
4. Soltys PA, Portman OW, O'Malley JP (1982) Biochim Biophys Acta 713: 300-314
5. Tamai T, Patsch W, Lock D, Schonfeld G (1983) J Lipid Res 24: 1568-1577
6. Schneider WJ, Beisiegel U, Goldstein JL, Brown MS (1982) J Biol Chem 257: 2664-2673
7. Russell DW, Yamamoto T, Schneider WJ, Slaughter CJ, Brown MS, Goldstein JL (1983) Proc Natl Acad Sci 80: 7501-7505
8. Dashti N, Wolfbauer G, Koren E, Knowles B, Alaupovic P (1984) Biochim Biophys Acta 794: 374-384
9. Leichtner AM, Krieger M, Schwartz AL (1984) Hepatology 4: 897-901
10. Cohen LH, Griffioen M, Havekes L, Schouten D, Van Hinsbergh V, Kempen HJ (1984) Biochem J 222: 35-39
11. Illingworth DR, Lindsey S, Hagemenas FC (1984) Exp Cell Res 155: 518-526
12. Mahley RW, Hui DY, Innerarity TL, Weisgraber K (1981) J Clin Invest 68: 1197-1206
13. Harders-Spengel K, Wood CB, Thompson GR, Myant NB, Soutar AK (1982) Proc Natl Acad Sci 79: 6355-6359
14. Hoeg JM, Demosky SJ, Schaefer EJ, Starzl TE, Brewer HB (1984) J Clin Invest 73: 429-436
15. Floren CH (1984) Scand J Gastroenterol 19: 473-479
16. Hoeg JM, Demosky SJ, Gregg RE, Schaefer EJ, Brewer HB (1985) Science 227: 759-761
17. Havel RJ, Eder HH, Bragdon JH(1955) J Clin Invest 34: 1345-1353
18. Mac Farlane AS (1958) Nature 182: 53
19. Bilheimer DW, Eisenberg S, Levy RI (1972) Biochim Biophys Acta 260: 212-221
20. Lowry OH, Rosebrough NJ, Farr AL, Randall RJ (1951) J Biol Chem 193: 265-275
21. Shepherd J, Bicker S, Lorimer AR Packard CJ (1979) J Lipid Res 19: 644-653
22. Kovanen PT, Basu SK, Goldstein JL and Brown MS (1979) Endocrinology 104: 610-616

Detection of LDL Receptors in Liver Membranes by Ligand Blotting with Biotin-Modified Plasma Lipoproteins

D. P. WADE, B. L. KNIGHT, and ANNE K. SOUTAR

MRC Lipoprotein Team, Hammersmith Hospital, Ducane Road, London W12 OHS, England

Introduction

Low density lipoprotein receptor (LDL-receptor) activity in hepatic tissues is difficult to identify and measure accurately by ligand-binding assays that depend upon separation of bound and free ligand by membrane filtration (Schneider et al., 1980) or centrifugation (Basu et al., 1978). With liver membranes, the proportion of non-specific binding relative to specific, saturable binding is high and saturable binding of LDL is less sensitive to EDTA, a potent inhibitor of LDL receptor activity, than in other tissues (Harders-Spengel et al., 1982). The LDL receptor protein in human skin fibroblasts and bovine adrenal cortex has been demonstrated by ligand blotting with LDL (Daniel et al., 1983). The native LDL receptor exhibits Ca^{++} dependent saturable binding of lipoproteins containing apoB and apoE and these properties are retained in the blotted protein if detergent-solubilised receptor is subjected to SDS-PAGE under non-reducing conditions. We have recently described a new method for the detection of bound lipoproteins based on the high affinity streptavidin-biotin interaction (Wade et al., 1985), and in this paper we report that a protein of MW approx. 130,000-150,000 can be detected in extracts of both adult dog liver and normal rat liver by ligand blotting with biotin-LDL. Binding of the lipoprotein was saturable and EDTA-sensitive, and thus the protein has the properties of the LDL-receptor of human skin fibroblasts or bovine adrenal cortex. Rat chylomicron remnants and rabbit ßVLDL, both modified with biotin, were also bound by the LDL-receptor protein in bovine adrenal cortex, dog liver and rat liver.

Methods

Human LDL was isolated from normal human plasma as previously described (Wade et al., 1985). Rabbit ßVLDL (d < 1.006 g/ml) was isolated from the plasma of cholesterol-fed New Zealand white rabbits. Chylomicron remnants were prepared by injecting rat intestinal lymph chylomicrons into functionally hepatectomised rats (Wade et al., 1984). Carbohydrate residues on the lipoproteins were modified with biotin by reacting periodate oxidised lipoproteins with biotin hydrazide (Wade et al., 1985). Biotin-LDL competed as effectively as unmodified LDL with ^{125}I-labelled unmodified LDL for binding to the LDL-receptor on human

Receptor-Mediated Uptake
in the Liver
Edited by H. Greten, E. Windler, U. Beisiegel
© Springer-Verlag Berlin Heidelberg 1986

skin fibroblasts (Wade *et al.*, 1985). The LDL-receptor protein from bovine adrenals was partially purified by DEAE-cellulose chromatography as described by Schneider *et al.* (1980). Liver membranes were prepared from the livers of adult mongrel dogs, normal rats and rats treated for 2 days with ethinyl estradiol (5 mg/kg body weight) (Kovanen *et al.*, 1979). Membranes, approx. 100 mg wet weight, were solubilised in 10 ml 50 mM tris-maleate pH 6.0 containing 2 mM $CaCl_2$, 1% triton X-100 and 1 mM PMSF by homogenisation in a glass homoge-

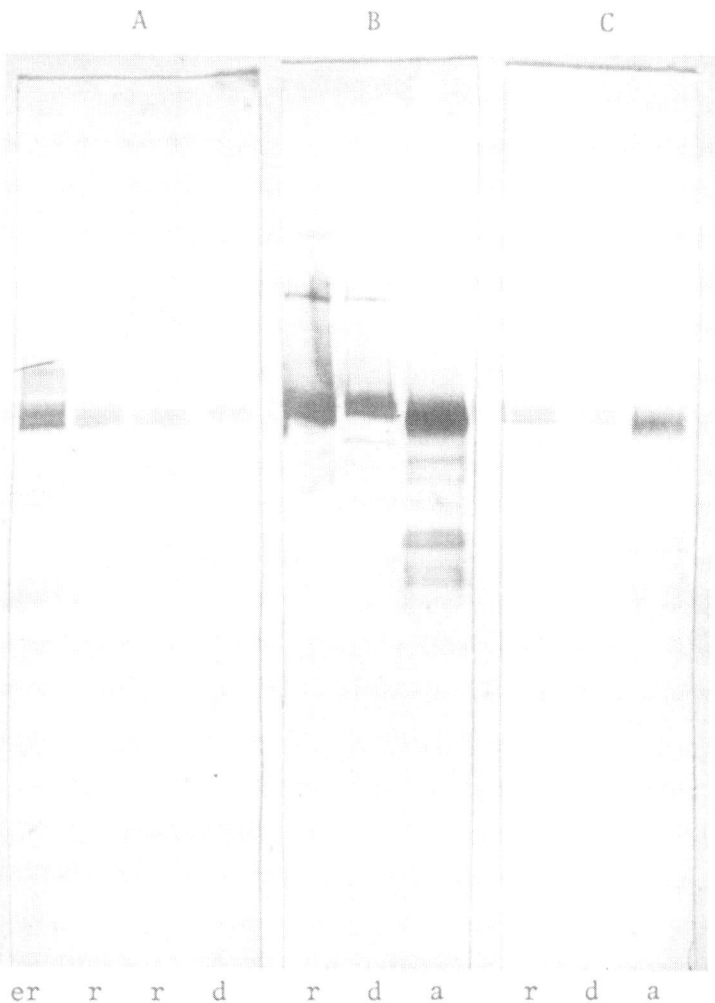

Fig. 1. Binding of biotin-modified lipoproteins by membrane proteins from liver and adrenals, separated on 10% polyacrylamide. Nitrocellulose strips containing transferred proteins were incubated with biotin-modified human LDL (20 µg protein/ml) (**a**), biotin-modified rat chylomicron remnants (20 µg protein/ml) (**b**), and biotin-modified rabbit ßVLDL (20 µg protein/ml) (**c**). The lanes contain protein from dog liver (d), rat liver (r), estrogen-treated rat liver (er) and bovine adrenal cortex (a). The approx. MW of the major lipoprotein binding protein in rat liver was 144,000, in dog liver 147,000 and in bovine adrenal cortex 130,000

niser. After 30 min at $0°$ C the extracts were cleared by centrifugation for 30 min at 50,000 rpm at $4°$ C in Beckman 50.3 rotor. Soluble proteins were incubated for 30 min at $4°$ C on a rotating platform with 0.8 ml packed DEAE-cellulose equilibrated in the same buffer. The DEAE-cellulose was pelleted by centrifugation, washed once with 5 ml of the same buffer and adsorbed proteins were eluted with 0.5 ml of the same buffer containing 0.5 M NaCl. Eluted proteins were desalted on small columns of Sephadex G25 equilibrated with SDS-PAGE sample buffer without 2-mercaptoethanol. (Laemmli, 1970). Samples were separated by SDS-PAGE, transferred to nitrocellulose membranes and incubated with biotin-modified lipoproteins as described previously (Wade *et al.*, 1985) and in the legends to figures.

Results and Discussion

Extracts of dog and rat liver membranes contained a protein of MW approx. 145,000 that bound human LDL, rat chylomicron remnants and rabbit ßVLDL

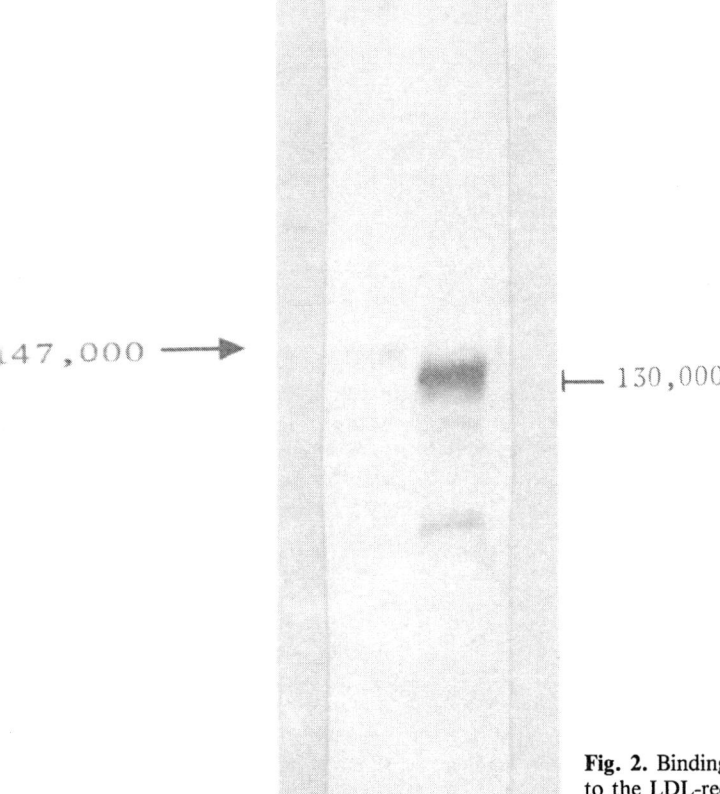

147,000 → |— 130,000

Fig. 2. Binding of biotin-modified human LDL to the LDL-receptor in dog liver (d) and bovine adrenal cortex (a) separated on 7.5% polyacrylamide

d   a

(Fig. 1). The MW of the lipoprotein-binding protein in each case was similar to but not identical with that of the LDL-receptor in bovine adrenal cortex (Fig. 1 and 2). Binding of rat chylomicron remnants to dog liver and rat liver membranes was inhibited by 10 mM EDTA and excess unlabelled human LDL (1.0 mg/ml) but not by human HDL (Fig. 3). Similar results were obtained with human LDL and rabbit ßVLDL (data not shown), suggesting that all the lipoproteins were binding to the same protein, probably the LDL-receptor. The results in Fig. 1 and 2 suggest that binding of rat chylomicron remnants and rabbit ßVLDL was greater than that of human LDL, but it is possible that the detection of these lipoproteins is more sensitive because they contain more biotin. The significance of the higher

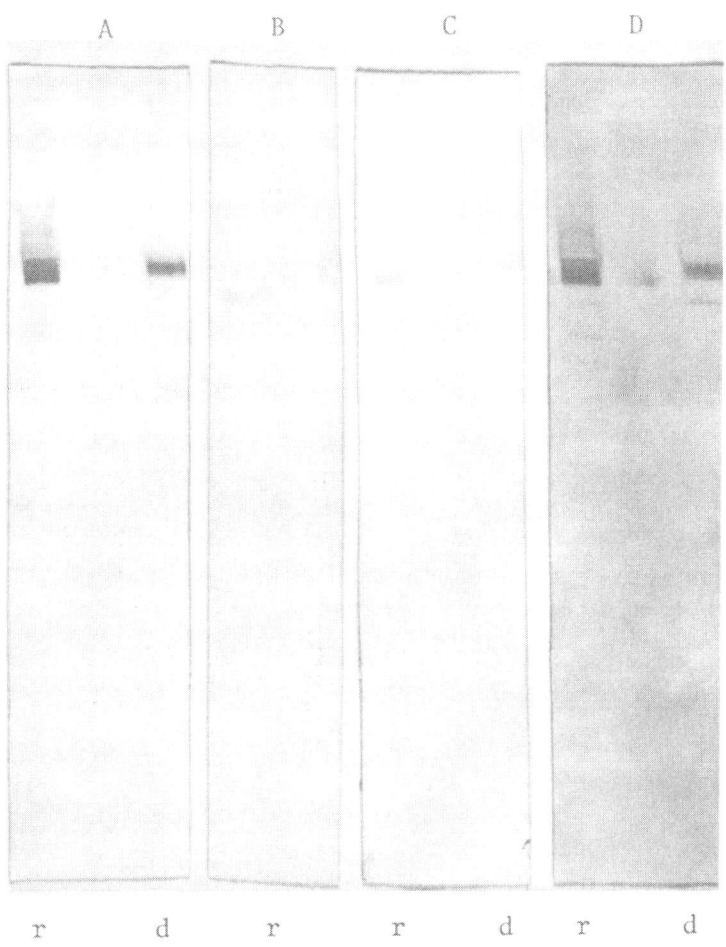

Fig. 3. Effect of EDTA, LDL and HDL on the binding of rat chylomicron remnants by rat liver and dog liver membrane proteins separated on 10% polyacrylamide. Nitrocellulose strips were incubated with rat chylomicron remnants (20 µg protein/ml) alone (a), or in the presence of 10 mM EDTA (b), human LDL (1.0 mg protein/ml) (c) and human HDL (1.0 mg protein/ml) (d). The lanes contain protein from rat liver (r); dog liver (d)

MW minor bands in rat liver extracts is not clear, but experiments are in progress to determine whether they result from aggregation of the native receptor, binding by different forms of the LDL receptor or binding by a distinct protein. It is of interest that the LDL-receptor in rat liver is able to bind biotin-modified human LDL, since it has been reported that the LDL receptor in rat fibroblasts does not recognise human LDL (Drevon *et al.*, 1981). It is possible that the properties of the receptor protein are modified by the solubilisation, separation or transfer procedures such that the binding specificity is altered, or that the receptor in the intact cells is inaccessible, but it is more likely that ligand blotting with biotin-modified lipoproteins is a cleaner and more sensitive technique.

Adult dogs have previously been reported to lack detectable LDL-receptor activity in the liver, as determined by binding of LDL to intact membranes (Mahley *et al.*, 1981) but to possess distinct receptors that recognise lipoproteins containing apoE. However, we have found that adult dog livers contain an LDL-binding protein with the properties of the LDL-receptor that can be detected by ligand blotting.

Detection of the LDL-receptor protein in bovine adrenal cortex membranes by ligand blotting with biotin-modified lipoproteins has been shown to be quantitative (Wade *et al.*, 1985). If detection of LDL-receptor activity in liver membranes by this technique can be shown to reflect accurately the activity and specificity of the receptor in intact tissues it will prove a useful method for measurement of lipoprotein receptor activity under different physiological conditions.

References

1. Basu SK, Goldstein JL, Brown MS (1978) J Biol Chem 253: 3852-3856
2. Daniel TO, Schneider WJ, Goldstein JL, Brown MS (1983) J Biol Chem 258: 4606-4611
3. Drevon CA, Attie AD, Pangburn SH, Steinberg D (1981) J Lipid Res 22: 37-45
4. Harders-Spengel K, Wood CB, Thompson GR, Myant NB, Soutar AK (1982) Proc Natl Acad Sci USA 79: 6355-6359
5. Kovanen PT, Brown MS, Goldstein JL (1979) J Biol Chem 254: 11367-11373
6. Laemmli UK (1970) Nature 227: 680-685
7. Mahley RW, Hui DY, Innerarity TL, Weisgraber KH (1981) J Clin Invest 68: 1197-1206
8. Schneider WJ, Goldstein JL, Brown MS (1980) J Biol Chem 255: 11442-11447
9. Wade DP, Soutar AK, Gibbons GF (1984) Biochem J 218: 203-211
10. Wade DP, Knight BL, Soutar AK (1985) Biochem J 229: 785-790

Cellular Localization of Lipoprotein Receptors in Liver

Theo. J. C. van Berkel, J. Kar Kruijt, J. Fred Nagelkerke, and Leen Harkes

Dept. of Biochemistry I, Erasmus University Rotterdam, P. O. Box 1738, 3000 DR Rotterdam, The Netherlands

Investigations on the quantitative role of the various cell types (parenchymal, Kupffer and endothelial cells) to the receptor-mediated uptake by the liver in vivo, were until recently hampered by the applied cell isolation procedures during which bound and/or internalized substances were processed and lost from the cells. The procedure as outlined in scheme 1 prevents such a processing because both liver perfusion, cell separation and cell purification are performed at a low temperature (at 8° C). In addition one is able to assess the recovery by comparing the radioactivity in the purified parenchymal, endothelial and Kupffer cells (all obtained from one liver) to the radioactivity originally present in the whole rat liver. The method was evaluated using ^{125}I-asialofetuin as the substrate (Fig. 1) and compared to quantitative autoradiographic data [1].

In accordance with the autoradiographic data of Hubbard et al. [1] we found that the great majority of ^{125}I-asialofetuin became associated to parenchymal

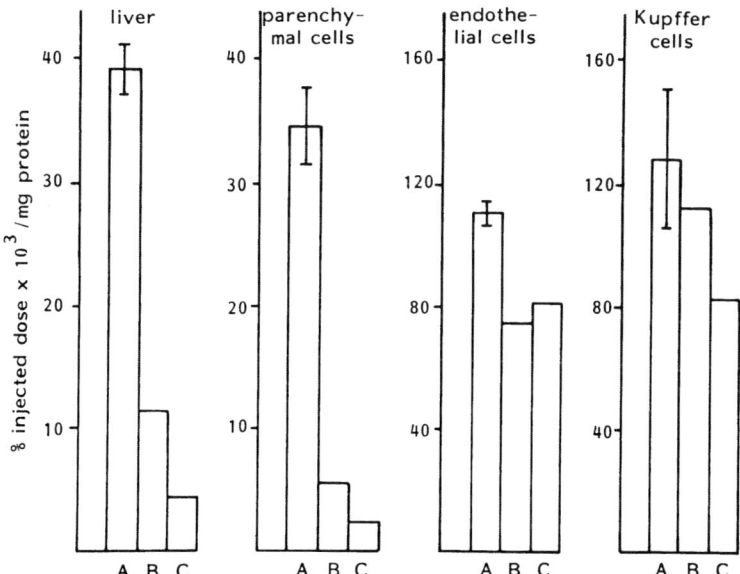

Fig. 1. The effect of unlabelled asialofetuin on the association of ^{125}I-asialofetuin to parenchymal, endothelial and Kupffer cells. Ten minutes after injection of 9 μg ^{125}I-asialofetuin the cells were isolated according to scheme 1. A control, B preinjection of 5 mg asialofetuin (-1 min), C preinjection of 25 mg asialofetuin (-1 min)

Receptor-Mediated Uptake
in the Liver
Edited by H. Greten, E. Windler, U. Beisiegel
© Springer-Verlag Berlin Heidelberg 1986

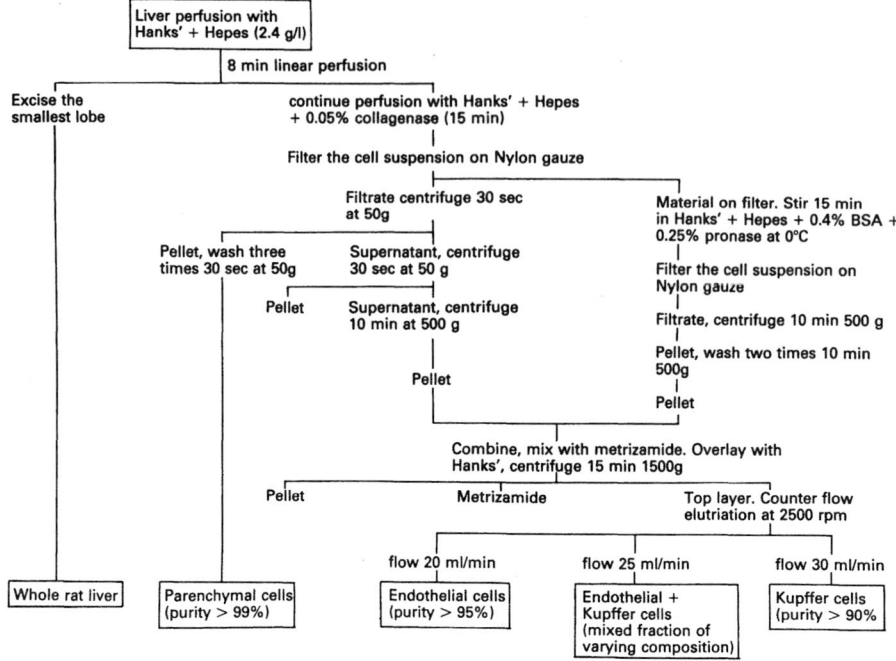

Scheme I. Procedure for the Isolation of Liver cells at a low Temperature (8° C)

cells. Preinjection of 5 and 25 mg of unlabelled asialofetuin inhibited the association of ^{125}I-asialofetuin to parenchymal cells for 84 and 93% respectively, while the association to endothelial and Kupffer cells was only inhibited for 22 and 28% respectively. (Hubbard et al [1] with 20 mg asialofetuin for parenchymal cells 99% and endothelial and Kupffer cells 24% inhibition).

Furthermore preinjection of N-acetyl galactosamine blocked specifically the uptake of ^{125}I-asialofetuin by parenchymal cells while the uptake by Kupffer and endothelial cells was specifically inhibited by preinjection of mannan (Fig. 2).

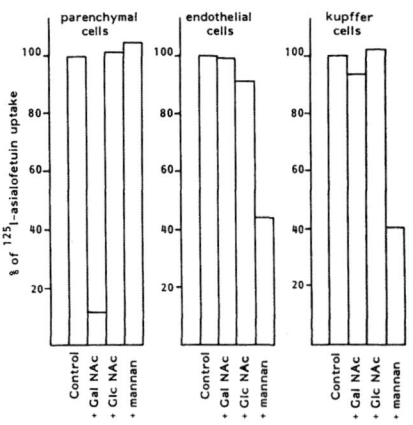

Fig. 2. The effect of preinjection of Gal-NAc, GlcNAc or mannan on the cell association of ^{125}I-asialofetuin to parenchymal, endothelial and Kupffer cells. Prior to the labelled asialofetuin, at -1 min, preinjection of 0.5 mmol of GalNAc, 0.5 mmol of GlcNAc or 5 mg mannan was performed

Fig. 3. Distribution of [^{14} C] sucrose-labelled LDL or methylated LDL between the various liver cell types at 4.5 h after injection. Screened lipoproteins were injected and 4.5 h after injection the cells were isolated. NPC is non-parenchymal cells, PC is parenchymal cells, EC is endothelial cells and KC is Kupffer cells. Values are means ± S.E.M. for 3 experiments

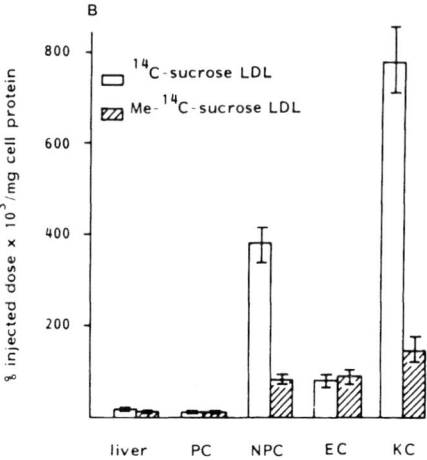

These data establish that the non-parenchymal cell preparations are free from any parenchymal cell derived material. The recovery calculations indicate a quantitative recovery in the isolated cells of the radioactivity originally present in the whole rat liver.

The above described method was applied in order to determine the cellular localization of lipoprotein receptors in liver. [^{14} C] sucrose-labelled human LDL (completely free from apo E and isolated according to [2] was injected into rats and 4.5 h after injection the various cell types were isolated (Fig. 3).

At this time interval after injection, approximately 35% of the injected dose is present in total liver while 50% is removed from serum. This indicates that the liver is responsible for 70% of the removal of LDL from blood. A comparison of the uptake of [^{14} C] sucrose-labelled LDL and reductive-methylated [^{14} C] sucrose-labelled LDL (Me-LDL) by the liver shows that methylation leads to a 65% decrease of the LDL uptake. This indicates that 65% of the LDL uptake by liver is mediated by a specific apo-B, E receptor. A comparison of the cellular uptake indicates that 79% of the uptake of LDL by non-parenchymal cells is receptor-dependent while with parenchymal cells no significant difference in uptake between LDL and Me-LDL was found. Within the non-parenchymal cells solely the Kupffer cells are responsible for the receptor-mediated uptake of LDL [2].

Chemically or biologically modified LDL forms a substrate for the so-called scavenger receptor [3, 4]. This receptor may mediate the deposition of cholesterol(esters) in the atherosclerotic plaque and therefore it is relevant to determine its distribution in the body. It can be argued that an adequate handling of substrates for this receptor by the liver could prevent the accumulation of cholesterol(esters) at other sites in the body.

After injection of acetylated LDL (acetyl-LDL) into rats, the particles are rapidly cleared by the liver (Table 1).

Isolated endothelial cells contained 5 times more acetyl-LDL per mg of cell protein than the Kupffer cells and 31 times more than the hepatocytes (Fig. 4). This uptake is mediated by the highly active receptor (scavenger receptor) on the

Table 1. Distribution of radioactivity between liver and serum 3, 10 and 30 min after intravenous injection of acetyl-LDL

Time after injection (min)	Radioactivity distribution (% of injected dose)	
	Liver	Serum
3	---	6.0 ± 0.8
10	83.4 ± 1.7	2.2 ± 0.2
30	18.0 ± 1.2	8.4 ± 0.3

Values are means of 3 different experiments

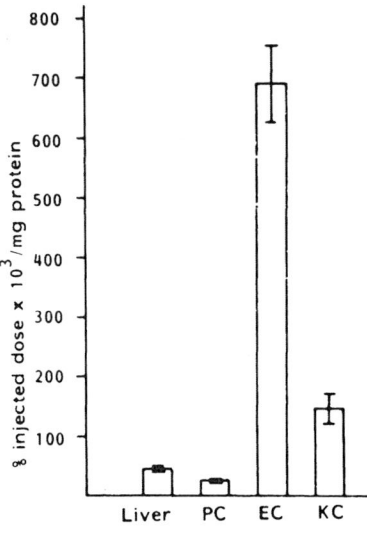

Fig. 4. Distribution of acetylated LDL between the various liver cell types at 10 min after injection. PC parenchymal cells, EC endothelial cells, KC Kupffer cells

liver endothelial cells [6]. Apparently the uptake by the liver cells prevents a quantitative important uptake in other tissues or cells. Recent morphological studies on the interaction of acetyl-LDL conjugated to 20 nm colloidal gold illustrate that the liver endothelial cells bind acetyl-LDL in coated pits, which is followed by rapid uptake [7]. Uptake proceeds through small coated vesicles and finally degradation of the apoprotein occurs in the lysosomes. An inadequate operation of this pathway may temporarily increase the serum concentration of the modified lipoprotein and thus allow deposition of cholesterol(esters) in the arterial wall. It is possible that a delicate balance between the formation of modified lipoproteins and the capacity of the liver to entrap them determines their pathological action.

The amount of radioactivity per mg cell protein in the isolated cell fractions was multiplied with the amount of protein that each cell type contributes to total liver protein. The values are the mean of 3 independent experiments.

In Table 2 the relative contribution of the different liver cell types to the total liver uptake of LDL and modified LDL is summarized and compared with asialofetuin. It will be clear that in studies on the receptor-mediated uptake in the liver, the presence of the various liver cell types must be taken into consideration (cf. also Kempen et al [8]). Non-parenchymal liver cells do contain 26.6% of the total liver plas-

Table 2. Relative contribution of the different liver cell types to the total liver uptake of LDL, Acetyl-LDL and asialofetuin

Cell type	LDL	Acetyl-LDL	Asialofetuin
Parenchymal cells (%)	29	38	82.5
Endothelial cells (%)	9	53	9.3
Kupffer cells (%)	62	9	8.2

ma membranes, 57.9% of the pinocytotic vesicles and 43.0% of the total amount of liver lysosomes [9]. These cellular compartments are specifically involved in receptor-mediated uptake. Therefore quantitative studies on the receptor-mediated uptake by the liver should include determination of the contribution of *all* liver cell types preferably by similar procedures as outlined in scheme 1.

Acknowledgements. The Dutch Heart Foundation is thanked for financial support (grants 31.014 and 82.053) and Martha Wieriks for the preparation of the manuscript.

References

1. Hubbard AL, Wilson G, Ashwell G, Stukenbrok H (1979) J Cell Biol 83: 47-64
2. Harkes L, Van Berkel TJC (1984) Biochem J 224: 21-27
3. Goldstein JL, Ho YK, Basu SK, Brown MS (1979) Proc Natl Acad Sci USA 76: 333-337
4. Henriksen T, Mahoney EM, Steinberg D (1981) Proc Natl Acad Sci USA 78: 6499-6503
5. Van Berkel TJC, Nagelkerke JF, Harkes L, Kruijt JK (1982) Biochem J 208: 493-503
6. Nagelkerke JF, Barto KP, Van Berkel TJC (1983) J Biol Chem 258: 12221-12227
7. Mommaas-Kienhuis AM, Nagelkerke JF, Vermeer BJ, Daems WT, Van Berkel TJC (1985) Eur J Cell Biol 38: 42-50
8. Kempen HJM, Spanjer HH, Van Berkel THJC (1985) Eur J Cell Biol in press
9. Van Berkel TJC (1982) in ,,Metabolic Compartmentation" (H. Sies, ed) Academic Press Inc London pp 437-482

Cell Density Dependent Uptake of LDL in Cultured Rat Hepatocytes

E. Jensen, C.-H. Florén, and Åke Nilsson

Department of Internal Medicine, Lund Hospital, 221 85 Lund (Sweden)

Abstract

An inverse relationship between low-density lipoprotein uptake and cell density was observed in rat hepatocyte monolayers incubated with lipoprotein-deficient serum. This was also true for cell association, binding and degradation of low-density lipoproteins. Compactin stimulated cell association and degradation of low-density lipoproteins at low cell densities.

Introduction

LDL is an independent risk factor in atherogenesis [1]. In man, about one third of LDL is catabolized by a receptor-mediated pathway and the rest by a receptor-independent pathway [2] and this probably occurs to a large extent in the liver [3]. The liver is the only organ where cholesterol can be removed from the circulation to be excreted [4]. It is therefore important to determine cellular mechanisms for hepatic uptake and degradation of LDL. For this purpose, hepatocyte monolayers were considered an appropriate model system [5].

Human LDL was considered suitable for use in this system because a saturable high-affinity binding of human LDL has been found in freshly isolated rat hepatocytes [6]. In trying to elucidate the effects of insulin on LDL uptake by rat hepatocytes in monolayer culture, we found that LDL uptake varied with cell density. It was therefore necessary to eliminate cell density as a variable, as has been done previously in experiments with LDL uptake in fibroblasts [7]. To vary LDL uptake in hepatocytes, a substance known to elevate the number of LDL receptors in pig hepatocytes [8], namely compactin [9], was used.

An account of this work has earlier been published [10].

Materials and Methods

(^{125}I) Iodide (carrier free, 100 mCi/ml) was obtained from the Radiochemical Center, Amersham, Bucks, U.K. Leibovitz L-15 medium, fetal calf serum and Hepes were purchased from Flow Laboratories, Irvine, Ayshire, U.K. Acid-soluble calf skin collagen was obtained from Sigma Chemical Co, Saint Louis, MO,

Receptor-Mediated Uptake
in the Liver
Edited by H. Greten, E. Windler, U. Beisiegel
© Springer-Verlag Berlin Heidelberg 1986

U.S.A., and collagenase (CLS 143-180 units per mg (one unit liberates one mole of amino acid from collagen in 5 h at 37° C, pH 7.4) from Millipore Corporation, Freehold, NY. Male white Sprague-Dawley rats weighing 250-350 g were obtained from Anticimex AB, Stockholm, Sweden. Compactin was a kind gift from Dr. A. Endo, Tokyo.

Rat hepatocytes were prepared by a collagenase procedure [11] using the conditions of Seglen [12]. The perfusate was buffered with 40 mM Hepes. Hepatocytes were cultured in primary monolayers [5, 13, 14] according to Lin and Snodgrass [15]. The culture medium was Leibovitz L-15 containing 28 mM Hepes (pH 7.4) 1.0 mM sodium succinate, 100 μg penicillin and 50 μg gentamicin per ml. Collagen coated [15] 60-mm Petri dishes (Falcon 1007) were used and 0.25-3,5 x 10^6 suspended hepatocytes were plated in each dish in a volume of 2.5 ml. The dishes were placed in humidified air at 37° C. 24 h after plating the cells had arranged themselves in monolayers in trabecular cell aggregates as described by others [5, 13, 15], and all the cells, except for a very small percentage that was not firmly attached to the dish, excluded Trypan blue.

LDL (1.019 < density < 1.063 kg/l) was isolated from human plasma by sequential preparative ultracentrifugation using a Beckmann L 5-65 ultracentrifuge with the 60 Ti rotor (Beckman Instruments, Inc., Fullerton, CA) [16]. The protein content of LDL was determined by the Lowry method [17], using human serum albumin as a standard. The LDL was then iodinated with ^{125}I by the iodine monochloride method as modified for lipoproteins [18]. The specific radioactivity was between 200 and 300 cpm per ng protein.

Lipoprotein-deficient serum was prepared from fetal calf serum by ultracentrifugation at d = 1.25 kg/l. After recentrifugation under identical conditions, the d > 1.25 kg/l fraction was extensively dialyzed against 0.15 M NaCl/l mM EDTA (pH 7.4). The cholesterol content in lipoprotein-deficient serum ranged between 0.10 and 0.18 mM (as determined by a commercial kit from Boehringer Mannheim, F.R.G.).

After incubation with lipoproteins, medium was collected and the cells were washed according to standard procedures [19]. When cell association was to be determined, the washed cells were incubated with 0.1 M NaOH for 4 h. The cells were then scraped off with a rubber policeman. Binding of LDL to hepatocytes was regarded as the trypsin-releasable radioactivity after the cells had been washed, and uptake as the remaining radioactivity in the cells [20, 21]. Degradation was measured as the trichloroacetic acid-soluble non-iodide ^{125}I radioactivity in the medium [20]. As a control, iodinated lipoproteins were also incubated in cell-free collagen-coated dishes in each experiment.

Results

When LDL was incubated with hepatocytes at different cell densities both binding, uptake and degradation of LDL was cell density dependent (Fig. 1). Binding and degradation of LDL were at lower cell densities (around 250 μg protein/dish) approximately 3-5 times as high per mg cell protein as that at higher cell densities (around 1.5 mg protein/dish) (Fig. 1).

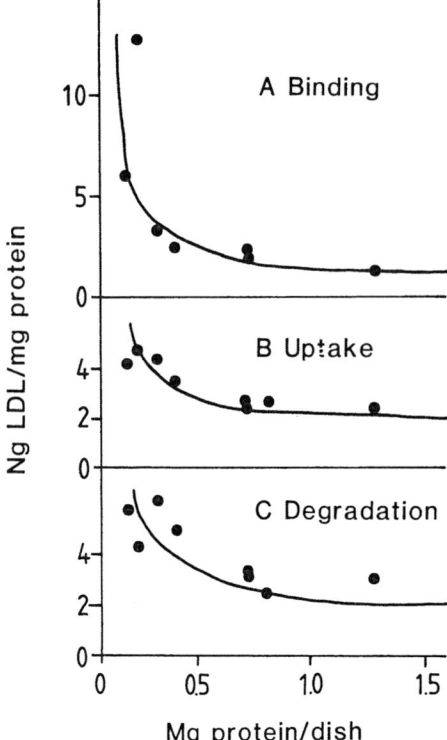

Fig. 1. Density dependency of LDL binding, uptake and degradation in rat hepatocytes. A, B and C represent one experiment in which binding, uptake and degradation were determined in cells at different densities. The hepatocytes were plated with 10% lipoprotein-deficient serum in a volume of 2 ml medium. After 24 h, new medium was added together with 10 μg LDL per ml, and the experiment was interrupted after another 4 h. Each point represents one dish

In order to compare metabolism of LDL in hepatocytes incubated under different conditions, it was necessary to eliminate cell density as a variable. Therefore, data were normalized according to the relationship observed in Fig. 2 to that which would be expected at a protein concentration of 1 mg per dish [7]. A double log plot makes it possible to decide the normalized values for each observation by drawing lines parallel with the main line through each point representing an observation. The intercept with the line x = 0, i. e., anti log x = 1 gives the normalized value. As long as the points are arranged fairly symmetrically around a common axis they will also have comparable normalized values and thus they will have the same K_m. Evaluation of the normalized values was done with Student's t-test.

When hepatocytes were cultured in medium with fetal calf serum containing lipoproteins, the cell association was low and did not vary with cell density (Fig. 3). However, when lipoprotein-deficient serum was used, the uptake was higher and varied inversely with cell density. Cells incubated with both lipoprotein-deficient serum and compactin had a higher cell association and degradation of iodinated LDL than cells which were only incubated with lipoprotein-deficient serum — both a low and high LDL concentrations (Fig. 4).

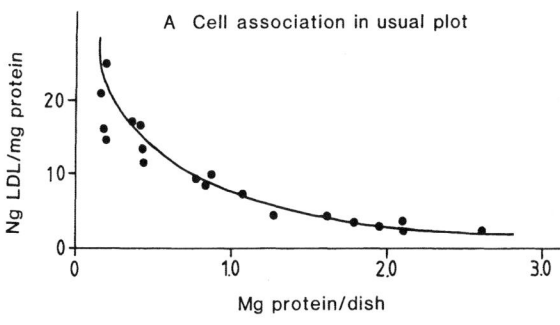

A Cell association in usual plot

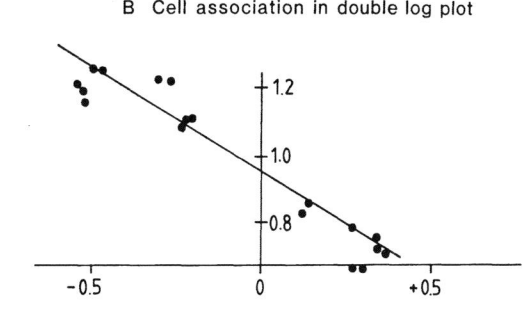

B Cell association in double log plot

Fig. 2. Double log transformation of cell association per mg protein vs. mg protein per dish. In this experiment, the conditions were the same as in Fig. 1, but only cell association was determined. In 2A, the mean of the observed cell associations in ng per mg cell protein was 10.27 ± 5.78 (S.D.) n = 19. The coefficient of variation was 0.56. After normalization, the mean value was 8.22 ± 1.34 (S.D.) and the coefficient of variation was 0.16. Each point represents one dish

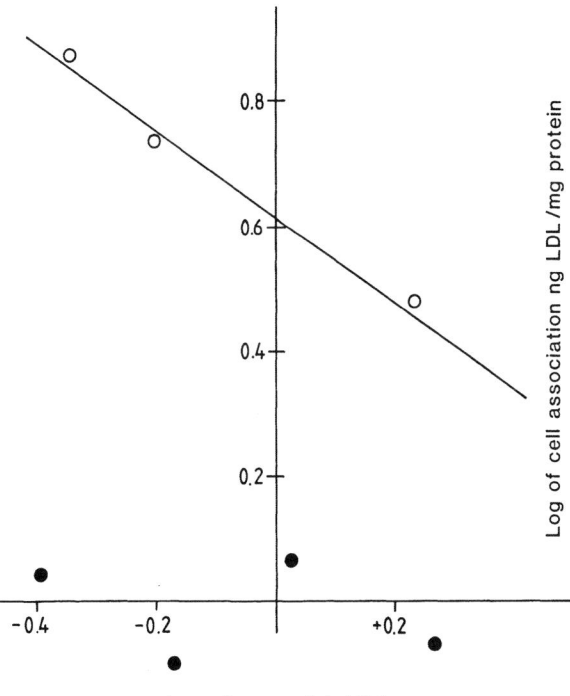

Fig. 3. The effect of lipoprotein-deficient serum on cell association of LDL to rat hepatocytes. The cells were incubated with 10% fetal calf serum (●) or with 10% lipoprotein-deficient calf serum (0). Cell association of LDL was determined after 44 h by incubating the hepatocytes with 2.5 μg ^{125}I-labelled LDL protein per ml for the last 4 h. Each point represents one dish. As for degradation, the same pattern was seen (data not shown)

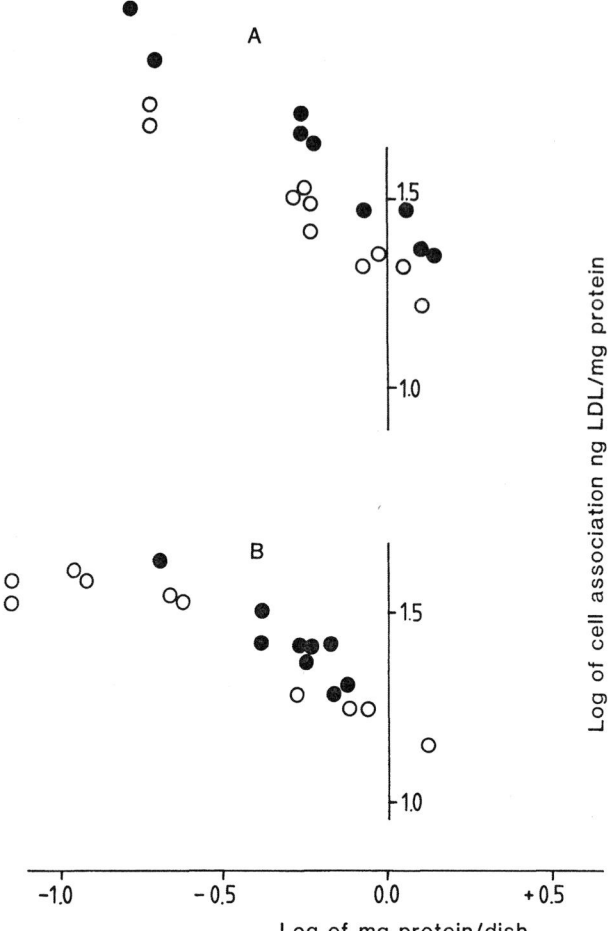

Fig. 4. The effect of compactin on cell association of LDL. The cells were incubated in medium with 10% lipoprotein-deficient calf serum with (●) or without (0) 20 nmol compactin per ml. After 48 h, ^{125}I-labelled LDL was added. In experiment B, 2.5 μg LDL protein was added per ml and, in experiment A, 25 μg LDL. After 4 h cell association was determined and normalization of data was then done. In Expt. B, compactin augmented cell association from 11.9 ± 1.43 (S.D.) (number of observations = 9) to 15.6 ± 2.2 (S.D.) (n = 9) i. e. +30% (P < 0.001). Degradation was augmented from 1.57 ± 0.50 (n = 7) to 2.04 ± 0.37 (S.D.) (n = 9) i. e. +30% (not statistically significant). In A, the normalized cell association increased from 21.1 ± 1.4 (S.D.) (n = 10) to 36.6 ± 7.3 (S.D.) (n = 9) i. e. +73% (p < 0.001). Degradation was augmented from 2.24 ± 0.49 (S.D.) (n = 8) to 3.31 ± 0.48 (S.D.) (n = 9)i. e. +48% (p < 0.001). Each point represents one dish

In Fig. 4a, it appears that the difference between the compactin-treated dishes and the control dishes becomes smaller at higher cell densities. This would imply that at high cell densities compactin has less effect on LDL uptake.

At low cell concentrations there is a tendency towards a constantly high LDL metabolizing activity. Further dilution of the cell concentration does not give any

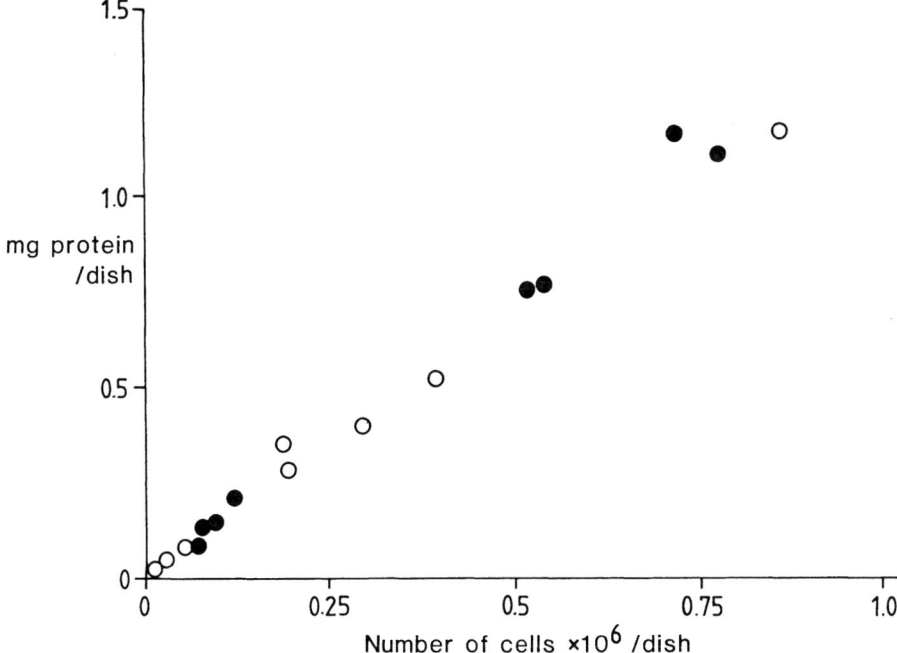

Fig. 5. Cell number and protein per dish in hepatocyte monolayers incubated with or without compactin. The cells were plated with (●) or without (0) 4 nmol/ml compactin in medium with 5% lipoprotein deficient serum. Medium was changed 4 and 24 hours after plating. After 48 hours the cells were washed four times with 2 mmol/l EDTA, 150 mmol/l NaCl, pH 7.4 at 4° C. Then 2 ml of the same buffer was added to each dish and the dishes were kept at 4● C for 12 hours. The cells could then easily be detached and counted in a Fuchs- Rosenthal chamber. Protein mass was measured on an aliquot [17]. The contents of protein per cell were in cells incubated with compactin 1.514 ± 0.113 ng (n = 8) and in control cells 1.389 ± 0.083 ng (n = 8), (non-significant difference)

dramatic augmentation of the cell association per mg protein. This is most clearly seen in the control dishes of Fig. 4b.

In order to ascertain that an increase in cell-protein per dish represented an increase in cell number per dish, even in compactin treated hepatocytes, the experiment shown in Fig. 5 was done. This figure shows that there is a close correlation (r = 0.99) between cell number and cell protein.

Discussion

This study shows that cell association and degradation of LDL in rat hepatocytes is cell density dependent and that it can be increased by preincubating cells with lipoprotein-deficient serum and compactin.

The fact that LDL uptake in cultured cells is cell density dependent have earlier been described in fibroblasts [7]. In that cell system it has clearly been shown that

LDL uptake is mediated through a LDL receptor [19, 21]. In fibroblasts it thus seems that the number of receptors per cell diminishes as the cell density increases [7]. The reasons for this to occur is obscure.

In cultured rat hepatocytes the uptake process of LDL is not elucidated. In freshly isolated rat hepatocytes there does, though, exist a saturable high affinity binding for human LDL [6] and presumably this means that LDL uptake is partly receptor dependent. Cell density dependent uptake of LDL in hepatocytes, as shown in this study, may then also depend on regulation of the receptor number per cell as the cell density varies.

Another question which arises is if all lipoprotein uptake in hepatocytes is cell density dependent. We have in preliminary experiments (Jensen, Florén and Nilsson, unpublished observations) shown that uptake and degradation of rat chylomicron remnants in rat hepatocyte monolayers is also cell density dependent. The uptake of this lipoprotein in hepatocytes has also been shown to be receptor mediated [22, 23].

Acknowledgements. The work was supported by grants from the Medical Faculty, University of Lund and The Swedish Medical Research Council (No. 03X-3969 and 03X-6802), and the Swedisch Diabetes Foundation.

References

1. Carlson LA (1982) in Metabolic Risk Factors in Ischemic Cardiovascular Disease (Carlsson LA and Pernow B eds) pp 1-3, Raven Press New York
2. Shepherd J, Bicker S, Lorimer AR, Packard CJ (1979) J Lipid Res 20: 999-1006
3. Steinberg D, Pittman RC, Attie AD, Carew TE, Pangburn S, Weinstein D (1980) in Atherosclerosis V. (Gotto AM ed) pp 800-803 Springer Verlag New York
4. Lindstedt S (1970) in Proceedings of the Second International Symposium on Atherosclerosis (Jones RJ ed) pp 262-271 Springer Verlag New York
5. Bonney RJ, Becker JE, Walker PR, Potter VR (1974) In Vitro 9: 399-413
6. Harkes L, Van Berkel TJC (1982) Biochim Biophys Acta 712: 677-683
7. Chait A, Bierman El, Albers JJ (1979) Diabetes 28: 914-918
8. Pangburn S, Newton RS, Chang CM, Weinstein DB, Steinberg D (1981) J Biol Chem 256: 3340-3347
9. Endo A, Kuroda M, Tanzawa K (1976) FEBS Lett 72: 323-326
10. Jensen E, Florén CH, Nilsson Å (1985) Biochim Biophys Acta 834: 279-283
11. Berry MN, Friend DS (1969) J Cell Biol 43: 506-520
12. Seglen PO (1973) Expl Cell Res 82: 391-398
13. Bisell DM, Hammaker LE, Meyer UA (1973) J Cell Biol 59: 722-734
14. Florén CH, Nilsson Å (1978) Biochem J 174: 827-838
15. Lin RC, Snodgrass PJ (1975) Biochem Biophys Res Commun 64: 725-734
16. Havel RJ, Eder HA, Bragdon JH (1955) J Clin Invest 34: 1345-1353
17. Lowry OH, Rosebrough NJ, Farr AL, Randall RJ (1951) J Biol Chem 193: 265-275
18. Bilheimer DW, Eisenberg S, Levy RI (1972) Biochim Biophys Acta 260: 212-221
19. Goldstein JL, Basu SK, Brunschede GY, Brown MS (1976) Cell 7: 85-95
20. Bierman EL, Stein O, Stein Y (1974) Circ Res 35: 136-150
21 Goldstein JL, Brown MS (1974) J Biol Chem 250: 7854-7862
22. Sherill BC, Innerarity TL, Mahley RW (1980) J Biol Chem 255: 1804-1807
23. Hui DY, Innerarity TL, Mahley RW (1981) J Biol Chem 256: 5646-5655

APO-B, E Receptor Binding of LDL: Evidence for Species-specific Segments of APO-B100 in the Binding Site Domain

M. J. Chapman, F. Loisay, and P. Forgez

Equipe de Recherches sur les Lipoprotéines, INSERM U-9, Hôpital de la Pitié, 75651 Paris Cedex 13, France

The low-density lipoprotein (LDL) is a complex macromolecule, about half of whose weight is represented by cholesterol, in both free and esterified forms. This quasi-spherical, pseudomicellar particle accounts for the transport of about two-thirds of the cholesterol in human plasma, assuring its delivery to diverse tissues and organs for eventual utilisation in cellular membrane synthesis. The specific interaction of LDL with cells occurs by way of a highly-specialised membrane receptor, the LDL (apo-B, E) receptor [1, 2]. Indeed, this receptor mediates a major portion of the catabolism of LDL, an essential process in the regulation of circulating LDL levels and of cholesterol homeostasis in the intact animal *in vivo* [1, 2]. Substantial progress has recently been made in our knowledge of the structure and biosynthesis of the LDL receptor protein, as well as in its gene structure [3, 4]. By contrast, we remain largely ignorant of the precise nature of the interaction of LDL with the receptor, although the specificity for this interaction is embodied in the major protein component of the lipoprotein particle, apolipoprotein B100 [5, 6]. Moreover, certain of these residues are located in the trypsin-accessible regions of apo-B100, their removal (or cleavage) diminishing the ability of LDL to bind to its receptor [7-9]. To further define the receptor binding site region on LDL/B100, and to evaluate the extent to which this domain may be species-specific, we have determined *i*) the characteristics of the high affinity binding of homologous (porcine) and heterologous (human) LDL to apo-B, E receptors of porcine adrenocortical membranes, and *ii*) the effect of limited proteolysis (using trypsin) of the heterologous (human) LDL on its interaction with the porcine receptor.

Methodological Approach

Low-density lipoproteins of d 1.024-1.050 g/ml were isolated from normolipidemic human and from porcine serum by sequential ultracentrifugal flotation as previously described [10]. The physicochemical and immunological characteristics of these lipoprotein preparations resembled those outlined earlier [10]. Their protein moieties contained the high molecular weight form of apo-B (termed "B100" by Kane *et al.* [11]), exclusively; indeed this protein represented > 98% of apo-LDL in each species. Limited proteolysis of apo-B100 was achieved by tryptic treatment of the native human LDL, using TPCK-trypsin to avoid chymotryptic cleavages [8, 9]. In this way, some 20% of human B100 was released into the incubation me-

Receptor-Mediated Uptake
in the Liver
Edited by H. Greten, E. Windler, U. Beisiegel
© Springer-Verlag Berlin Heidelberg 1986

dium as small peptides ($M_r < 5000$), while B100 remaining in the protein-deficient particles was extensively cleaved into a series of polypeptide fragments of $M_r \sim$ 10,000-95,000; no intact human B100, B74 or B26 was detected upon electrophoresis in SDS-polyacrylamide gels (3% monomer and 5-20% gradient gels [7, 8, 9].

Following separation of the protein-deficient, trypsinised human LDL (T-LDL) from the enzymic digest by gel filtration chromatography, aliquots of the native porcine and human and of the trypsinised human LDL were radio-iodinated with I^{125} by the iodine monochloride procedure [12]. I^{125}-LDL and I^{125}-T-LDL preparations displayed specific activities of 100-300 cpm/ng protein; > 95% of the radioactivity was typically precipitable in 5% trichloroacetic acid.

Adrenal cortex membranes (100,000 x g) were prepared from fresh porcine adrenals essentially as described by Kovanen et al. [13] for the bovine tissue. The binding of porcine and of human I^{125}-LDL's, and of human I^{125}-T-LDL to such porcine adrenocortical membranes was determined essentially by the method of Basu et al. [14], with some modifications [15]. Protein contents of lipoprotein and membrane samples were measured by the Lowry [16] procedure, using bovine serum albumin as standard. Lipoprotein concentrations are expressed exclusively in terms of their protein content.

Results

Binding of homologous LDL

A linear relationship was found between the total binding at 4° C of porcine I^{125}-LDL (added in fixed amount) and increasing concentrations of adrenocortical membrane protein (Fig. 1), to a maximum of $\sim$ 100 μg membrane protein. Non-specific binding, assessed in the presence of an excess of unlabelled porcine LDL, typically represented $\sim$ 20% of total binding. Unlabelled LDL and I^{125}-LDL thus appear to compete for binding to a limited number of sites of high affinity. Specific binding of I^{125}-LDL to high affinity sites then was proportional to membrane concentration. Time course studies showed that specific binding reached completion after $\sim$ 60 min incubation at 4° C; a period of 120 min was used subsequently.

Having evaluated the basic conditions for equilibrium binding in this system, we proceeded to determine the concentration dependence of specific I^{125}-porcine LDL binding (Fig. 2). At a fixed concentration of membrane protein (50 μg), specific binding plateaud at $\sim$ 15 μg I^{125}-LDL/ml. In subsequent studies, a working concentration of $\sim$ 10 μg/ml of I^{125}-LDL was used, as this fell on the linear portion of the binding curve. Specific binding was maximal at 90-100 μg I^{125}-LDL/ml.

The saturation kinetics of I^{125}-porcine LDL binding were analysed according to Scatchard [17], and gave a straight line plot (not shown), indicative of the presence of a single type of saturable, high affinity binding site. The apparent K_d was typically $\sim$ 15 μg LDL protein/ml, and the binding capacity 2.5 μg I^{125}-porcine LDL/mg membrane protein. Such binding parameters resemble those of bovine I^{125}-LDL in the bovine adrenocortical membrane system [13].

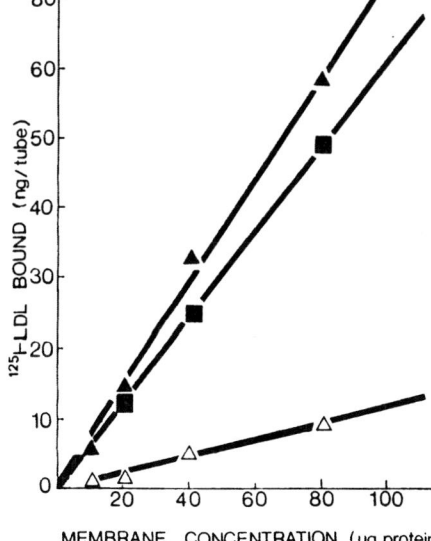

Fig. 1. Relationship of I^{125}-porcine LDL binding to the concentration of adrenocortical membrane protein. I^{125}-LDL (10.2 μg/ml) was incubated for 2 h at 4° C with increasing amounts of membrane protein, and specific binding determined at each concentration. Specific binding (■) was assessed as total binding (▲) less that due to non-specific binding (△), the latter being determined in the presence of 500 μg/ml of unlabelled porcine LDL

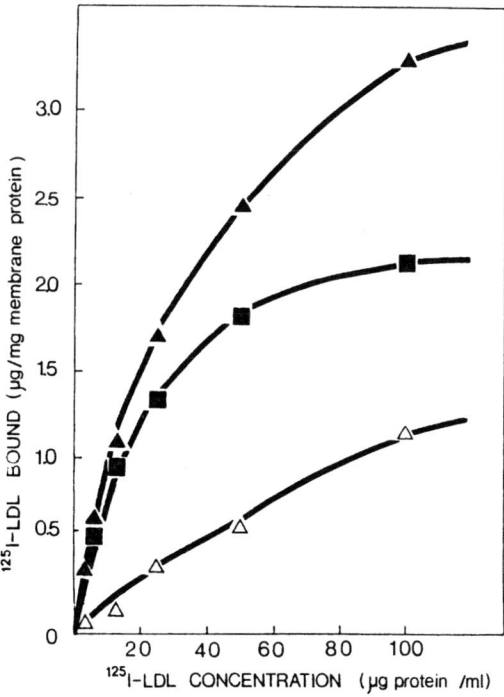

Fig. 2. Concentration dependence of I^{125}-porcine LDL binding to porcine adrenocortical membranes at 4° C. Each assay tube contained 50 μg membrane protein (100,000 x g_{ave} pellet) and the indicated concentrations of I^{125}-porcine LDL in the absence (▲) or presence (△) of 550 μg/ml unlabelled porcine LDL. The specific, high affinity binding component (■) was determined from the total binding (▲) after substraction of the non-specific binding (△), estimated in the presence of unlabelled LDL

Binding of heterologous LDL

The interaction of native human I^{125}-LDL with high affinity binding sites on porcine adrenocortical membranes was evaluated in a similar fashion to that for the homologous labelled ligand. Again, binding was time- and temperature-dependent. Indeed, maximal specific binding was some 1.4 fold higher at 37° C than 4° C, and reached completion more rapidly at the higher temperature; nonetheless, incubations in subsequent studies were performed at 4° C, in part to diminish any potential proteolysis of LDL-B100 by membrane-associated proteases, and in part to limit any possible exchange between membrane lipids and the trace amounts of labelled phospholipids in I^{125}-human LDL.

The receptor binding activity of the heterologous ligand was assessed in direct binding studies, in which I^{125}-human LDL displayed high affinity, saturable binding activity (Fig. 3). Upon data analysis by the method of Scatchard, a straight line plot was obtained (not shown). The equilibrium dissociation constant (K_d) calculated from such plots was ~ 19 µg/ml, and the binding capacity 1.7 µg I^{125}-human LDL/mg membrane protein.

Our direct binding data with labelled homologous and heterologous native LDL's suggested that both the binding affinity and binding capacity of porcine LDL for the high affinity receptor sites on porcine adrenocortical membranes were superior to those of human LDL. This postulate was indeed confirmed in competitive displacement experiments (Fig. 4 and 5), in which the ability of native porcine and of native human LDL to displace either I^{125}-porcine LDL or I^{125}-human LDL were compared. Thus, some 7-fold more human than porcine LDL were required to displace 50% of I^{125}-porcine LDL from membrane receptors (*i. e.* 15.3 ± 10.3 µg/ml (n = 5) of porcine LDL as compared to 110 µg/ml (n = 2) of human LDL). Furthermore, pig LDL was some two-fold more efficient in displacing its heterologous labelled counterpart, I^{125}-human LDL, from high affinity binding sites than unlabelled human LDL (*i. e.* 22 µg/ml (n = 2) of pig LDL was needed for displacement of 50% of the labelled ligand, versus 50.6 ± 16.1 µg/ml (n = 7) of human LDL). These data clearly attest to the higher affinity of the homologous LDL for the porcine apo-B, E membrane receptor.

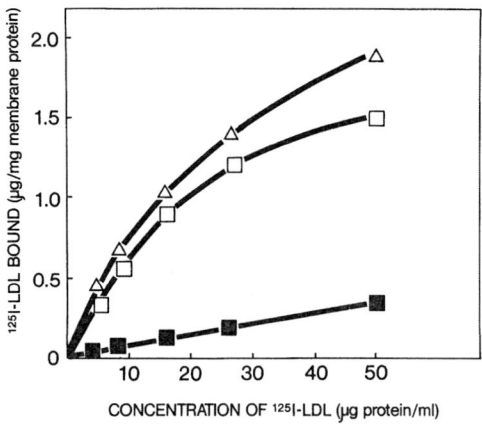

Fig. 3. Concentration dependence of I^{125}-human LDL binding to porcine adrenocortical membranes at 4° C. Increasing amounts of I^{125}-LDL were incubated for 90 min with 145 µg of membrane protein per tube. Specific binding (□) was determined as the total binding ( ) after subtraction of the non-specific binding (■), estimated in the presence of an excess (1 mg protein/ml) of unlabelled LDL

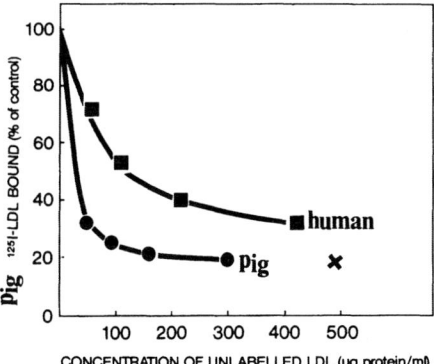

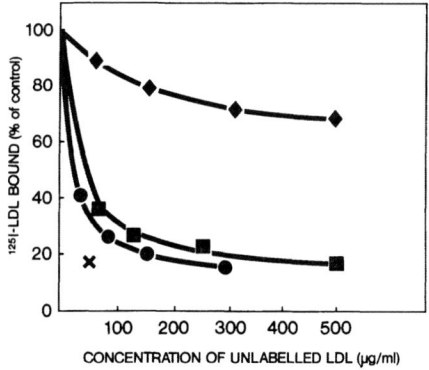

Fig. 4. Ability of unlabelled porcine and human LDL to compete with I[125]-porcine LDL for binding to membranes from porcine adrenal cortex. I[125]-porcine LDL (12.9 μg/ml) were incubated with membranes (100 μg protein/tube) for 2 h at 4° C in the presence of increasing concentrations of unlabelled porcine (●) or human LDL (■); the LDL fraction from each species was of d 1.024-1.050 g/ml. The labelled ligand was also incubated in the presence of 30 mM EDTA (X) to determine the total EDTA-resistant binding

Fig. 5. Competitive displacement of I[125]-human LDL from high affinity binding sites on porcine adrenocortical membranes by unlabelled human or by unlabelled porcine LDL. I[125]-human (8 μg/ml) was incubated with membranes (116 μg protein/tube) for 2 h at 4° C in the presence of increasing concentrations of unlabelled pig (●) or human LDL (■), or of human HDL (◆). The labelled ligand was also incubated in the presence of membranes and 30 mM EDTA (X), but in the absence of unlabelled LDL

It was of some interest to evaluate whether limited proteolysis of the heterologous, human LDL would be of any consequence to its binding activity in our porcine system. This question was prompted by the following observations:

a) that tryptic treatment of human LDL reduces its ability to bind to the apo-B, E receptor in a (homologous) human fibroblast system [7],

b) that tryptic treatment of porcine LDL diminishes its capacity to displace its native counterpart from high affinity sites in the presently-described membrane binding system (data not shown), and

c) it is established that porcine and human apo-B100 exhibit structural differences which concern surface-exposed regions of both particles (10, 18); might such differences be accentuated or reduced then, at least in the region of the B, E receptor binding domain, by limited proteolysis?

Indeed, the ability of human LDL to bind to the porcine receptor was enhanced after tryptic treatment, as illustrated by the greater efficiency of human T-LDL to separately displace both I[125]-human LDL and I[125]-human T-LDL (Fig. 6). On the basis of the amount of unlabelled ligand required for 50% displacement of I[125]-human LDL, T-LDL was more than two-fold more efficient in competing for high affinity binding than LDL (21.7 ± 9.8 μg/ml (n = 4) of T-LDL versus 50.6 ± 16.1 (n = 7) of LDL). These findings were entirely consistent with competition studies of I[125]-human T-LDL binding in the presence of either unlabelled T-LDL

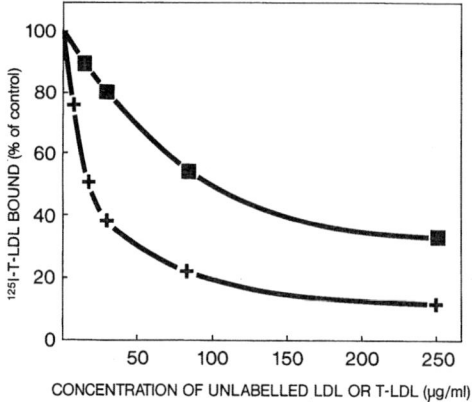

Fig. 6. Competitive displacement of I^{125}-human T-LDL from high affinity binding sites on porcine adrenocortical membranes by unlabelled human LDL or human T-LDL. Human I^{125}-T-LDL (8 μg/ml) was incubated for 2 h at 4° C with membranes (53 μg protein/tube) in the presence of increasing concentrations of native LDL (■) and of T-LDL (+)

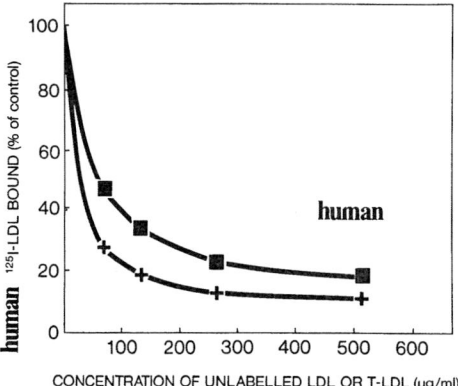

Fig. 7. Competitive displacement of human I^{125}-LDL from high affinity binding sites on porcine adrenocortical membranes by unlabelled native human LDL or human T-LDL. Human I^{125}-LDL (11.4 μg/ml) was incubated for 2 h at 4° C with the membranes (130 μg protein/tube) in the presence of increasing concentration of unlabelled human native LDL (■) or human T-LDL (+)

or LDL (Fig. 7), in which T-LDL was again superior in its ability to displace the labelled ligand as compared to native LDL (50% displacement points: 21.4 ± 12.3 μg/ml (n = 4) for T-LDL versus 130.2 ± 18.3 (n = 4) for LDL). Moreover in direct binding experiments (not shown), the equilibrium dissociation constant of human T-LDL (8.3 μg/ml) was less than half that of the native (human) LDL (19.2 μg/ml), illustrating the elevated binding affinity of the trypsinised particle.

We interpret these studies to confirm that surface-exposed trypsin-accessible segments of apo-B100 in LDL contribute to the apo-B, E receptor binding domain(s) on this complex macromolecule [7]. In addition, they raise the interesting possibility that such segments of B100 may exhibit some degree of species-specificity, and may thus have been subject to evolutionary modification. This hypothesis is consistent with studies of the structural evolution of animal LDL's using monoclonal antibodies to the human lipoprotein, in which marked variation was seen in the degree of binding of two monoclonal antibodies (each of which blocked the binding of human LDL to apo-B, E receptors on human fibroblasts), to the LDL of a wide range of mammalian species [19].

Acknowledgements. F. Loisay and P. Forgez were supported by Research Fellowships from ICI-Pharma Ltd. We thank Drs D.C.N. Earl and A. Rossi for their continued interest and support.

References

1. Brown MS, Kovanen PT, Goldstein JL (1981) Science 212: 628-635
2. Mahley RW, Innerarity TL (1983) Biochim Biophys Acta 737: 197-222
3. Yamamoto T, Davis CG, Brown MS, Schneider WJ, Casey ML, Goldstein JL, Russell DW (1984) Cell 39: 27-38
4. Lehrman MA, Schneider WJ, Sudhof TC, Brown MS, Goldstein JL, Russell DW (1985) Science 227: 140-146
5. Mahley RW, Innerarity TL, Pitas RE, Weisgraber KH, Brown JA, Gross E (1977) J Biol Chem 252: 7279-7287
6. Weisgraber KH, Innerarity TL, Mahley RW (1978) J Biol Chem 253: 9053-9062
7. Chapman MJ, Innerarity TL, Arnold KS, Mahley RW in "Latent Dyslipoproteinemias and Atherosclerosis" ed JL de Gennes et al Raven Press NY (1984) pp 93-99
8. Chapman MJ, Millet A, Lagrange D, Goldstein S, Blouquit Y, Taylaur CE, Mills GL (1982) Eur J Biochem 125: 479-489
9. Chapman MJ, Goldstein S, Mills GL (1978) Eur J Biochem 87: 475-488
10. Chapman MJ, Goldstein S (1976) Atherosclerosis 25: 267-291
11. Kane JP, Hardman DA, Paulus HE (1980) Proc Natl Acad Sci USA 7: 2465-2469
12. Mc Farlane AS (1958) Nature 182: 53-56
13. Kovanen PT, Basu SK, Brown MS (1979) Endocrinology 104: 610-616
14. Basu SK, Goldstein JL, Brown MS (1978) J Biol Chem 253: 3852-3856
15. Chapman MJ, Loisay FYM, Forgez P, Cadman H (1985) Biochem Biophys Acta 835: 258-272
16. Lowry OH, Rosebrough NJ, Farr AL, Randall RJ (1951) J Biol Chem 193: 265-275
17 Scatchard G (1949) Ann NY Acad Sci 51: 660-672
18. Chapman MJ (1980) J Lipid Res 21: 789-853
19. Nelson CA, Tasch MA, Tikkanen M, Dargar R, Schonfeld G (1984) J Lipid Res 25: 821-830

Effect of the Phorbol Esters on the Receptors for LDL on U-937 Monocyte-Like Cells and Acetyl-LDL on Mouse Peritoneal Macrophages

S. GOLDSTEIN[1], M. ROUIS[2], D. ERLICH[1], M. BERTHELIER[1], C. CHERIER[2], and P. THOMOPOULOS[2]

[1] INSERM, Laboratoire de Biochimie, Faculté de Médecine Saint-Antoine,
  F-75012 Paris, France
[2] INSERM U-282, Hôpital Henri Mondor, F-94010 Créteil, France

Tumor-promoting phorbol diesters exhibit a wide variety of effects on cultured cells [1], which are probably mediated by the activation of protein kinase C [2]. In particular they induce an acute reduction of the binding ability of the membrane receptors for epidermal growth factor [3-5], thyrotropin-releasing hormone, somatostatin [6], insulin [7, 8], insulin-like peptides [9], colony-stimulating factor [10, 11] and transferrin [12]. It has been demonstrated that the receptors for insulin, somatomedin [13], transferrin [14], epidermal growth factor [15, 16] and catecholamines [17, 18] are phosphorylated by the phorbol esters. Finally, these tumor promoters induce a rapid internalization of the transferrin receptors [14, 19]. In this study we demonstrate that the phorbol esters are able to decrease acutely and reversibly the binding ability of the receptors for LDL and acetyl-LDL.

Materials and Methods

U-937 human monocyte-like cells were grown in suspension in RPMI-1640 medium containing 10% fetal calf serum at 37° C under 95% air − 5% CO_2 humidified atmoshpere. Mouse peritoneal macrophages were isolated as previously described [20]. The iodination and the binding assays of LDL and acetyl-LDL were performed as already reported [21].

Results and Discussion

U-937 cells possess specific LDL receptors [21]. Incubation with the phorbol esters induced a rapid inhibition of the binding ability of the cells (Fig. 1). The phenomenon was reversible. After removal of the promoters, treated cells recovered their ^{125}I-LDL-binding activity in 60 min (Fig. 2). Inhibition appeared to be due to a reduction of the number of available LDL receptors rather than a decrease in receptor affinity.

The action of the phorbol esters on acetyl-LDL receptors was studied on mouse peritoneal macrophages, because of the lack of such "scavenger" receptors on the U-937 cells. The binding and degradation of ^{125}I-acetyl-LDL was inhibited by the

Receptor-Mediated Uptake
in the Liver
Edited by H. Greten, E. Windler, U. Beisiegel
© Springer-Verlag Berlin Heidelberg 1986

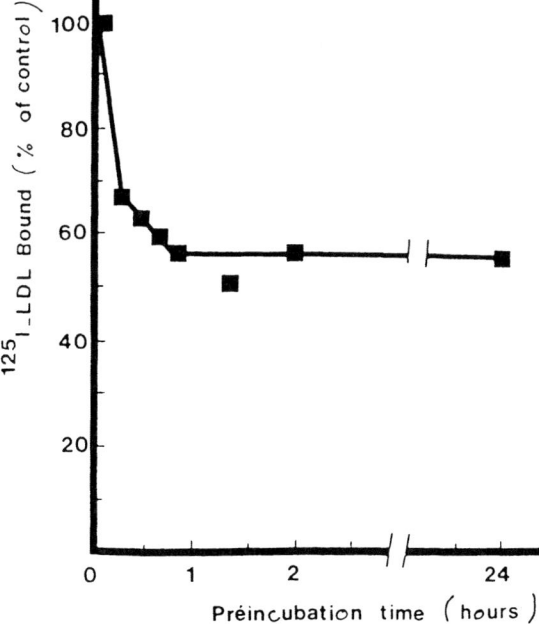

Fig. 1. Kinetics of TPA inhibition of ^{125}I-LDL binding. U-937 cells were incubated for the indicated time intervals in the absence or presence of TPA (10^{-7}M) at 37° C. Following TPA treatment, cells were washed and the specific binding of ^{125}I-LDL was measured for 60 min at 4° C. The results are expressed as the percentage of the binding on the control (acetone-treated) cells measured at the same time intervals

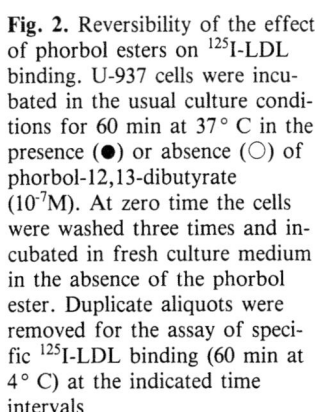

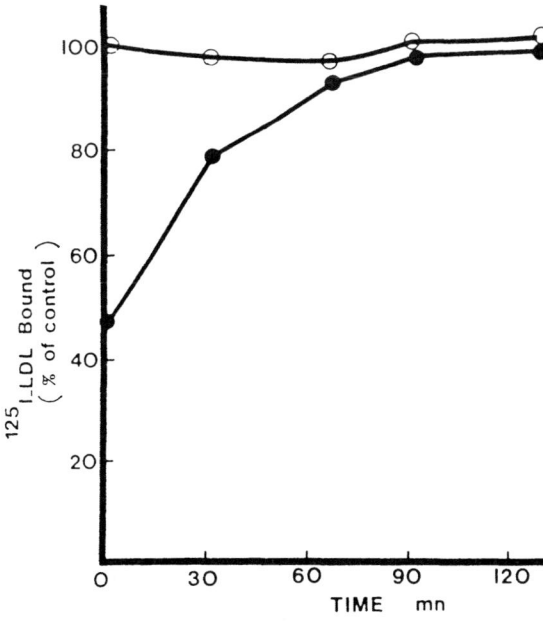

Fig. 2. Reversibility of the effect of phorbol esters on ^{125}I-LDL binding. U-937 cells were incubated in the usual culture conditions for 60 min at 37° C in the presence (●) or absence (○) of phorbol-12,13-dibutyrate (10^{-7}M). At zero time the cells were washed three times and incubated in fresh culture medium in the absence of the phorbol ester. Duplicate aliquots were removed for the assay of specific ^{125}I-LDL binding (60 min at 4° C) at the indicated time intervals

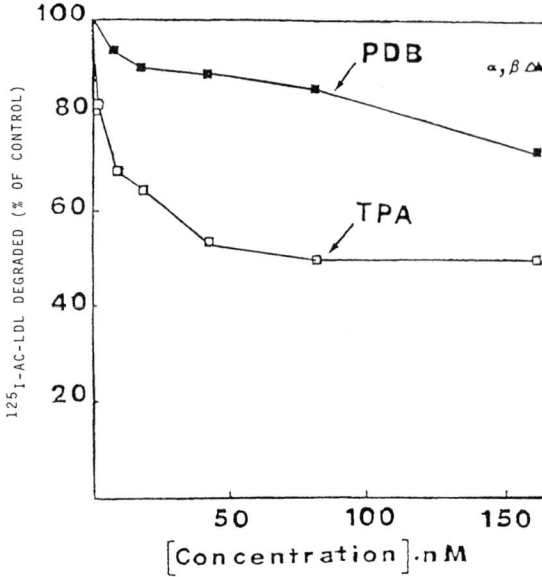

Fig. 3. Effect of phorbol derivatives on ^{125}I-acetyl-LDL degradation by mouse peritoneal macrophages. Macrophages were incubated for 5h with ^{125}I-acetyl-LDL (3 $\mu g/ml$) in the presence of the indicated concentrations of 12-0-tetradecanoyl-phorbol-13 acetate ($\square$), phorbol-12,13-dibutyrate $\blacksquare$), α or β phorbol ($\triangle$ $\blacktriangle$). The degradation of the tracer was measured as described in (20)

phorbol esters (Fig. 3) and this phenomenon was rapidly reversible in 15 min (data not shown).

Our data demonstrate that the tumor promoting phorbol esters inhibit the binding of LDL and of acetyl LDL to U-937 cells and to mouse peritoneal macrophages, respectively. This effect is cell-specific since it has not been observed on fibroblasts [22]. Its mechanism remains to be elucidated, but we suggest that these receptors might be a target for the phorbol ester-activated protein kinase C.

References

1. Weinstein IB, Lee LS, Fisher PB, Mufson A, Yamasaki H (1979) J Supramolec Struct 12: 195-208
2. Nishizuka Y (1984) Nature 308: 693-698
3. Lee LS, Weinstein IB (1978) Science 202: 313-315
4. Brown KD, Dicker P, Rozengurt E (1979) Biochem Biophys Res Commun 86: 1037-1043
5. Shoyab M, DeLarco JE, Todaro GJ (1979) Nature 279: 387-391
6. Osborne R, Tashjian AH (1982) Cancer Res 42: 4375-4381
7. Thomopoulos P, Testa U, Gourdin MF, Hervy C, Titeux M, Vainchenker W (1982) Eur J Biochem 129: 389-393
8. Robert A, Grunberger G, Carpentier JL, Dayer JM, Orci L, Gorden P (1984) Endocrinology 114: 247-253
9. Rouis M, Thomopoulos P, Postel-Vinay MC, Testa U, Guyda HJ, Posner BI (1984) Mol Physiol 5: 123-130
10. Chen BDM, Lin HS, Hsu S (1983) J Cell Physiol 116: 207-212
11. Guilbert LJ, Nelson DJ, Hamilton JA, Williams N (1983) J Cell Physiol 115: 276-282
12. Pelicci PG, Testa U, Thomopoulos P, Tabilio A, Vainchenker W, Titeux M, Rochant H (1984) Leukemia Res 8: 597-609
13. Jacobs S, Sahyoun NE, Saltiel A, Cuatrecasas P (1983) Proc Natl Acad Sci USA 80: 6211-6213

14. May WS, Jacobs S, Cuatrecasas P (1984) Proc Natl Acad Sci USA 81: 2016-2020
15. Cochet C, Gill GN, Meisenhelder J, Cooper JA, Hunter T (1984) J Biol Chem 259: 2553-2558
16. Iwashita S, Fox CF (1984) J Biol Chem 259: 2559-2567
17. Sibley DR, Nambi P, Peters JR, Lefkowitz RJ (1984) Biochem Biophys Res Commun 121: 973-979
18. Kelleher DJ, Pessin JE, Ruoho AE, Johnson GL (1984) J Biol Chem 81: 4316-4320
19. Klausner RD, Harford F, VanRenswoude J (1984) Proc Natl Acad Sci USA 81: 3005-3009
20. Goldstein JL, Ho YK, Basu SK, Brown MS (1979) Proc Natl Acad Sci USA 76: 333-337
21. Rouis M, Goldstein S, Thomopoulos P, Berthelier M, Hervy C, Testa U (1984) J Cell Physiol 121: 540-546
22. Shoyab M, De Larco JE, Todaro GJ (1979) Nature 279: 387-391

Regulation of Low Density Lipoprotein Levels in Animals and Man with Particular Emphasis on the Role of the Liver

J. M. DIETSCHY and D. K. SPADY

University of Texas Health Science Center at Dallas, Southwestern Medical School, Dallas, Texas 75235 USA

During the past few years, there has been considerable progress in understanding the physiology involved in the regulation of circulating LDL levels. Much of this progress has been made possible by the development of techniques for measuring rates of cholesterol synthesis and rates of receptor-dependent and receptor-independent LDL uptake in the live animal. These techniques have provided the means for unraveling the complex interactions that exist in the intact animal between the rates of cholesterol uptake and synthesis, and that determine sterol balance across individual organs and across the whole animal.

Rates of cholesterol synthesis in the intact animal

In the past, rates of cholesterol synthesis were measured largely in vitro by assessing either the activity of microsomal 3-hydroxy-3-methylglutaryl (HMG) CoA reductase or the rates of incorporation of various ^{14}C-labeled substrates such as acetate, octanoate and glucose [1]. While useful in a relative sense, neither method yields rates of sterol synthesis that equal those found in vivo [2, 3]. Furthermore, because of relatively greater dilution of the specific activity of the precursor pool of acetyl CoA in the extrahepatic tissues [4], the importance of the liver to whole-animal synthesis has been grossly overestimated [5]. More recently, several laboratories have begun using [^{3}H]water to assess rates of sterol synthesis under both in vitro and in vivo conditions. This substrate rapidly penetrates nearly all cell membranes and its specific activity is essentially not subject to dilution [6]. Furthermore, when the number of ^{3}H atoms incorporated into each sterol molecule is known, rates of [^{3}H]water incorporation into cholesterol can be converted into the mass of cholesterol actually synthesized per unit time [7, 8].

   Using this substrate, rates of cholesterol synthesis have been measured in all major tissues of a number of different species of both sexes [5, 9] and three major findings have become apparent. First, rates of cholesterol synthesis are much higher in all extrahepatic organs than previously believed. Second, the contribution of hepatic synthesis to whole-animal cholesterol synthesis is much less than earlier work suggested. Third, and most important, there are major differences in the rates of cholesterol synthesis by the liver in different animal species under conditions of a very low dietary cholesterol intake [10]. Thus, for example, the basal rates of cholesterol synthesis seen in the rat (1500-2300 nmol/hr per g), monkey

Receptor-Mediated Uptake
in the Liver
Edited by H. Greten, E. Windler, U. Beisiegel
© Springer-Verlag Berlin Heidelberg 1986

(500-900), female hamster (180-500), rabbit (150-250), guinea pig (75-150), and male hamster (30-60) vary over a 50-fold range when these animals are fed the same low-cholesterol diet. Several lines of evidence also suggest that the liver of man synthesizes at the low rates found in the male and female hamster [10-12].

Rates of LDL uptake in various organs

Methods also have recently become available for measuring rates of LDL uptake in all of the major organs of the experimental animal in vivo. By labeling the homologous LDL molecule with markers such as [14C]sucrose [13] and using a primed-continuous infusion technique [12, 14, 15], it is possible to assess absolute rates of LDL clearance in every major organ under circumstances where the rates of uptake are a linear function of time, where differential losses of the radioactive label are minimized and where the circulating levels of LDL can be essentially instantaneously altered. Such measurements have now been made in a number of species, both male and female, including the rat, hamster, rabbit and dog, and essentially three findings have been seen in all species. First, the liver manifests a high rate of LDL uptake with clearance rates equaling approximately 100 μl/hr per g in most animals. This organ accounts for the uptake of 60-75% of all LDL cleared from the plasma in the species that have been studied thus far. The gastrointestinal tract is the only other tissue that clears significant amounts of LDL. Second, LDL uptake by most other extrahepatic organs is very low and is quantitatively of little importance. Third, LDL uptake by the endocrine glands is highly variable from species to species [16]. For example, some species rely primarily on cholesterol that is newly synthesized for hormone production while other species use sterol acquired from HDL or LDL [16].

Thus, unlike rates of cholesterol synthesis, there is relatively little variation among different species in the importance of the liver for the clearance of plasma LDL. This important observation is emphasized by the data summarized in Fig. 1. As shown in the lower panel, the rate of hepatic sterol synthesis in animals fed

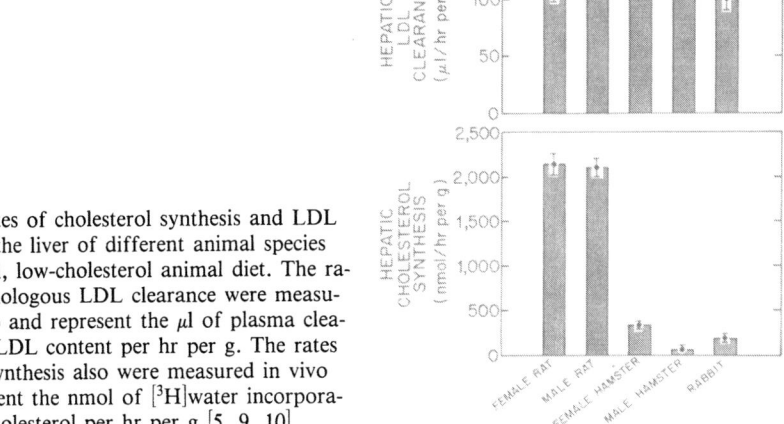

Fig. 1. Rates of cholesterol synthesis and LDL uptake in the liver of different animal species fed control, low-cholesterol animal diet. The rates of homologous LDL clearance were measured in vivo and represent the μl of plasma cleared of its LDL content per hr per g. The rates of sterol synthesis also were measured in vivo and represent the nmol of [3H]water incorporated into cholesterol per hr per g [5, 9, 10]

a low-cholesterol diet may vary as much as 50-fold (the rat versus the male hamster, for example) yet the liver is the primary site for LDL uptake in all of these species. There is no relationship between the rate of cholesterol synthesis and the rate of LDL transport in the basal state. Indirect evidence also suggests that the liver is the primary site for LDL removal from the circulation in man [17].

Mechanisms of LDL uptake in various organs

The transport of LDL into various tissues is generally considered to take place by either receptor-dependent [18] or receptor-independent mechanism. Since the LDL receptors on a given species do not interact well with LDL from a second species and since methylation of the LDL molecule further blocks this binding reaction, methylated human LDL (methyl-hLDL) has been used to quantitate the receptor-independent component of LDL transport in the tissues of various animal species [14]. When labeled with [14C]sucrose and administered to animals as a primed-continuous infusion, the receptor-independent clearance of this molecule takes place in every organ at rates varying from 1-10 μl/hr per g. Only the spleen manifests a significantly higher rate of receptor-independent clearance.

Thus, as shown in Fig. 2 in the case of the rat, and as has been found in all other species that have been examined, receptor-independent LDL transport occurs in all organs while receptor-dependent LDL uptake is primarily localized to those few tissues like the liver, intestine and endocrine glands that have high rates of total LDL transport per g of tissue. When such data are calculated in terms of whole-organ uptake, the liver and intestine in most species not only account for the clearance of 70-80% of the circulating LDL, but these same two organs contain nearly 90% of the receptor-dependent LDL transport that occurs in these species.

Thus, in the rat, hamster, rabbit and man, about two-thirds of the circulating LDL pool is cleared by receptor-mediated means [19]. Probably 90% of this is accounted for by transport into the liver and intestine. In contrast, about one-third of the LDL in the plasma pool is cleared by receptor-independent mechanisms, and this transport activity is distributed in a number of different organs other than the liver and intestine. It should also be emphasized that these two transport pro-

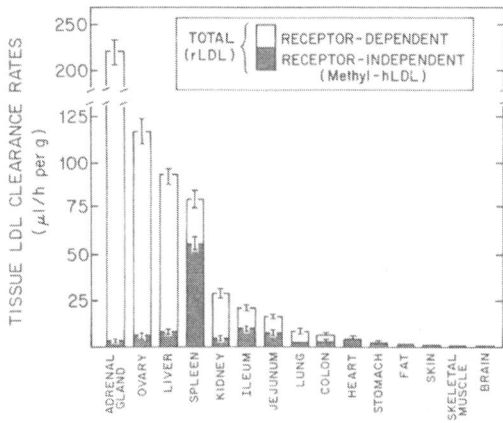

Fig. 2. Rates of LDL uptake per g of tissue in 15 organs of the rat. The rates of total LDL clearance in each organ were measured using homologous LDL while the receptor-independent component was measured using methylated human LDL (methyl-hLDL) [14]

cesses are probably localized on the same parenchymal cells in each organ and not on some other cell type such as phagocytes. The same profile of transport activity found in the whole organ (Fig. 2) is seen when the cells of that organ are isolated [20].

Kinetics of receptor-dependent and receptor-independent LDL transport

These quantitative relationships, however, are true only in normal animals and man with normal circulating levels of LDL-cholesterol. Under circumstances where the plasma LDL concentration is either lowered or elevated, the relative importance of receptor-dependent and receptor-independent uptake in each organ changes depending upon the kinetic characteristics of each of the transport processes in that organ. By adding mass qualities of LDL to the primed-continuous infusion, it is possible to abruptly elevate the circulating plasma concentration of either the homologous LDL or the methyl-hLDL in a given species. In this manner the rate of clearance and LDL-cholesterol uptake can be measured in every organ as a function of the plasma LDL-cholesterol concentration. It should be emphasized that during the 4-6 hr interval over which such measurements are made, infusion of mass qualities of LDL does not down-regulate LDL receptor activity in any tissue [21].

Such detailed kinetic curves are now available for a number of species and an example is shown in Fig. 3 for the liver of the hamster. As is apparent in panel

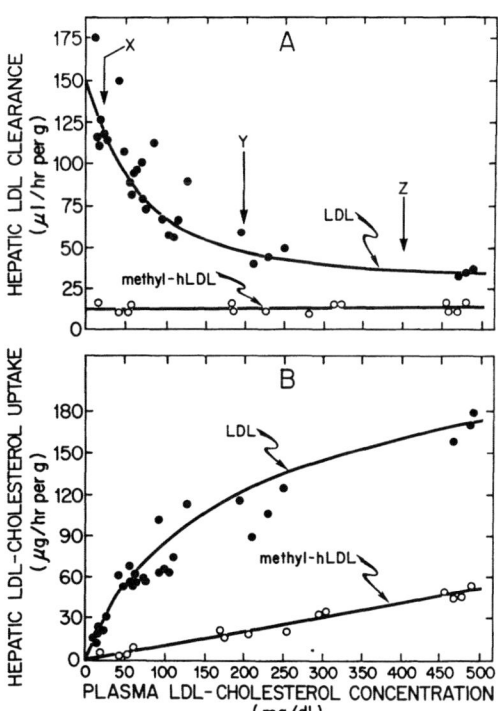

Fig. 3. Kinetics of LDL transport by the liver of the hamster. The upper panel shows the rates of both total and receptor-independent LDL clearance by the liver under circumstances where the plasma cholesterol level was abruptly increased from normal values (about 20 mg/dl) to nearly 500 mg/dl. The lower panel shows the total μg of LDL-cholesterol taken up into the liver per hr per g. The receptor-independent component of this uptake process also is shown (methyl-hLDL) [21]

A, the clearance of LDL by the receptor-independent mechanism is constant at about 10 μl/hr per g. Thus, the rate of uptake of LDL-cholesterol by this process is a linear function of the plasma LDL concentration, as shown in panel B. In contrast, total LDL clearance, which contains a large receptor-dependent component, decreases as the plasma LDL level is elevated and the LDL receptors become relatively more saturated. At very high plasma LDL-cholesterol levels, the rate of receptor-dependent LDL transport becomes quantitatively much less important, even if there is no suppression of LDL-receptor activity. This is also illustrated in Fig. 3. The point labeled X represents the normal plasma LDL-cholesterol level in the hamster. At this concentration about 90% of hepatic LDL uptake is receptor-dependent. However, if there is overproduction of LDL and the plasma LDL-cholesterol rises, the receptor-independent component of total hepatic LDL uptake becomes progressively more important as shown at points Y and Z.

Another important point illustrated by this curve is that equal amounts of cholesterol can be taken up into the liver by the receptor-independent process as by the receptor-dependent transport system, although the plasma cholesterol level must be increased to accomplish this. For example, at a plasma LDL-cholesterol concentration of 25 mg/dl, about 30 μg/hr per g of LDL-cholesterol is taken up by the normal liver by predominantly receptor-dependent transport. Essentially the same amount of cholesterol can be taken up by the receptor-independent system if the plasma LDL-cholesterol concentration is raised to about 300 mg/dl. The importance of receptor-independent LDL transport in the liver also can be shown in the receptor-deficient rabbit, as illustrated in Fig. 4. The liver of the control rabbit takes up about 600 μg/hr of LDL-cholesterol, predominantly by receptor-dependent transport. The liver of the WHHL rabbit, on the other hand, actually takes up twice as much cholesterol by the receptor-independent pathway and this is associated with a proportionate suppression in the rate of cholesterol synthesis in the liver of these animals [22].

Thus, because of these kinetic differences in the receptor-dependent and receptor-independent pathways, the receptor-independent transport system becomes the predominant mechanism for LDL removal from the plasma under any circumstance where there is marked overproduction of LDL or where LDL receptor activity is reduced below normal levels by genetic or environmental factors. Ne-

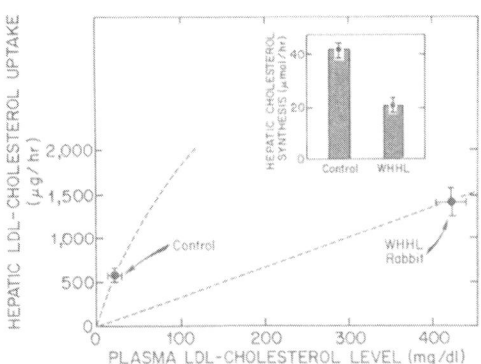

Fig. 4. Rates of hepatic LDL uptake and cholesterol synthesis in the normal and receptor-deficient (WHHL) rabbit. The dashed lines represent the kinetic curves for total LDL transport in control animals and for the receptor-independent component in both the control and WHHL rabbits. The insert shows the rate of hepatic cholesterol synthesis measured in vivo in the two groups of animals and synthesis is expressed as the μmol of [³H]water incorporated into cholesterol per hr by the whole organ [22]

vertheless, under these conditions cholesterol balance across individual tissues and across the whole-animal is maintained, but this balance is achieved by a marked elevation in the circulating levels of LDL-cholesterol.

Interrelation between hepatic cholesterol synthesis and receptor-mediated LDL uptake

Receptor-independent LDL clearance is not only constant at all plasma LDL-cholesterol concentrations (Fig. 3) but, in addition, it is constant under different nutritional states and under circumstances where rates of sterol synthesis in the various organs have been changed [20]. In contrast, the rate of receptor-dependent LDL transport can, in a few experimental situations, be altered. Since the great majority of receptor-mediated LDL transport demonstrated in the whole animal resides in the liver, it follows that regulation of hepatic receptor-mediated LDL transport should be of greatest importance in regulation of plasma LDL-cholesterol levels.

Unlike isolated cells, however, there is no relationship between the rate of sterol synthesis in the liver and LDL uptake. As illustrated in Fig. 5, for example, in both the rat and female hamster the rate of cholesterol synthesis in the liver can be in-

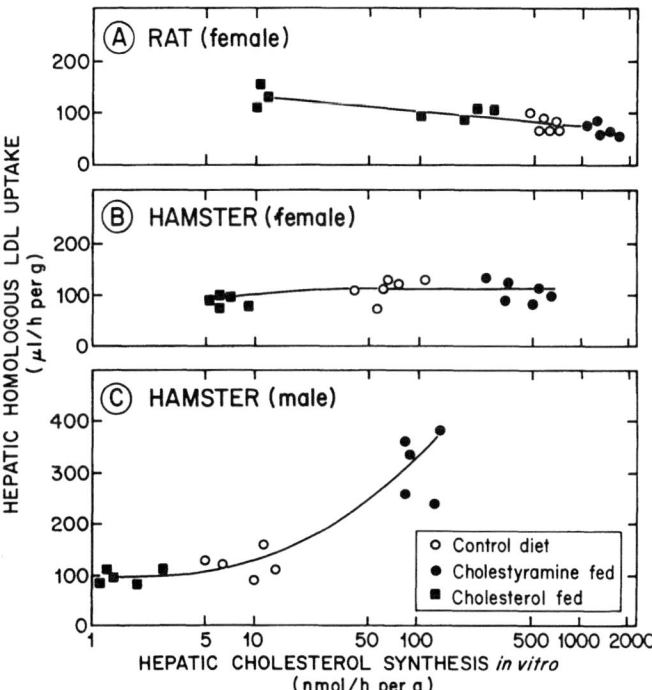

Fig. 5. Rates of hepatic LDL uptake as a function of the rate of hepatic cholesterol synthesis. Groups of each of these three species were fed either control diet or diets containing cholesterol or cholestyramine in order to vary the rate of sterol synthesis over a very large range [19]

creased or decreased over a very large range without altering the rate of LDL transport. As long as the change in sterol synthesis fully compensates for the induced change in cholesterol flux across the liver, the rate of LDL transport (and the circulating level of LDL-cholesterol) remains constant. This compensatory capacity is much lower in an animal like the male hamster that, in the basal state, synthesizes cholesterol at a rate that equals only 1-2% of the rate seen in the rat. Thus, feeding cholestyramine to this animal induces a loss of sterol from the liver that cannot be compensated for by an increase in sterol synthesis and, hence, receptor-dependent (but not receptor-independent) LDL clearance increases. Receptor activity may also be suppressed by feeding this animal relatively large amounts of cholesterol (not shown in Fig. 5). Thus, whether or not a given manipulation alters hepatic LDL clearance (and circulating LDL-cholesterol levels) critically depends upon the capacity of that particular animal (or man) to compensate for the maneuver by a change in hepatic cholesterol synthesis [20, 21].

Regulation of hepatic receptor-mediated LDL uptake

With these interrelations defined and with complete kinetic curves available for both the receptor-dependent and receptor-independent transport system, it is now possible to explore quantitatively some of the major factors that regulate circulating LDL-cholesterol levels. First, however, there are several important considerations concerning whole-animal LDL turnover data that must be understood. Fig. 6 represents the theoretical curves for LDL turnover in the whole animal or man.

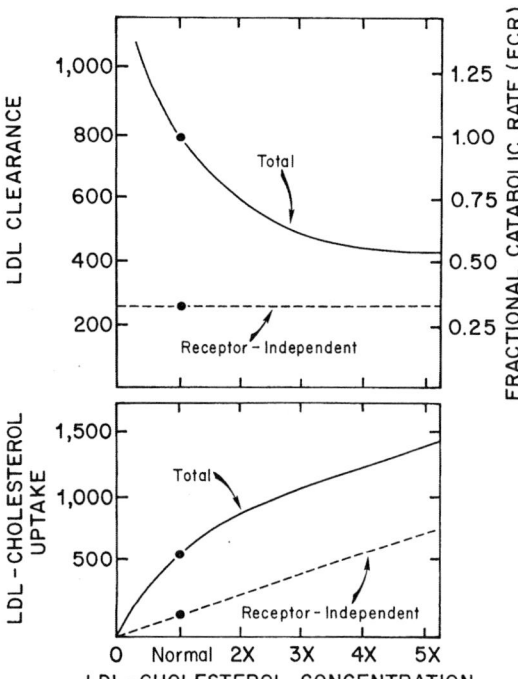

Fig. 6. Theoretical relationship between whole-animal LDL clearance, fractional catabolic rate and LDL transport out of the plasma. The lower panel shows the rate of LDL-cholesterol transport out of the plasma while the upper panel shows the same data expressed as clearance values and as fractional catabolic rates. The solid lines represent the curves for total LDL transport while the dashed lines show the receptor-independent component of this transport process. The solid points represent the values for total and receptor-independent LDL transport in normal animals and man where approximately two-thirds of LDL clearance is receptor-dependent and one-third is receptor-independent. the numbers on the scales are only relative and have no absolute meaning

The two curves in the lower panel show the rate of total LDL transport out of plasma and into all of the tissues in the body and the receptor-independent component as a function of the concentration of plasma LDL-cholesterol. In the upper panel, these same data are presented as LDL clearance or as the fractional catabolic rate of the LDL molecule. These curves represent the rates of whole-body LDL transport (expressed as uptake, clearance or FCR) as the plasma LDL-cholesterol level is varied from 0 to 5 times the normal level and under circumstances where there has been no change in LDL-receptor activity in any organ. The solid points show the situation in the normal animal or man where about two-thirds of LDL transport is receptor-mediated and one-third is receptor-independent. If the animal or man is subjected to a maneuver that raises the plasma LDL-cholesterol level, it necessarily follows that the clearance or FCR must decrease. Conversely, if the manipulation lowers the plasma LDL-cholesterol level, the clearance or FCR must increase. These changes take place even though there has been no change in receptor-mediated LDL transport in the body. The point to be emphasized is that a change in LDL clearance or FCR *cannot* be interpreted as a change in receptor-mediated LDL transport. Such changes would also be evident if the LDL production rate were altered. Data on LDL clearance or FCR can only be interpreted if superimposed upon the kinetic curves constructed for each experimental animal. If the experimental data fall above or below this curve at a particular LDL-cholesterol concentration, then there has been an increase or decrease, respectively, in the receptor-mediated component of LDL transport.

Specific data of this type are illustrated in Fig. 7. In this case, the kinetic curves for total and receptor-independent LDL uptake in the liver of the control hamster are shown as the shaded areas. The data in panels A and B show the effect of feeding cholesterol to this animal for 3 and 30 days. At 30 days the clearance rate is below the kinetic curve indicating that there was an approximate 30% reduction in receptor-mediated LDL transport by the liver as the plasma LDL-cholesterol concentration increased nearly 3-fold. The addition of polyunsaturated triglyceride to the diet had no additional effect on LDL transport. However, when saturated triglyceride was fed, there was essentially 90% suppression of receptor-mediated LDL transport in the liver. Thus, as shown in panel F, in the control hamster about 30 μg/hr per g of LDL-cholesterol was taken up by the liver and this was 90% mediated by the receptor-dependent process. After feeding cholesterol and saturated triglyceride for 30 days, the liver took up approximately the same amount of LDL-cholesterol but this was 90% mediated by the receptor-independent process and the plasma LDL-cholesterol concentration had risen nearly 7-fold. Using this type of quantitative analysis it is possible to define very precisely how any dietary addition or drug therapy actually alters plasma LDL-cholesterol levels.

Conclusions

In summary, in all species that have been examined, including probably man, about two-thirds of LDL clearance from the plasma is receptor-dependent and most of this activity is localized to the liver. The other third of LDL clearance takes place by receptor-independent mechanisms and this transport system is widely distri-

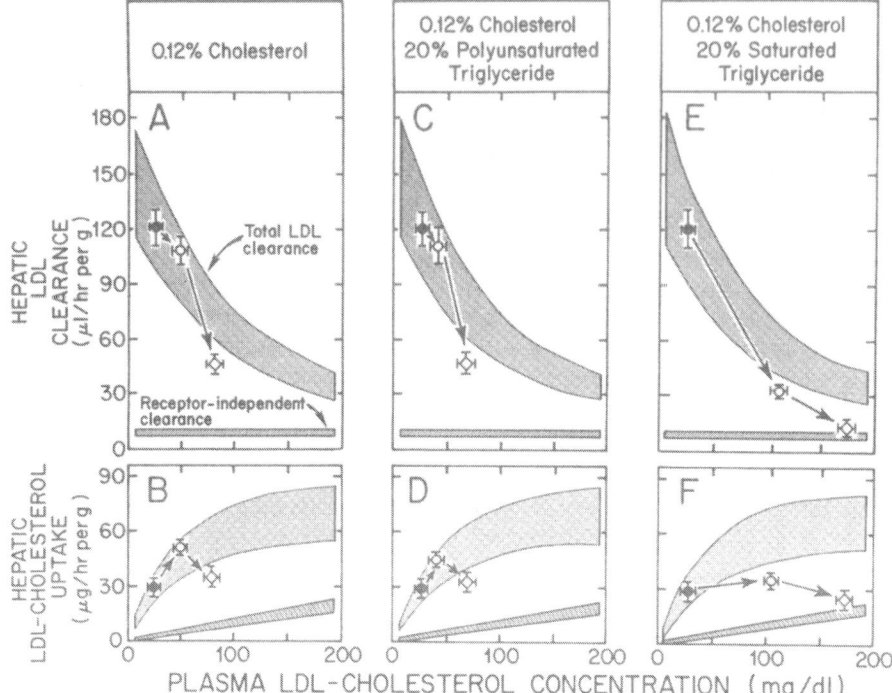

Fig. 7. Regulation of hepatic LDL receptor activity by cholesterol and triglyceride feeding. The individual points show the experimental results obtained after feeding the three experimental diets for 0 days (●), 3 days (○) or 30 days (□). These points are superimposed upon the standard kinetic curves for LDL transport in the liver of the hamster, and a decrease in receptor-dependent activity is indicated in those situations where the experimental points fall below the standard kinetic curves [21]

buted throughout the body. Receptor-independent LDL uptake can compensate for loss of receptor-dependent transport but the plasma LDL-cholesterol level must rise to achieve similar rates of uptake. Clearly techniques are now available to examine in detail how LDL metabolism in individual organs and in the whole animal is altered by various dietary, environmental and pharmacological manipulations.

Acknowledgements. The various experiments reviewed in this section were supported by U.S. Public Health Service Research Grants HL-09610 and AM-19329 and by grants from the Moss Heart Fund. Dr. Spady is a recipient of Clinical Investigator Award Am-01221 from the U.S. Public Health Service.

References

1. Dietschy JM, Wilson JD (1970) Regulation of cholesterol metabolism. N Engl J Med 282: 1128-1138 1179-1183 1241-1249

 2. Brown MS, Goldstein JL, Dietschy JM (1979) Active and inactive forms of 3-hydroxy-3-methylglutaryl coenzyme A reductase in the liver of the rat. J Biol Chem 254: 5144-5149
 3. Stange EF, Dietschy JM (1983) Absolute rates of cholesterol synthesis in rat intestine in vitro and in vivo: A comparison of different substrates in slices and isolated cells. J Lipid Res 24: 72-82
 4. Andersen JM, Dietschy JM (1979) Absolute rates of cholesterol synthesis in extrahepatic tissues measured with ^{3}H-labeled water and ^{14}C-labeled substrates. J Lipid Res 20: 740-752
 5. Spady DK, Dietschy JM (1983) Sterol synthesis in vivo in 18 tissues of the squirrel monkey, guinea pig, rabbit, hamster, and rat. J Lipid Res 24: 303-315
 6. Jeske DJ, Dietschy JM (1980) Regulation of rates of cholesterol synthesis in vivo in the liver and carcass of the rat measured using [^{3}H]water. J Lipid Res 21: 364-376
 7. Turley SD, Andersen JM, Dietschy JM (1981) Rates of sterol synthesis and uptake in the major organs of the rat in vivo. J Lipid Res 22: 551-569
 8. Dietschy JM, Spady DK (1984) Measurement of rates of cholesterol synthesis using tritiated water. J Lipid Res 25: 1469-1476
 9. Spady DK, Turley SD, Dietschy JM (1983) Dissociation of hepatic cholesterol synthesis from hepatic low-density lipoprotein uptake and biliary cholesterol saturation in female and male hamsters of different ages. Biochem Biophys Acta 753: 381-392
10. Turley SD, Dietschy JM (1982) Cholesterol metabolism and excretion. In The Liver: Biology and Pathobiology. I Arias, Popper H, Schachter D, Shafritz DA, editors. Raven Press New York pp 467-492
11. Dietschy JM, Gamel WG (1971) Cholesterol synthesis in the intestine of man: Regional differences and control mechanisms. J Clin Invest 50: 872-880
12. Spady DK, Bilheimer DW, Dietschy JM (1983) Rates of receptor-dependent and -independent low density lipoprotein uptake in the hamster. Proc Natl Acad Sci USA 80: 3499-3503
13. Pittman RC, Attie AD, Carew TE, Steinberg D (1979) Tissue sites of degradation of low density lipoprotein: Application of a method for determining the fate of plasma proteins. Proc Natl Acad Sci USA 76: 5345-5349
14. Dietschy JM, Turley SD, Spady DK (1983) The role of the liver in lipid and lipoprotein metabolism. In Liver in Metabolic Diseases. Bianchi L, Gerok W, Landmann L, Sickinger K and Stalder GA, editors. MTP Press Limited, Boston/The Hague/Dordrecht/Lancaster. pp 25-39
15. Stange EF, Dietschy JM (1984) Age-related decreases in tissue sterol acquisition are mediated by changes in cholesterol synthesis and not low density lipoprotein uptake in the rat. J Lipid Res 25: 703-713
16. Spady DK, Dietschy JM (1985) Rates of cholesterol synthesis and low density lipoprotein uptake in the adrenal glands of the rat, hamster and rabbit in vivo. Biochim Biophys Acta 836: 167-175
17. Bilheimer DW, Goldstein JL, Grundy SM, Starzl TE, Brown MS (1984) Liver transplantation to provide low-density-lipoprotein receptors and lower plasma cholesterol in a child with homozygous familial hypercholesterolemia. N Engl J Med 311: 1658-1664
18. Yamamoto T, Davis CG, Brown MS, Schneider WJ, Casey ML, Goldstein JL, Russell DW (1984) The human LDL receptor: A cysteine-rich protein with multiple ALU sequences in its mRNA. Cell 39: 27-38
19. Spady DK, Turley SD, Dietschy JM (1985) Rates of low density lipoprotein uptake and cholesterol synthesis are regulated independently in the liver. J Lipid Res 26: 465-472
20. Stange EF, Dietschy JM (1983) Cholesterol synthesis and low density lipoprotein uptake are regulated independently in rat small intestinal epithelium. Proc Natl Acad Sci USA 80: 5739-5743
21. Spady DK, Dietschy JM (1985) Dietary saturated triglycerides suppress hepatic low density lipoprotein receptors in the hamster. Proc Natl Aca Sci USA 82: 4526-4530
22. Dietschy JM, Kita T, Suckling KE, Goldstein JL and Brown MS (1983) Cholesterol synthesis in vivo and in vitro in the WHHL rabbit, an animal with defective low density lipoprotein receptors. J Lipid Res 24: 469-480

Turnover of Light and Heavy Fractions of Human LDL in Normal and WHHL Rabbits

M. KANO, J. KOIZUMI, A. JADHAV, and G. R. THOMPSON

MRC Lipoprotein Team, Hammersmith Hospital, London, England

Introduction

In humans light (L) LDL is catabolised faster than heavy (H) LDL, of which it is the precursor (Thompson et al., 1982). In familial hypercholesterolaemia (FH) this relationship is lost and the catabolism of L-LDL is decreased more markedly than that of H-LDL. However, the catabolic defect, especially of L-LDL, can be partly reversed by therapeutic measures which stimulate LDL receptors. This suggests that catabolism of L-LDL is normally more dependent on LDL-receptor-mediated mechanisms than is catabolism of H-LDL (Thompson et al., 1984).

Methods

To investigate this hypothesis L-LDL and H-LDL were isolated from human plasma by density gradient centrifugation (Teng et al., 1983) and labelled with ^{125}I or ^{131}I. In some instances the labelled fractions were treated with cyclohexanedione (CHD). Pairs of contrastingly labelled LDL preparations were then injected into normal or WHHL rabbits, so as to enable the fractional catabolic rate (FCR) of L- and H-LDL to be compared in rabbits with and without LDL receptors (WHHL) and to observe the effects of CHD, which blocks receptor-mediated uptake of LDL. In some instances the liver was removed and perfused with saline at the end of the experiment and aliquots were homogenised and counted for radioactivity, as described previously in Rhesus monkeys (Spengel et al., 1982).

Results

As shown in Table 1 there was no difference between the FCR of L- and H-LDL in either normal or WHHL rabbits but the FCR of both fractions was much lower in WHHL rabbits.

In normal rabbits, as shown in Fig. 1 and 2 the difference between the FCRs of L-LDL and L-LDL-CHD was greater than the difference between the FCRs of H-LDL and H-LDL-CHD. In WHHL rabbits, however, the FCRs of all 4 LDL preparations were similar, as shown in Fig. 3 and 4.

Also, as shown in Table 2, the percentage of radioactivity in the liver was greater 48 hours after injection of L- than of H-LDL, as was the corresponding liver:plas-

Receptor-Mediated Uptake
in the Liver
Edited by H. Greten, E. Windler, U. Beisiegel
© Springer-Verlag Berlin Heidelberg 1986

Table 1. Simultaneous turnover of ^{125}I- or ^{131}I-labelled human LDL fractions in rabbits

| | FCR/day | |
	L-LDL	H-LDL
Normal rabbit (3)	1.93	1.87
WHHL rabbit (3)	0.54	0.62

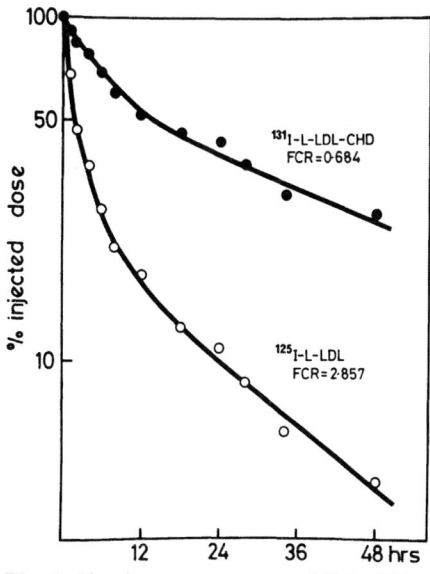

Fig. 1. Simultaneous turnover of light LDL and light LDL-CHD in normal rabbit

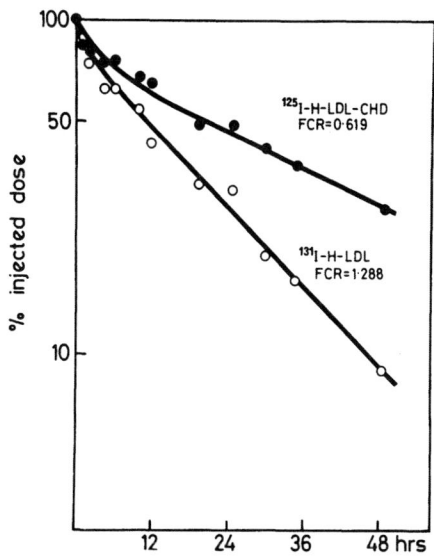

Fig. 2. Simultaneous turnover of heavy LDL and heavy LDL-CHD in normal rabbit

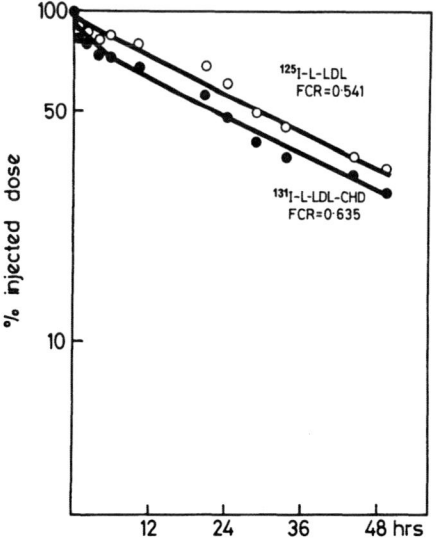

Fig. 3. Simultaneous turnover of light LDL and light LDL-CHD in WHHL rabbit

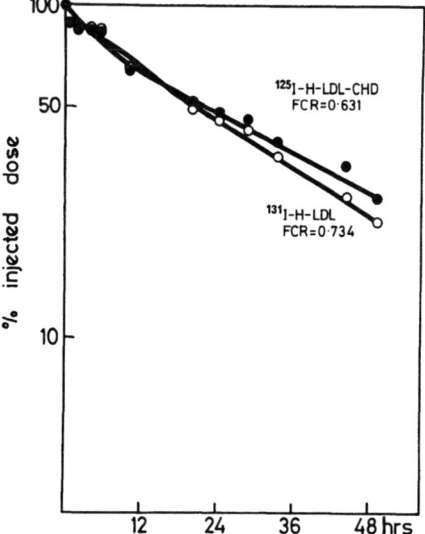

Fig. 4. Simultaneous turnover of heavy LDL and heavy LDL-CHD in WHHL rabbit

Table 2. Plasma and hepatic radioactivity at 48 hours after injecting native and cyclohexanedio-ne-blocked (CHD) human LDL fractions into normal rabbits

LDL fraction	Liver	Plasma	Liver
		% dose	plasma
^{125}I-L-LDL ⎫	3.65	1.39	2.63
^{131}I-H-LDL ⎬	2.46	1.29	1.91
^{125}I-L-LDL-CHD ⎫	3.04	9.36	0.33
^{131}I-H-LDL-CHD ⎬	2.41	10.27	0.24

ma radioactivity ratio. Much lower liver: plasma ratios occurred after injection of CHD blocked L- and H-LDL, indicating reduced rate of uptake of both fractions by the liver.

Conclusions

Total FCR of both fractions of human LDL was similar in normal rabbits but receptor-mediated FCR of L-LDL, calculated as the difference between FCR of native and CHD-blocked preparations, appeared greater for L- than for H-LDL. No such difference was observed in WHHL rabbits, in which the turnover of native and CHD-blocked LDL fractions was almost identical; similar findings have been observed using unfractionated LDL in patients with homozygous FH (Thompson *et al.,* 1981), who also lack LDL receptors. These data, together with the higher liver: plasma radioactivity ratio of L-LDL, suggest that removal of L-LDL from plasma is mediated to a proportionately greater extent by hepatic LDL receptors than is removal of H-LDL. To what extent removal of L-LDL reflects conversion to H-LDL as opposed to irreversible degradation is currently being studied in humans, since density gradient centrifugation of plasma obtained during the current studies has shown no evidence that labelled human L-LDL is converted to H-LDL after injection into normal rabbits.

References

1. Spengel FA, Harders-Spengel K, Duffield R, Wood C, Myant NB, Thompson GR (1982) The effect of partial ileal bypass on receptor-mediated uptake and catabolism of low density lipoprotein in the Rhesus monkey. Res Exp Med 180: 263-270
2. Teng B, Thompson GR, Sniderman AD, Forte TM, Krauss RM, Kwiterovich PO (1983) Composition and distribution of low density lipoprotein fractions in hyperapobetalipoproteinemia, normolipidemia and familial hypercholesterolemia. Proc Natl Acad Sci USA 80: 6662-6666
3. Thompson GR, Soutar AK, Spengel FA, Jadhav A, Gavigan SJP, Myant NB (1981) Defects of receptor-mediated low densitiy lipoprotein catabolism in homozygous familial hypercholesterolemia and hypothyroidism *in vivo. Proc Natl Acad Sci USA* 78: 2591-2595
4. Thompson GR, Teng B, Sniderman A (1982) Metabolic conversion of 'light' to 'heavy' low density lipoprotein (LDL) in subjects with normal and increased plasma LDL-apoB levels *Circulation 66* Supp II, 158
5. Thompson GR, Teng B, Sniderman AD (1984) Preferential catabolism of light LDL by the receptor-mediated pathway *Circulation 70* Supp II 268

Regulation of LDL Receptor Activity in Human Hepatocytes

L. HAVEKES, E. de WIT, and H. PRINCEN

Gaubius Institute TNO, Herenstraat 5d, 2313 AD Leiden, The Netherlands

Introduction

In extra-hepatic cells the LDL receptor activity is strongly reduced after incubation of the cells with LDL [1]. Although in vivo hepatocytes are exposed to physiological concentrations of LDL [2], the liver LDL receptor activity is responsible for the catabolism of the main portion of the total amount of plasma LDL [3]. This suggests that in hepatocytes the LDL receptor activity is regulated differently from that in extra-hepatic cells. We studied the regulation of the LDL receptor activity in the human hepatoma cell line Hep G2. The results are compared with those obtained with fibroblasts.

Results

Preincubation of Hep G2 cells with 20% whole serum instead of 20% LPDS resulted in an about 70% inhibition of the LDL receptor activity (90% inhibition in fibroblasts) (Fig. 1). A further increase in the concentration of whole serum (up to 100%) resulted in an increase of the LDL association as compared with preincubation with 20% whole serum (Fig. 1a). This increase in LDL association was not observed with fibroblasts (Fig. 1b).

In order to investigate which serum fraction is responsible for the observed stimulation of the LDL association in Hep G2 cells at high concentrations of whole serum, Hep G2 cells and fibroblasts were incubated with various serum density fractions (Fig. 2). Incubation with physiological concentrations of LDL reduced the LDL receptor activity in Hep G2 cells only to about 50% (15% in fibroblasts) whereas incubation with HDL with density between 1.16 and 1.20 g/ml (heavy HDL) displayed a strong stimulation (no stimulation in fibroblasts).

In Hep G2 cells the LDL association and degradation continued to increase by up to 7- and 4-fold respectively, upon increasing the concentration of heavy HDL during the preincubation (Fig. 3). In fibroblasts this increase was low as compared with that in Hep G2 cells. Scatchard plot analyses showed that the heavy HDL-mediated stimulation of the LDL receptor in Hep G2 cells is due to an increase in the number of LDL receptors rather than to an increase in the affinity of the receptor for LDL.

Receptor-Mediated Uptake
in the Liver
Edited by H. Greten, E. Windler, U. Beisiegel
© Springer-Verlag Berlin Heidelberg 1986

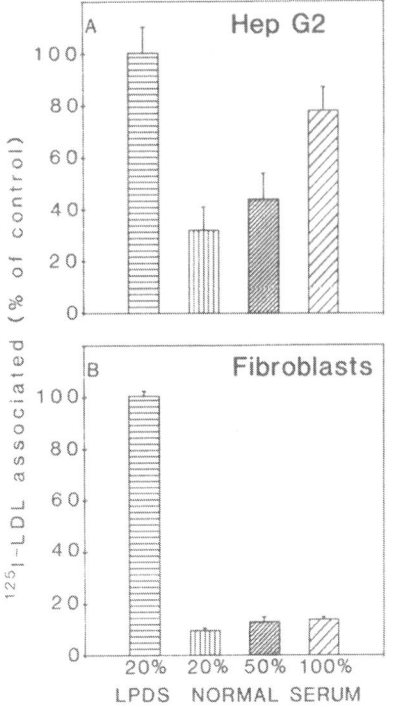

Fig. 1. High-affinity association of ^{125}I-LDL after preincubation of the cells for 20 h in medium containing 20% LPDS and 20, 50 and 100% normal whole serum

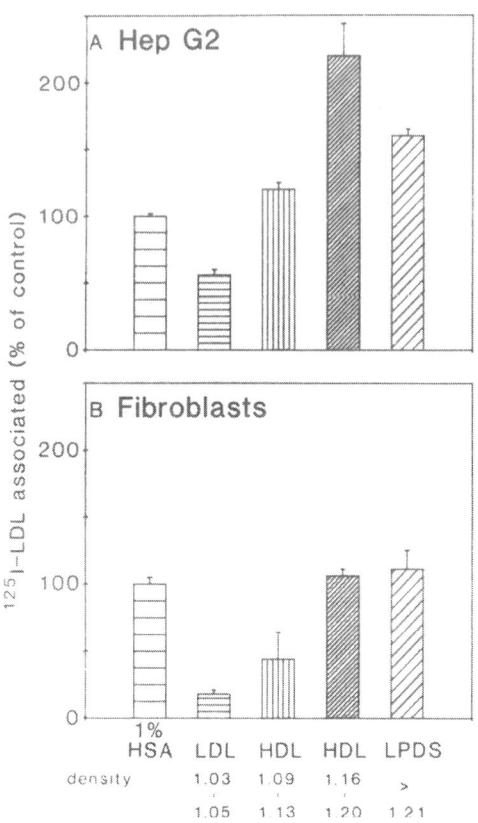

Fig. 2. High-affinity association of ^{125}I-LDL after preincubation of the cells for 20 h in medium containing physiological concentrations of different serum density fractions as indicated

With both cell types the down-regulation by preincubation with LDL in the presence of heavy HDL is less pronounced as compared with the down-regulation by preincubation with LDL alone (Fig. 4). Strikingly, in Hep G2 cells, even after incubation with 200 µg per ml LDL protein, there is still a 3-fold stimulation of the LDL association by simultaneous incubation with heavy HDL. In fibroblasts, on the contrary, the effect of simultaneous incubation with heavy HDL on the LDL cell-association is already prevented at 100 µg/ml LDL protein.

We wondered whether the stimulation of the LDL receptor activity by heavy HDL was specifically due to the action of LCAT. Therefore, freshly isolated heavy HDL was incubated at 37° C in order to obtain LCAT-modified HDL. DTNB-treated heavy HDL was used as control. Our results (Fig. 5) show that, with Hep G2 cells, LCAT-modified heavy HDL is a more potent stimulator than unmodified heavy HDL. Furthermore, the presence of active LCAT in the preincubation medium is not a requirement for the heavy HDL-mediated stimulation. With fibroblasts, heavy HDL is a weak stimulator irrespective of whether it is modified by LCAT or not.

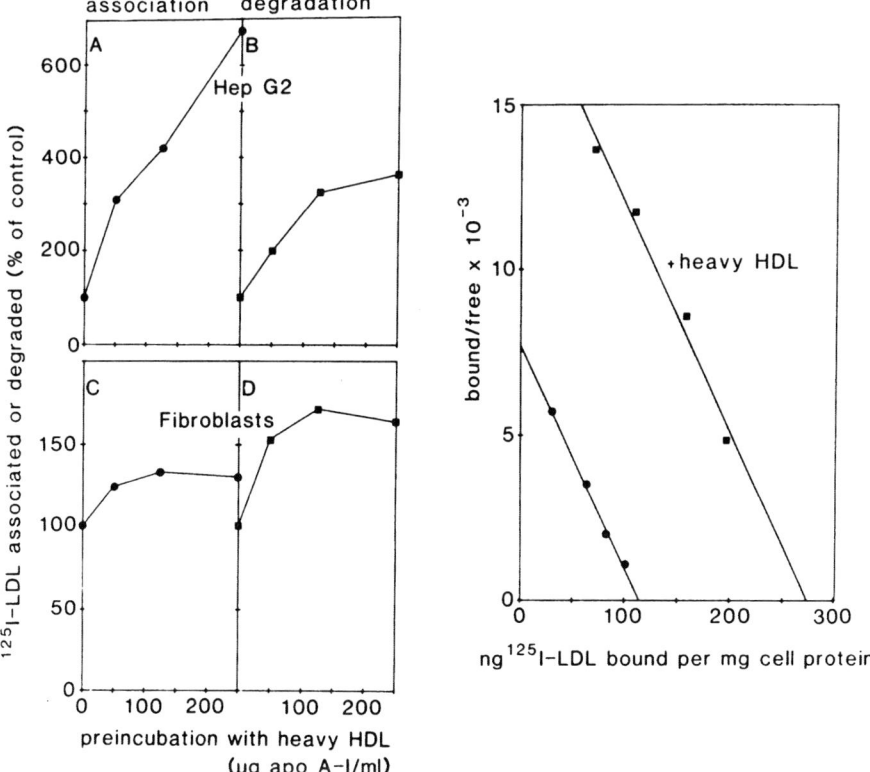

Fig. 3. High-affinity association and degradation of ^{125}I-LDL after preincubation of the cells for 20 h with increasing amounts of heavy HDL. Scatchard plot analysis represents the high-affinity binding of ^{125}I-LDL to Hep G2 cells preincubated in the presence or in the absence of heavy HDL

Discussion

The weak (50%) down-regulation of the LDL receptor in Hep G2 cells after incubation with LDL at fairly high concentrations (Fig. 2 and 4), together with the observation that in Hep G2 cells the number of LDL receptors is increased by up to 7-fold after incubation with heavy HDL (Fig. 2 and 3), could explain our observation that the LDL receptor activity in Hep G2 cells is increased after incubation of the cells with high concentrations of normal whole serum (Fig. 1), provided that in normal whole serum heavy HDL particles are present. Although several groups of investigators [4-6] have reported that very high density apo A-I containing particles are artifactually generated during extensive ultracentrifugation, other reports [7-9] strongly suggest that, also in whole human sera, there are relatively low molecular weight apo HDL containing compounds.

It is concluded from the results reported by Oram et al. [10] that apo A-I-containing particles present in the HDL 3 and very high density lipoprotein fractions are able to increase the LDL receptor activity in fibroblasts by promoting net

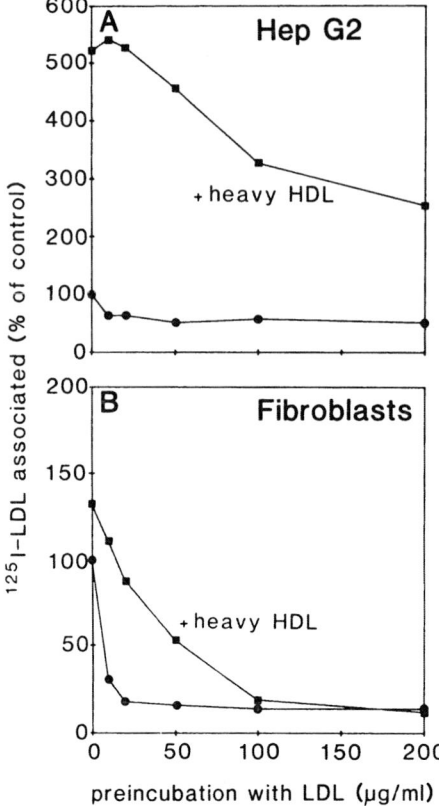

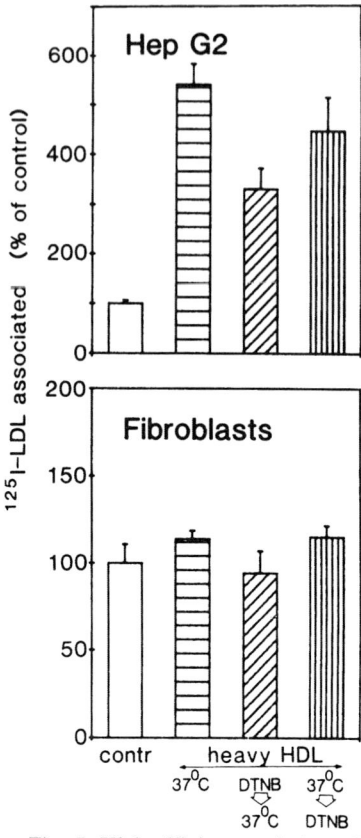

Fig. 4. High-affinity association of ^{125}I-LDL after preincubation of the cells for 20 h with increasing amounts of unlabelled LDL in the absence or in the presence of heavy HDL

Fig. 5. High-affinity association of ^{125}I-LDL after preincubation of the cells for 20 h with different heavy HDL samples treated as indicated

transport of cholesterol from the cells into the medium. Strikingly, our results show that, in this respect, the Hep G2 cells are far more sensitive than fibroblasts. In fibroblasts the heavy HDL-mediated stimulation of the LDL receptor activity is already prevented by the simultaneous addition of 100 μg per ml, whereas in Hep G2 cells this stimulation is not eliminated when more than 200 μg per ml LDL is added simultaneously (Fig. 4).

It has been proposed that LCAT activity, which is associated primarily with the HDL density fraction [11], may play a role in cholesterol removal from the cells [12, 13]. Our results show that the action of LCAT during the incubation of the cells is not a requirement for the observed stimulation. However, modification by LCAT enhances the capacity of heavy HDL to stimulate the LDL receptor activity.

Very recently, we found that the regulation of LDL receptor activity in isolated human hepatocytes is similar to that in Hep G2 cells:

1. an increase upon incubation of the cells with increasing amounts of normal serum;
2. a weak down-regulation after incubation of the cells with LDL (30% decrease at 200 μg/ml LDL); and
3. a 3- to 4-fold stimulation by incubation of the cells with heavy HDL which could not be prevented by a simultaneous addition of LDL.

These observations strongly support our previous conclusion [14, 15] that the use of the human hepatoma cell line Hep G2 offers a potentially helpful tool for studying the metabolism of LDL in primary cultures of human hepatocytes.

If the observed regulation of the LDL receptor activity in Hep G2 cells in vitro, holds true for human hepatocytes in vivo, our results could explain why, in vivo, the liver still displays LDL receptor activity notwithstanding the exposure of the hepatocytes to physiological concentrations of LDL.

References

1. Goldstein JL, Brown MS (1977) Ann Rev Biochem 46: 897-930
2. Wisse D (1977) in Kupffer Cells and other Liver Sinusoidal Cells (E Wisse and DL Knook eds) pp 33-60, Elsevier/North Holland, Amsterdam
3. Bilheimer DW, Goldstein JL, Grundy SM, Starzl TE, Brown MS (1984) New Engl J Med 311: 1658-1664
4. Scanu A, Granda JL (1966) Biochemistry 5: 446-455
5. Fainaru M, Havel RJ, Imaizumi K (1977) Biochem Med 17: 347-355
6. Patsch W, Schonfeld G, Gotto AM, Patsch JR (1980) J Biol Chem 255: 3178-3185
7. Stein O, Fainaru M, Stein Y (1979) Biochim Biophys Acta 574: 495-504
8. Slater HR, Smith EB, Robertson FW (1980) Atherosclerosis 35: 41-49
9. Fielding CJ, Fielding PE (1981) Proc Natl Acad Sci USA 78: 3911-3941
10. Oram JF, Albers JH, Chung MC, Bierman EL (1981) J Biol Chem 256: 8348-8356
11. Glomset JA (1972) in Blood lipids and lipoproteins: Quantitation, Composition and Metabolism (GJ Nelson ed) pp 754-787, Wiley-Interscience New York NY
12. Glomset JA (1968) J Lipid Res 9: 155-167
13. Aron L, Jones SJ, Fielding CJ (1978) J Biol Chem 253: 7220-7226
14. Havekes L, Van Hinsbergh V, Kempen HJ, Emeis J (1983) Biochem J 214: 951-958
15. Cohen LH, Griffioen M, Havekes L, Schouten D, Van Hinsbergh V, Kempen HJ (1984) Biochem J 222: 35-39

Non-Genetic Regulation of LDL Metabolism: Role of Lipid Transfer Proteins and Hypertriglyceridemia

S. Eisenberg

Lipid Research Laboratory, Department of Medicine B, Hadassah University Hospital Jerusalem, Israel

Introduction

Since the initial discovery of the LDL (B, E) receptor by Brown and Goldstein, it has been amply demonstrated that genetic control of the synthesis of normal receptor protein determines LDL metabolic rates [1-3]. The outstanding example of the consequences of lack of normal receptors is familial hypercholesterolemia (FH), a disease where one or both genes responsible for the synthesis of the receptor protein are defective [3]. The impact of this discovery on current concepts of LDL metabolism cannot be over-emphasized. Yet, only recently has it been realized that environmental factors can greatly influence the levels of the LDL receptor activity, presumably by regulation of the number of receptor protein molecules synthesized by cells. The purpose of the present text is to describe and discuss one mechanism that appears to be responsible for major alterations of LDL degradation by the receptor pathway. This mechanism operates in hypertriglyceridemia, is non-genetic and can be modulated by changing plasma triglyceride levels.

Hypothesis

The working hypothesis predicts that intraplasma metabolic events affect LDL cholesterol content, and thereby regulate the rate of LDL degradation and of cellular cholesterol synthesis. This hypothesis is based on the known events that regulate LDL (B, E) receptor protein synthesis and cholesterol synthesis [1-3] and on the effects of lipid transfer proteins on LDL [4-6]. The regulation of the LDL receptor and cellular sterol synthesis by lipoproteins is well known [1-3]. For the sake of the present text, it is sufficient to comment that whereas the initial event of LDL degradation depends on recognition of amino acid sequences of the apo B (or apo E) protein by specific sites on the receptor protein, the consequences of lysosomal degradation of apo B (and apo E) containing lipoproteins reflect the number of cholesterol molecules that reach the lysosomes with the lipoprotein. Thus, cholesterol-poor LDL may interact with the receptor similarly to normal LDL, but its effect on the regulation of cellular metabolic processes is considerably reduced.

Plasma pathways that cause loss of cholesterol from LDL (predominantly cholesteryl ester) have been identified in the last few years. These pathways are dependent on the activity of lipid transfer proteins (LTP) that circulate in the plasma

Receptor-Mediated Uptake
in the Liver
Edited by H. Greten, E. Windler, U. Beisiegel
© Springer-Verlag Berlin Heidelberg 1986

of human subjects and several other mammalian species. The proteins catalyze transfer of hydrophobic molecules — triglycerides and cholesteryl esters — between lipoproteins. When the reaction occurs between two lipoproteins with similar core composition (e. g., LDL and HDL), it causes predominantly exchange of molecules [7]. When, however, a cholesteryl ester rich lipoprotein (e. g., LDL) interacts with a triglyceride-rich lipoprotein (e. g., VLDL), transfer of molecules occurs. For example, we showed that as much as 50% of the cholesteryl ester molecules in normal human plasma LDL can be replaced by triglycerides when the LDL is incubated with VLDL and lipid transfer proteins [6]. Of the different VLDL population, the large-sized, lighter and triglyceride-rich particles seem to be the preferred acceptors of transferred cholesteryl esters and preferred donors of triglycerides [8]. Of interest, the cholesterol-depleted LDL (modified, M-LDL) appears to possess lower capacity to down-regulate LDL receptor activity and cholesterol synthesis in cultured human skin fibroblasts [9]. While these observations support our hypothesis, they do not directly predict the situation in vivo, where many other reactions and receptors are present. This lack of knowledge prompted us to carry out investigations on the structure, composition and metabolism of LDL in patients with hypertriglyceridemia [10, 11]. Our assumption was that accelerated transfer of cholesteryl esters from LDL would occur when the plasma VLDL levels are greatly increased. To avoid the possibility that the basic defect responsible for the hypertriglyceridemic state may affect the LDL independently of plasma triglyceride levels, we chose to investigate LDL from the same patient twice: once at the height of hypertriglyceridemia (HTG), and later, after two or four weeks of treatment with the hypolipidemic drug, bezafibrate (BZ).

Structure and Composition of HTG-LDL

Several abnormalities are consistently found in HTG-LDL [11]. When separated on a zonal ultracentrifugation system, HTG-LDL (d 1.006-1.063 g/ml) always includes an abnormally higher proportion of IDL, and is composed of several populations (Fig. 1). The main LDL fraction, corresponding to N-LDL, was further analyzed. HTG-LDL (main fraction) is denser than N-LDL, relatively enriched with protein and triglycerides and contains significantly less cholesteryl ester and free cholesterol (Fig. 2).

As well, HTG-LDL is smaller (by electron microscopy) than N-LDL and diameters smaller than 170 A (N = 210-220 A) are found (Fig. 1). All these abnormalities are strongly and significantly related to the degree of triglyceridemia, and most tend to revert towards normal when plasma triglycerides are reduced. These abnormalities of HTG-LDL are best explained by continued activity of the core-lipid transfer proteins [4-6], followed by partial hydrolysis of the transferred triglycerides [6]. According to our view, LDL and HDL in hypertriglyceridemia are exposed to a greatly increased mass of VLDL and chylomicrons and therefore exchange very significant amounts of their cholesteryl esters for triglycerides [11]. Once the LDL and HDL acquire triglycerides (by the transfer reaction), however, these molecules are partially hydrolyzed by endothelial bound lipases and thus a net loss of core-molecules occurs and the particle becomes smaller and denser [6, 11]. The

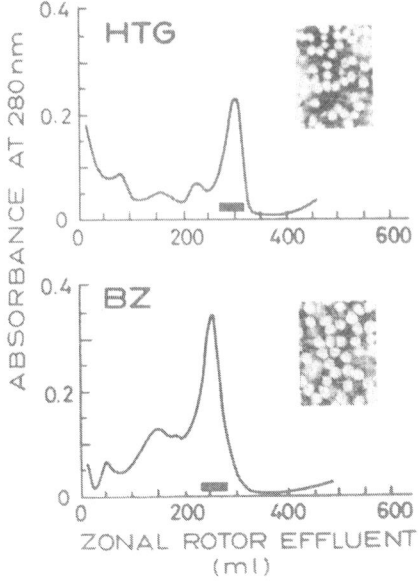

Fig. 1. Zonal ultracentrifugation elution profile of HTG- and BZ-LDL obtained from the same patient. Inserts in each frame are electron micrographs of the main LDL fraction (solid bar)

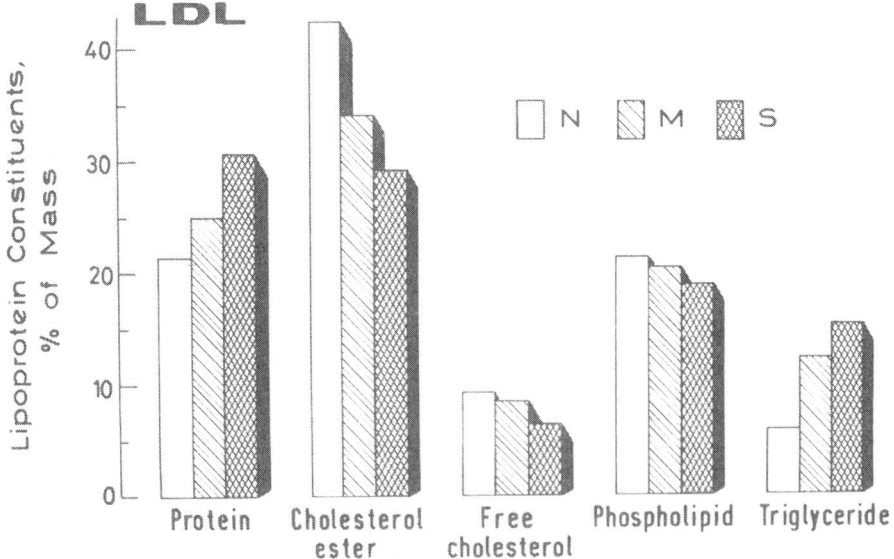

Fig. 2. Chemical composition of LDL (homogenous zonal fraction) from human subjects with normotriglyceridemia (N), moderate hypertriglyceridemia (M), and severe hypertriglyceridemia (S)

basis for free cholesterol redistribution in hypertriglyceridemia is unclear, as is that of the presence of several LDL populations.

Cholesteryl ester and triglyceride redistribution among hypertriglyceridemic lipoproteins appears to have important metabolic consequences . For HTG-LDL, the reduced cholesterol content (per particle) is possibly of utmost importance. It can be calculated (from the regression analysis [11]) for example, that at plasma triglyceride levels of 500 mg/dl single LDL particles contain about half the number of cholesterol molecules (free and ester) than at plasma triglyceride levels of 100 mg/dl [11]. That calculation prompted us to begin an extensive study of the metabolic behavior of HTG-LDL. The initial part of the study was carried out in cultured human skin fibroblasts and is briefly described below.

Defective Metabolism of HTG-LDL

In this study we compared the metabolic behavior of HTG-LDL, BZ-LDL (obtained at the end of two weeks therapy of the patients with bezafibrate), and N-LDL in cultured human skin fibroblasts [12]. Eleven studies were carried out on LDL's obtained from seven HTG-patients. Binding, internalization and degradation of HTG-LDL was found to be lower than N-LDL in all studies, and treatment appeared to correct these abnormalities. We believe that the basic defect is lower affinities of HTG-LDL preparations towards the receptor protein. While the reason for that decreased binding of HTG-LDL is unclear, it appears to reflect changes of the apo B conformation due to the changed size, structure or composition of the lipoprotein. Regulation of B, E receptor protein synthesis and of sterol synthesis was investigated in up-regulated cells, grown for 48 and 6 hours, respectively, in media containing either N-, HTG- or BZ-LDL. Not unexpectedly, HTG-LDL was considerably less efficient than N-LDL in down-regulating these activities while BZ-LDL restored normal, or close to normal activity. Of particular interest was the observation that sterol synthesis by the cells was strongly but negatively correlated with the content of cholesteryl esters in LDL, estimated by the cholesteryl ester to apo B ratio. Thus, the lower this ratio is (as seen in HTG), the higher are the rates of sterol synthesis. Similar observations were found for LDL receptor activity. Because cholesteryl ester to apo B ratios of LDL's used in the study spanned the range commonly observed in human subjects (1.0-2.5), we believe that our observations uncovered a phenomenon that operates in general and regulates LDL and cholesterol metabolism in populations.

Conclusions and Perspectives

The mechanisms responsible for non-genetic regulation of LDL and cholesterol metabolism as elucidated by our studies, are diagrammatically represented in Fig. 3. In hypertriglyceridemia, the LDL contains appreciably less cholesterol than N-LDL. In addition, the binding of HTG-LDL to the receptor is less effective than N-LDL. Therefore, delivery of cholesterol to the cells with HTG-LDL is considerably less than N-LDL. As a consequence, cells exposed to HTG-LDL do not

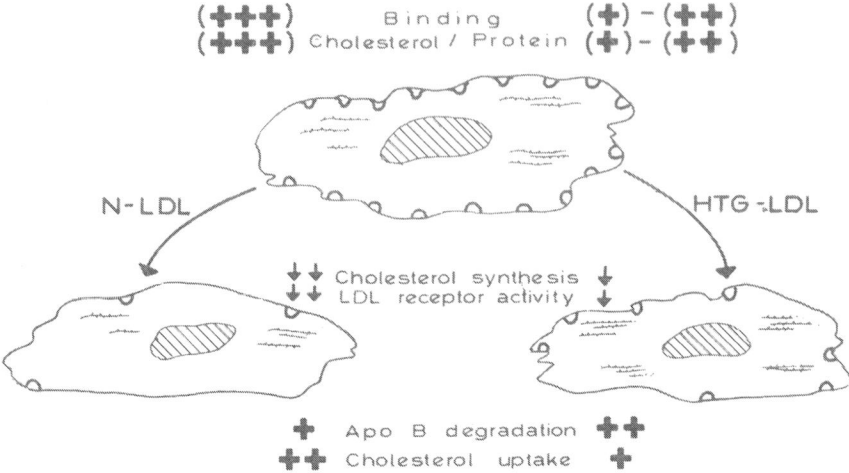

Fig. 3. Schematic representation of the regulation of LDL degradation and cellular cholesterol synthesis by normal and hypertriglyceridemic LDL

down regulate the synthesis of the B, E receptor protein as effectively as cells exposed to N-LDL. That might cause increased LDL degradation in hypertriglyceridemia, in spite of the lower affinity of HTG-LDL towards the receptor. Yet, in spite of the higher receptor activity, the amount of cholesterol that enters the cells with HTG-LDL is still lower than normal. Therefore, both LDL apo B degradation *and* cellular cholesterol synthesis would be higher than normal, as indeed has been found by several investigators [13-15]. We suggest that these abnormalities of LDL and cholesterol metabolism that are an essential part of the Hypertriglyceridemia state operate also in other conditions where variant LDL populations exist. That suggestion, however, remains to be tested.

References

1. Brown MS, Goldstein JL (1975) Regulation of the activity of the low density lipoprotein in human fibroblast. Cell 6: 307-316
2. Brown MS, Kovanen PT, Goldstein JL (1981) Regulation of plasma cholesterol by lipoprotein receptors. Science (Wash DC) 212: 628-635
3. Goldstein JL, Brown MS (1982) LDL receptor defect in familial hypercholesterolemia. Med Clin N AM 66: 335-362
4. Nichols AV, Smith L (1965) Effect of very low density lipoproteins on lipid transfer in incubated serum. J Lipid Res 6: 206-210
5. Zilversmit DB, Hughes LB, Balmer J (1975) Stimulation of cholesterol ester exchange by lipoprotein-free rabbit plasma. Biochim Biophys Acta 409: 393-398
6. Deckelbaum RJ, Eisenberg S, Oschry Y, Butbul E, Sharon I, Olivecrona T (1982) Reversible modification of human plasma low density lipoproteins toward triglyceride-rich precursors. J Biol Chem 257: 6509-6517

7. Morton RE, Zilversmit DB (1983) Inter-relationship of lipids transferred by the lipid-transfer protein isolated from human lipoprotein-deficient plasma. J Biol Chem 258: 11751-11757

8. Eisenberg S (1985) Preferential enrichment of large-sized very low density lipoprotein populations with transferred cholesteryl esters. J Lipid Res 26: 487-494

9. Chait A, Eisenberg S, Steinmetz A, Albers J, Bierman EL (1984) Low density lipoprotein modified by cholesterol ester transfer proteins have altered biological activity. Biochim Biophys Acta 795: 314-325

10. Deckelbaum RJ, Granot E, Oschry Y, Rose L, Eisenberg S (1984) Plasma triglyceride determines structure-composition in low and high density lipoproteins. Arteriosclerosis 4: 224-231

11. Eisenberg S, Gavish D, Oschry Y, Fainaru M, Deckelbaum RJ (1984) Abnormalities in very low, low, and high density lipoproteins in hypertriglyceridemia. Reversal toward normal with bezafibrate treatment. J Clin Invest 74: 470-482

12. Kleinman Y, Eisenberg S, Oschry Y, Gavish D, Stein O, Stein Y (1985) Defective metabolism of hypertriglyceridemic low density lipoprotein in cultured human skin fibroblasts. Normalization with bezafibrate therapy. J Clin Invest 75: 1796-1803

13. Sigurdsson G, Nicoll A, Lewis B (1976) The metabolism of low density lipoprotein in endogenous hypertriglyceridemia. Eur J Clin Invest 6: 151-158

14. Janus ED, Nicoll AM, Turner PR, Magill P, Lewis B (1980) Kinetic bases of the primary hyperlipidaemias: studies of apolipoprotein B turnover in genetically defined subjects. Eur J Clin Invest 10: 161-172

15. Sodhi HS, Kudchodkar BJ (1973) Correlating metabolism of plasma and tissue cholesterol with that of plasma lipoproteins. Lancet 1: 513-519

The Control of Cholesterol Homeostasis: Regulation of HMG CoA Reductase

K. L. LUSKEY

University of Texas Health Science Center, Department of Molecular Genetics, Dallas, TX USA

Cholesterol homeostasis within cells is regulated so as to provide adequate cholesterol without building up excessive stores. Two regulated pathways account for this cholesterol. The LDL receptor pathway mediates the uptake of cholesterol-containing lipoproteins from the plasma by receptor-mediated endocytosis. The endogenous cholesterol synthetic pathway which converts acetyl CoA to cholesterol via a multi-enzyme pathway is regulated by changes in the activity of HMG CoA reductase. Changes in the expression of HMG CoA reductase have been shown to affect the expression of LDL receptors both in cultured cells as well as in intact animals [1, 2]. To better understand the mechanisms that control cholesterol homeostasis, the means by which HMG CoA reductase is regulated have been studied. In cells, suppression of HMG CoA reductase activity by cholesterol is accomplished by at least two mechanisms:

1. decreased transcription of the HMG CoA reductase gene
2. enhanced degradation of the reductase protein.

The elements responsible for mediating these effects have been exposed by studying the structure and expression of the HMG CoA reductase gene and protein.

The HMG CoA reductase gene is 25 kilobases long and consists of 20 exons that are spliced together to form a mRNA of ~ 5.3 kilobases [3]. At the 3' end of the gene, at least three different polyadenylation sites are utilized. Although the significance of this heterogeneity is unknown, multiple polyadenylation sites have been found in many other eukaryotic mRNAs. In contrast, the 5' untranslated region is unique compared to the structure of other eukaryotic mRNAs [3, 4]. At the 5' end of the reductase gene, multiple transcription initiation sites are utilized followed by multiple sites where the 3' end of first exon can be spliced to join the second exon. This heterogeneity of both initiation and splicing results in mRNAs that can have from 68 to 670 nucleotides upstream of the AUG codon that initiates translation of the reductase protein. Many of these mRNA species have AUG codons upstream of the initiation methionine for the reductase protein and might interfere with the translation of the reductase mRNA.

The region upstream of the initiation sites is also different from many eukaryotic genes. Sequences such as the TATA box and CCAAT box are not found, however GC-boxes containing the sequence CCGCCC or its complement are repeated five times [3]. Such GC-boxes are found in the SV40 promoter, the herpes thymidine kinase promoter and cellular genes such as superoxide dismutase and hypoxanthine-guanine phosphoribosyl transferase. Studies by Osborne, et al., have

Receptor-Mediated Uptake
in the Liver
Edited by H. Greten, E. Windler, U. Beisiegel
© Springer-Verlag Berlin Heidelberg 1986

shown that a 513 bp fragment from the promoter region of the HMG CoA reductase gene can function independently as a promoter and that transcription from this region is subject to regulation by sterols [5].

Changes in the rate of degradation of the enzyme are mediated at the protein level and require a unique membrane-bound domain of the enzyme. This domain is found in the amino-terminal 339 amino acid residues of the 887 residue protein and contains seven stretches of hydrophobic amino acids that are predicted to span the membrane of the endoplasmic reticulum seven times [6]. The carboxy-terminal portion of the enzyme projects into the cytoplasm of the cell and is responsible for the catalytic activity of the enzyme. Expression studies have shown that when HMG CoA reductase is expressed as a soluble enzyme lacking the membrane-bound domain, the degradation of the enzyme is retarded and no longer regulated by cholesterol [7, 8]. The relative importance of the membrane-bound domain is illustrated by comparing amino acid sequence of the human and hamster enzyme. This region is the most highly conserved region of the protein with only a 2% amino acid substitution rate, whereas the remainder of the protein has a 10% amino acid substitution rate [9]. Further studies are underway to determine the mechanism by which this part of the reductase protein can modulate the rate of degradation of the enzyme.

Understanding the molecular mechanisms that regulate HMG CoA reductase are critical to understanding the cellular signals that regulate LDL receptor activity. Both of these proteins are key elements in regulating the different pathways by which cells obtain cholesterol. In addition, as both of these proteins are coordinately regulated common molecular mechanisms might exist for control of the LDL receptor and HMG CoA reductase.

References

1. Brown MS, Goldstein JL (1980) Multivalent feedback regulation of HMG CoA reductase, a control mechanism coordinating isoprenoid synthesis and cell growth. J Lipid Res 21: 505-517
2. Goldstein JL, Brown MS (1984) Progress in understanding the LDL receptor and HMG CoA reductase, two membrane proteins that regulate the plasma cholesterol. J Lipid Res 25: 1450-1461
3. Reynolds GA, Basu SK, Osborne TF, Chin DJ, Gil G, Brown MS, Goldstein JL, Luskey KL (1984) HMG CoA reductase: A negatively regulated gene with unusual promoter and 5' untranslated regions. Cell 38: 275-286
4. Reynolds GA, Goldstein JL and Brown MS (1985) Multiple mRNAs for 3-hydroxy-3-methylglutaryl coenzyme A reductase determined by multiple transcription initiation sites and intron splicing sites in the 5' untranslated region. J Biol Chem 260: 10369-10377
5. Osborne TF, Goldstein JL, Brown MS (1985) 5' End of HMG CoA reductase gene contains sequences responsible for cholesterol-mediated inhibition of transcription. Cell 42: 203-212
6. Liscum L, Finer-Moore J, Stroud RM, Luskey KL, Brown MS, Goldstein JL (1985) Domain structure of 3-hydroxy-3-methylglutaryl coenzyme A reductase, a glycoprotein of the endoplasmic reticulum. J Biol Chem 260: 522-530
7. Chin DJ, Gil G, Faust JR, Goldstein JL, Brown MS, Luskey KL (1985) Sterols accelerate degradation of HMG CoA reductase encoded by a constitutively expressed cDNA. Mol Cell Biol 5: 634-641

8. Gil G, Faust JR, Chin DJ, Goldstein JL, Brown MS (1985) Membrane-bound domain of HMG CoA reductase is required for sterol-enhanced degradation of the enzyme. Cell 41: 249-258

9. Luskey KL, Stevens B (1985) Human 3-hydroxy-3-methylglutaryl coenzyme A reductase: Conserved domains responsible for catalytic activity and sterol-regulated degradation. J Biol Chem 260: 10271-10277

Cholesterol and Bile Acid Synthesis as Related to Receptor and Non-receptor Mediated Degradation of LDL in Man

Y. Antero Kesäniemi and Tatu A. Miettinen

Second Department of Medicine, University of Helsinki, SF-00290 Helsinki, Finland

The activity of hepatic cholesterol and bile acid synthesis has a powerful role in the overall regulation of plasma lipoprotein metabolism. Enhanced elimination of cholesterol from the body as bile acids by ileal dysfunction, e. g. ileal bypass surgery, is one of the most effective means to lower plasma low density lipoprotein (LDL) concentrations [1]. The LDL lowering is supposed to happen through the stimulation of specific hepatic receptors that remove LDL from the plasma to cover hepatic cholesterol depletion caused by enhanced bile acid synthesis [2, 3]. The latter results finally in proportionately increased cholesterol synthesis. However, in quantitative terms cholesterol and bile acid synthesis have not been related to the catabolism of LDL by the specific LDL receptor-mediated and the receptor-independent mechanisms in man. Therefore, the present studies were carried out to determine LDL metabolism in patients with various degree of bile acid malabsorption. Some of the patients were normolipidemic control subjects but patients with a selective disorder in expressing the specific LDL receptors (familial hypercholesterolemia = FH) [4] were also recrueted.

The studies were performed in controls, in controls with ileal dysfunction (includes patients with ileal resections or jejunoileal bypass), in patients with heterozygous FH (FH het), in FH het patients with ileal bypass and in a patient with homozygous FH treated with ileal bypass and portacaval shunt (FH hom). All the patients underwent measurements of fecal outputs of bile acids and neutral steroids and the determinations of the percentage of intestinal cholesterol absorption [5-7]. Total, receptor-mediated and receptor-independent catabolism of LDL were also quantitated using the injections of radioiodinated native and glucosylated autologous LDL [8].

The controls with ileal dysfunction had 2.9 times higher cholesterol synthesis than the controls due to a 7.1 fold increase in fecal bile acid loss (equals synthesis in Table 1)

Similarly, ileal bypass stimulated cholesterol and bile acid synthesis in FH het patients 340 and 860%, respectively, the corresponding synthesis rates being 272 and 795% of the controls. FH hom also had markedly enhanced cholesterol and bile acid synthesis.

The controls with ileal dysfunction had a 55 and 93% increase in the total and receptor-dependent fractional removal of LDL compared to the controls (Table 2). This was associated with a 44% decrease in LDL cholesterol concentration (Table 1). Ileal bypass increased total and receptor-mediated clearance of LDL by 36 and 59% in FH het and reduced LDL cholesterol level by 30%. The corresponding

Receptor-Mediated Uptake
in the Liver
Edited by H. Greten, E. Windler, U. Beisiegel
© Springer-Verlag Berlin Heidelberg 1986

Table 1. Bile acid and cholesterol synthesis and LDL cholesterol concentration; percent of control

Group	Bile acid synthesis	Cholesterol synthesis	LDL cholesterol
Control	100	100	100
Control with ileal dysfunction	710[a]	290[a]	56[a]
FH het	93	80	235
FH het with	795[a]	272[a]	165[a]
ileal bypass	860[b]	340[b]	70[b]
FH hom	748	310	368

a Significantly different from control (p $<$ 0.05 or less)
b Percent of FH het

values of total and receptor-mediated catabolism of LDL in FH het with ileal by-pass were 70 and 78% of the values in the controls. In FH het and FH het with ileal bypass 62 and 72% of LDL was cleared by the receptor pathway, values very similar to 65 and 75% in the controls and the controls with ileal dysfunction.

As compared to the controls LDL cholesterol transport through the receptor-independent pathway was decreased by 53% in the controls with ileal dysfunction (Table 2). Similarly, the receptor-independent mechanism transported 30% less LDL cholesterol in FH het with ileal bypass than in FH het. In the controls without and with ileal dysfunction cholesterol synthesis was significantly correlated with the LDL cholesterol transport through the nonreceptor (r $=$ -0.78; p $<$ 0.05) but not with the receptor pathway (r $=$ 0.51, NS). In the combined FH het groups cholesterol synthesis tended to correlate negatively with the LDL cholesterol transport via the nonreceptor mechanism (r $=$ -0.61; NS) and positively with the LDL cholesterol transport through the receptor pathway (r $=$ 0.77; NS). With the exception of FH hom the LDL receptor-mechanism transported surprisingly similar amounts of LDL cholesterol in each group.

These studies show that the threefold stimulation of cholesterol synthesis due to bile acid depletion in both normals and FH het patients increases the fractional removal of LDL by the LDL receptor pathway 90-60%. However, in quantitative

Table 2. The fractional catabolic rate (FCR) and LDL cholesterol transport values for total, receptor-dependent and non-receptor-mediated removal of LDL; percent of control

Group	FCR			LDL cholesterol transport		
	total	receptor	non-receptor	total	receptor	non-receptor
Control	100	100	100	100	100	100
Control with ileal dysfunct.	155[a]	193[a]	84	78	94	47[a]
FH het	51	49	56	118	112	129
FH het with	70	78	55	113	124	90
ileal bypass	136[b]	159[b]	99[b]	95[b]	111[b]	70[b]
FH hom	31	-	88	111	—	317

a Significantly different from control (p $<$ 0.05 or less)
b Percent of FH het

terms the major effect of the stimulated hepatic cholesterol synthesis was a decrease in the receptor-independent LDL cholesterol transport in both controls and FH het patients whereas at various LDL levels the LDL receptor-pathway seemed to transport surprisingly similar amounts of cholesterol. These fingings suggest that the LDL receptor pathway tries to cover a certain almost fixed amount of cholesterol transport to maintain cellular cholesterol homeostasis. Calculations revealed, however, that in the patients with high bile acid and cholesterol synthesis the transport of LDL cholesterol through the combined receptor-mediated and receptor-independent mechanisms is much less than the overall cholesterol synthesis. This suggests that most of the newly synthesized hepatic cholesterol was converted directly to bile acids without preceeding release into the bloodstream as VLDL. Alternatively, part of VLDL could be picked up effectively by the activated B, E receptors without conversion to LDL. However, VLDL cholesterol transport appears to be similar in the FH subjects with and without ileal bypass (Koivisto P, Miettinen TA, unpublished observation).

Two of the controls with ileal dysfunction had a jejunoileal bypass. In these patients markedly increased cholesterol synthesis was due to two factors: first, low intestinal absorption of cholesterol resulting in 2.2 times higher fecal output of neutral sterols than in the controls, and second, depletion of bile acids. In these few patients a remarkable 135% increase was noticed in the fractional removal of LDL by the receptor mechanism and as compared to the controls was associated with a 62% decrease in the LDL cholesterol level. Also, LDL cholesterol transport through the receptor-independent pathway(s) in these patients was only 28% of that of the controls. Interestingly, the lowering of LDL cholesterol by cholesterol malabsorption seems to be even more efficient than that by bile acid malabsorption [9], but the mechanism for this phenomenon is not clear. It is possible that a combination of cholesterol malabsorption to bile acid malabsorption further increases the LDL receptor activity. On the other hand in cholesterol malabsorption without loss of bile acids as in patients with coeliac disease and in subjects under neomycin treatment the major mechanism for lowered LDL levels seems to be a decrease in LDL synthesis rate [10, 11]. At any rate, an additional loss of cholesterol as neutral sterols together with bile acid depletion is remarkably effective in LDL lowering.

In conclusion, these studies show that the quantity of the receptor-independent pathway(s), presumably crucial in the development of atherosclerosis, can also be modified. Ileal dysfunction stimulates cholesterol synthesis due to bile acid depletion, has virtually no effect on the LDL cholesterol transport through the receptor-mediated pathway but results in a remarkable decrease in the transport of LDL cholesterol via the receptor-independent pathways in the subjects presumably with no genetic lipid abnormalities. In heterozygous FH patients the high nonreceptor-mediated transport of LDL cholesterol is normalized after ileal bypass to the level observed in the controls with no treatment. However, in FH homozygous subjects who cannot express the LDL receptor activity the nonreceptor-mediated mechanism remains high even after ileal bypass and portacaval shunt.

References

1. Miettinen TA, Lempinen M (1977) Eur J Clin Invest 7: 509
2. Spengel FA, Jadhav A, Duffield RGM, Wood CB, Thompson GR (1981) Lancet 2: 768
3. Kovanen PT, Bilheimer DW, Goldstein JL, Jaramillo JJ, Brown MS (1981) Proc Natl Acad Sci USA 78: 1194
4. Brown MS, Goldstein JL (1974) Proc Natl Acad Sci USA 71: 788
5. Miettinen TA, Ahrens EH Jr, Grundy SM (1965) J Lipid Res 6: 411
6. Grundy SM, Ahrens EH Jr, Miettinen TA (1965) J Lipid Res 6: 397
7. Crouse JR, Grundy SM (1978) J Lipid Res 19: 967
8. Kesäniemi YA, Witztum JL, Steinbrecher UP (1983) J Clin Invest 71: 950
9. Miettinen TA (1979) J Clin Invest 64: 1485
10. Kesäniemi YA, Vuoristo M, Miettinen TA (1984) In Treatment of hyperlipoproteinemia. eds. LA Carlson, AG Olsson, Raven Press, New York 49-53
11. Kesäniemi YA, Grundy SM (1984) Arteriosclerosis 4: 41

The Reticuloendothelial System and Low Density Lipoprotein Metabolism

J. Shepherd, C. J. Packard, and S. A. W. Gibson

Department of Biochemistry, Royal Infirmary, Glasgow G4 OSF, UK

The foam cells which characterise many early subendothelial arterial fatty lesions are generally thought to derive from wandering monocytes which invade the arterial wall from the bloodstream and adopt their typical histological appearance by accumulating lipid in their cytoplasm. Despite their apparently central role in the pathogenesis of atherosclerosis, both the biological mechanism responsible for the localisation of these cells in the lesions and their quantitative importance in the metabolism of plasma lipoproteins remain to be established. The greatest impediment to performing such studies in intact animals lies in the difficulties inherent in producing selective ablation of the reticuloendothelial system. Sublethal whole body irradiation or cyclophosphamide therapy can temporarily abolish the supply of monocytes from the bone marrow but neither approach is selective in its choice of target, and both leave mature macrophages unaffected [1, 2].

Reticuloendothelial suppression with ethyl oleate emulsions

In 1961, Stuart et al. [3] described an alternative approach to reticuloendothelial suppression. In a series of studies they documented the suppressant action of long chain fatty acid monoesters (eg ethyl oleate) on the phagocytic activity of macrophages. Administration of an ethyl oleate emulsion to rabbits (1 ml of lipid per kg body weight stabilised with 0.7% Tween 20 and given intravenously) reduced their ability to clear colloidal carbon from the bloodstream by about 50%. We have shown [4] that, following injection, the agent is rapidly and quantitatively taken up by the liver and spleen where its hydrolysis results in suppression of macrophage activity without producing either cell death or gross morphological or biochemical changes. Within hours of treatment, however, there is a significant increment in plasma cholesterol (Table 1) and in the circulating concentration of low density lipoprotein (LDL); and kinetic studies of LDL metabolism (4, Table 1) suggested that this resulted from direct interference with LDL catabolism, both via the high affinity LDL receptor pathway and by receptor independent processes. The response of the receptor path was variable and may have arisen from receptor downregulation secondary to the increase in plasma LDL or from a direct toxic effect of ethyl oleate on reticuloendothelial cells (which are known to express LDL receptor activity [5, 6]). By contrast, the ethyl oleate induced fall in receptor-independent LDL catabolism occurred in all animals, implicating the reticuloendothelial system in LDL clearance by this mechanism.

Receptor-Mediated Uptake
in the Liver
Edited by H. Greten, E. Windler, U. Beisiegel
© Springer-Verlag Berlin Heidelberg 1986

Table 1. Effects of ethyl oleate on the plasma concentration and metabolism of LDL in rabbits

Treatment	Plasma Cholesterol mmol/l	LDL Cholesterol mmol/l	Fractional Clearance Rate of LDL (pools/d)	
			Receptor Mediated	Receptor Independent
None[a]	2.12 ± 0.95	1.03 ± 0.92	0.84 ± 0.13[b]	0.66 ± 0.19[b]
Ethyl oleate[a]	2.40 ± 0.95	1.37 ± 0.89	0.55 ± 0.09	0.46 ± 0.27
Paired t test, control vs ethyl oleate treatment	< 0.02	< 0.01		
Unpaired t test, control vs ethyl oleate treatment a n = 11 b n = 14			< 0.05	< 0.001

Immunomodulation with muramic acid peptide conjugates

Bacterial cell walls contain peptide conjugates of N-acetyl muramic acid (Fig. 1) which are responsible for the endotoxic effects produced by the organisms. The active agent in this process, muramyl peptide, can be targeted selectively to cells

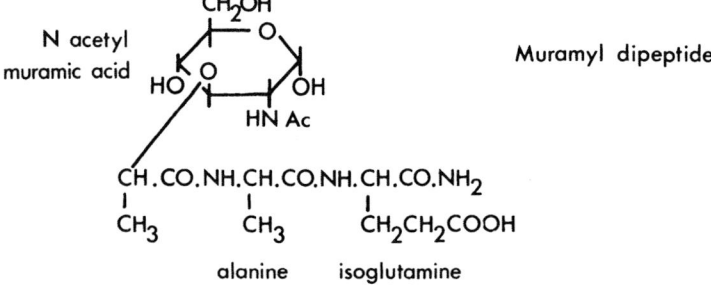

Fig. 1. Muramic acid peptide conjugates. The active agent, muramyl dipeptide (upper panel) requires to be targeted selectively to cells of the reticuloendothelial system by complexing it with phospholipid or acetylated albumin (lower panel)

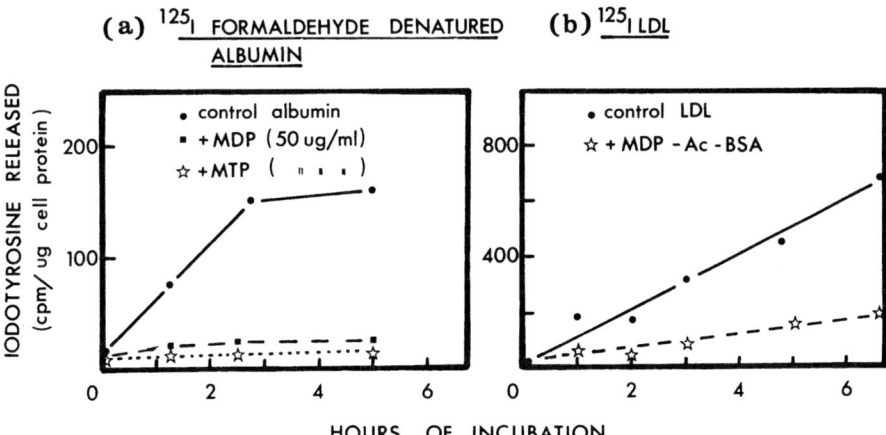

Fig. 2. Suppression of J774 macrophage phagocytic activity by muramyl dipeptide. Treatment of the cells with muramyl dipeptide-Ac albumin (50 μg/ml) significantly suppressed their ability to ingest and hydrolyse denatured albumin and human LDL

of the reticuloendothelial system by complexing it with phospholipid or acetylated albumin. We tested its potency against cultured J774 macrophages and found that it inhibited their ability to ingest and degrade both LDL and denatured rabbit serum albumin (Fig. 2). In a series of *in vivo* studies we have confirmed that it has a similar effect on plasma lipids as ethyl oleate, raising circulating cholesterol and LDL concentrations. An examination of the mechanism involved in the production of these acute changes was made in rabbits. The animals were injected with ^{125}I-LDL and ^{131}I-cyclohexanedione-treated LDL (which is not recognized by

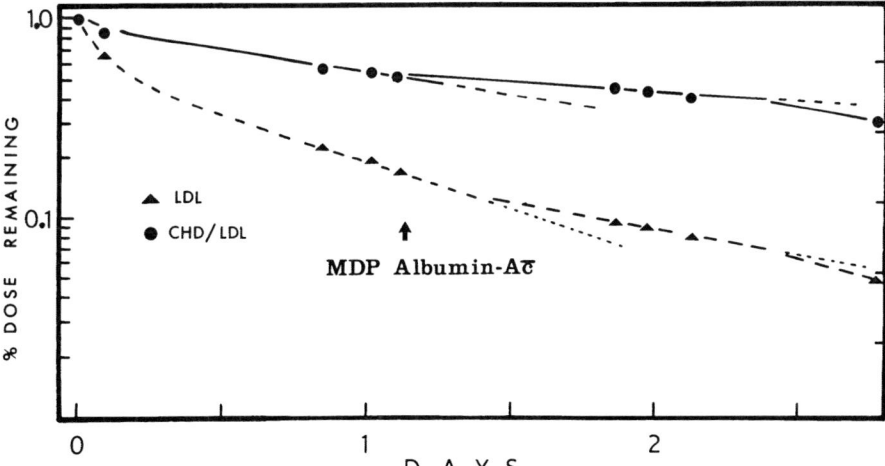

Fig. 3. Delayed clearance of human LDL from rabbit plasma following intravenous administration of muramyl dipeptide complexes. The suppressant retarded the catabolism of both native and receptor-blocked LDL. Kinetic analysis showed that the treatment selectively downregulated receptor-independent catabolic processes

the high affinity LDL receptor and is therefore channelled exclusively into other pathways) and the plasma clearance rates of the two tracers followed until they had reached their terminal monoexponential phase. At this point, intravenous administration of acetyl-albumin complexed muramyl dipeptide produced an abrupt change in the slope of both decay curves (Fig. 3), and kinetic analysis of the data revealed, in support of the earlier study with ethyl oleate, that LDL clearance into receptor-independent pathways had been reduced.

These studies with reticuloendothelial suppressants demonstrate that the monocyte/macrophage system plays a significant role in the catabolism of LDL. The detailed mechanism involved in the interaction remains to be elucidated.

Acknowledgements. This study was performed during tenure of grants from the Scottish Hospital Endowments Research Trust (HERT 673) and the Cancer Research Campaign (SP 1671).

References

1. Volkman A, Collins FM (1968) Recovery of delayed-type hypersensitivity in mice following suppressive doses of x-radiation. J Immunol 101: 846-859
2. Bach JF (1975) "The Mode of Action of Immunosuppressive Agents". North-Holland, Amsterdam
3. Stuart AE, Biozzi G, Stiffel C, Halpern BN, Mouton D (1960) The stimulation and depression of reticuloendothelial phagocytic function by simple lipids. Br J Exp Pathol 41: 599-604
4. Slater HR, Packard CJ, Shepherd J (1982) Receptor-independent catabolism of low density lipoprotein: involvement of the reticuloendothelial system. J Biol Chem 257: 307-310
5. Fogelman AM, Shechter I, Seager V, Hokum M, Child JS, Edwards PM (1980) Malondialdehyde alteration of low density lipoproteins leads to cholesteryl ester accumulation in human monocyte-macrophages. Proc Natl Acad Sci USA 77: 2214-2218
6. Traber MG, Kayden HJ (1980) Low density lipoprotein receptor activity and its relation to atheromatous lesions. Proc Natl Acad Sci USA 77: 5466-5470

Removal of Chylomicron Remnants by the Hepatic LDL Receptor Liver — Possible Contribution of the Low Densitiy Lipoprotein Receptor

E. E. T. WINDLER, W. H. DÄRR, and H. GRETEN

Medizinische Kernklinik und Poliklinik, Universitätskrankenhaus Eppendorf, Hamburg, West Germany

Introduction

Triglyceride-rich lipoproteins as very low density lipoproteins and chylomicrons are snythesized by liver and intestine. After their secretion into the bloodstream they are catabolized in two steps. Firstly the triglyceride moiety is hydrolized and tissues are supplied with the released fatty acids. The triglyceride hydrolysis leads to a decrease in particle size and is accompanied by various changes in the chemical composition (Fig. 1).

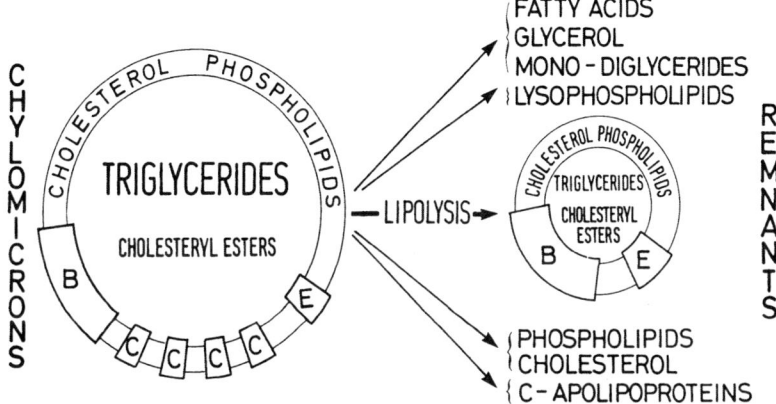

Fig. 1. Changes of lipid and apolipoprotein constituents during remnant formation by lipolysis of chylomicrons

A relative increase in the content of lysophosphatidylcholine in the formed remnant particles reduces the affinity for the C-apolipoproteins, which are transfered to high density lipoproteins [1]. As the C-apolipoproteins exert an inhibitory effect on the binding of remnants to cell surface receptors, at this point the second step of catabolism can take place: Apolipoprotein E mediates the binding of the particles to hepatic receptors followed by internalization [2, 3, 4].

This research was supported by the Deutsche Forschungsgemeinschaft SFB 232

Receptor-Mediated Uptake
in the Liver
Edited by H. Greten, E. Windler, U. Beisiegel
© Springer-Verlag Berlin Heidelberg 1986

At least two kinds of receptors may be involved in the process of uptake: the classical low-density-lipoprotein-receptor and the apolipoprotein E-receptor, both of which are able to bind lipoproteins containing apolipoprotein E [5, 6]. From studies in humans and animals that lack the low-density-lipoprotein-receptor it is known that other mechanisms but the low-density-lipoprotein-receptor are sufficient for the chylomicron remnant removal by the liver [6]. However, it is not known if and to which extent the low-density-lipoprotein-receptor takes part in the binding and uptake of remnants under normal conditions. Therefore we started to investigate the binding of chylomicrons and their remnants to hepatic receptors in an attempt to assess the contribution of the various mechanisms.

Methods

Sprague-Dawley rats of 250-350 g were kept on a standard rat chow and tap water. Lymph was obtained by cannulation of the mesenteric lymph duct and intraduodenal infusion of 10% glucose in saline as described [2]. For radioactive labelling of chylomicrons ^{3}H-cholesterol (Amersham-Buchler, Braunschweig, FRG) was added to the infusion. Small chylomicrons were isolated from lymph by two centrifugations at 4° C with 100,000 g for 4 hours. To obtain postheparin plasma free of very low density lipoproteins, rats were bled 10 min. after injection of 60 IU of heparin (Thrombophob, Nordmark, Hamburg, FRG)) per kg bodyweight, and the plasma was centrifuged at 4° C with 100,000 g at a density of 1.019 g/ml for 24 hours. Remnants of small chylomicrons were prepared by incubating small chylomicrons in postheparin plasma at 37° C for 15 min. and centrifuging the plasma twice as above for 20 hours. An average of 72.2% of triglycerides were hydrolized and the ratio of triglycerides over cholesteryl esters fell to 7.3 ± 0.7 (w/w). Serum chylomicrons were produced by incubation of small chylomicrons in serum free of very low density lipoproteins, prepared from serum by centrifugation as described for postheparin plasma, at room-temperature for 1 hour. Serum chylomicrons were isolated by two centrifugations at 1.019 g/ml under conditions as above. Low density lipoproteins were isolated from normal human serum by centrifugation twice at 1.024 g/ml and at 1.050 g/ml for 20 hours as above. Low density lipoproteins were further concentrated by ultrafiltration (Amicon-Diaflow UM 30) and dialyzed against multiple changes of Tris-HCl-buffer (50 mM NaCl, 1 mM CaCl$_2$, 20 mM Tris, pH 7.4). Apolipoprotein E was not detectable in low density lipoproteins by SDS- or isoelectric focussing polyacrylamide gel electrophoresis.

For the preparation of hepatic membranes, rat livers were homogenized with a Teflon-pestle in Tris-buffer at 4° C 5 times for 10 sec., and centrifuged with 500 g at 4° C for 20 min. The supernatant was centrifuged with 8000 g for 15 min. ånd recentrifuged with 100,000 g for 1 hour, both times at 4° C. The pellet of the latter centrifugation was used for binding-experiments and stored in liquid nitrogen. For binding-assays 100 μg membrane protein were incubated with lipoproteins and Tris-buffer made up to 100 μl at 37° C in Polyallomer tubes (Beckman Instr., Munich, FRG; 7 x 20 mm) for 90 min. 75 μl Tris-buffer were added and the samples centrifuged in a LP 42-Ti rotor (Beckman Instr., Munich, FRG) at 4° C with 100,000 g for 30 min. The pellets were washed with 175 μl Tris-buffer and recentrifuged under the same conditions. The upper phase was discarded and the lower parts of the tubes were cut and the radioactivity counted in 5 ml of scintillation solvents (Rotiszint, Roth Comp., Karlsruhe, FRG). To enable subtraction of background radioactivity, for each sample a control was prepared in the same way but without membrane added. All data are the mean of duplicate assays and multiple experiments as indicated. Determinations of protein and lipids in lipoproteins and thin-layer chromatography of lipids were performed by standard procedures as previously described [2, 7].

Results

When ^{3}H-small chylomicron remnants were incubated with rat hepatic membranes at 37° C for various length of time, the bound fraction increased and reached its maximum value within 90 min. (not shown). Therefore this time of incubation was chosen for all experiments. About 80% of ^{3}H in chylomicrons or their remnants was recovered with the cholesteryl esters and about 20% with free cholesterol on thin layer chromatography. The same ratio was found in lipoproteins bound to hepatic membranes. Thus whole ^{3}H-counts could be used as a measure for the lipoproteins in binding assays.

Binding of ^{3}H-small chylomicron remnants increased with higher concentrations of remnants curvilinearly (Fig. 2). Binding in the presence of a tenfold excess of unlabelled small chylomicron remnants was little, presumably due to nonspecific, not receptor-mediated absorption. When this portion was subtracted from total binding, the resultant saturation-curve should represent receptor-mediated binding, which became saturated at a concentration of about 100 μg cholesteryl esters per ml and 35 ng cholesteryl esters bound per μg of membrane protein (Fig. 2).

The high affinity binding of small chylomicron remnants was in contrast to that of small chylomicrons from lymph and serum (Fig. 3). Lymph chylomicrons exhibited very little or no binding, while serum chylomicrons that had absorbed the apolipoproteins E and C during incubation with serum showed some binding (Fig. 3).

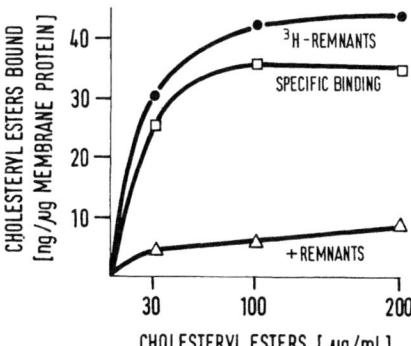

Fig. 2. Binding of ^{3}H-chylomicron remnants in the absence (●, n = 3) and presence (Δ, n = 2) of a tenfold excess of unlabeled chylomicron remnants to hepatic membranes. Specific binding resuleted from subtraction of the two values (□)

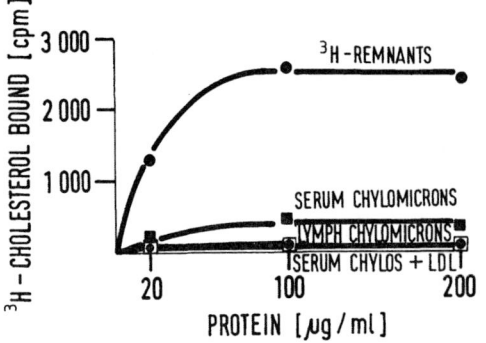

Fig. 3. Binding of labeled chylomicron remnants (●, n = 2), serum chylomicrons (■, n = 3), lymph chylomicrons (□, n = 2), and serum chylomicrons in the presence of a fiftyfold excess of low density lipoproteins (●, w/w of cholesteryl esters, n = 2) to hepatic membranes

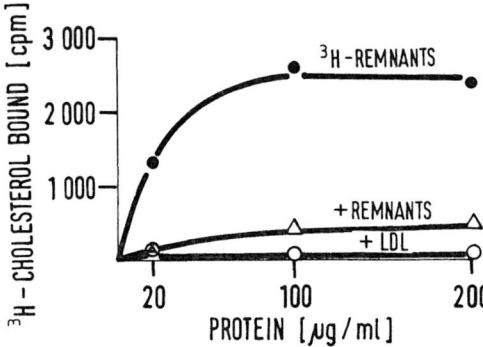

Fig. 4. Binding of ^{3}H-chylomicron remnants in the absence (●) or presence of a tenfold excess of unlabeled chylomicron remnants (Δ) and of a fiftyfold excess of unlabeled low density lipoproteins (○) (w/w cholesteryl esters) to hepatic membranes (n = 2 each)

Unlabelled low density lipoproteins competed with the binding of both, serum small chylomicrons and their remnants (Fig. 3 and 4). A fiftyfold excess of low density lipoproteins reduced the binding of serum chylomicrons virtually to zero (Fig. 3). The same was true for a fiftyfold excess of low density lipoproteins in the case of small chylomicron remnants, which was as or even more efficient than a tenfold excess of unlabelled small chylomicron remnants (Fig. 4).

Discussion

The results of this investigation are consistent with the view that chylomicrons and their remnants bind through the action of apolipoprotein E to hepatic cell surface receptors and that this binding is inhibited by the C-apolipoproteins [3]. Lymph chylomicrons which contain none or only very little apolipoprotein E and some C-apolipoproteins do not bind to hepatic receptors. Chylomicron remnants, however, which are rich in apolipoprotein E but poor in C-apolipoproteins bind with high affinity. Serum chylomicrons contain both, apolipoprotein E and C-apolipoproteins and show some binding. According to these experiments the apolipoproteins A-I, A-IV and especially B-48 are no ligands of hepatic receptors, as these are the predominant apolipoproteins of lymph chylomicrons, which do not show any affinity for hepatic membranes, as has been similarly found by others [5]. The results are only partially in agreement with previous studies [2]. Isolated perfused rat livers took up lymph chylomicrons more readily than serum chylomicrons. Thus these in vitro binding studies do not necessarily reflect all aspects that contribute to the behaviour of the various lipoproteins in vivo.

The competition of low density lipoproteins with the binding of chylomicron remnants suggest that both these lipoproteins may be a ligand of a common receptor. Former experiments clearly demonstrate that remnants of very low density lipoproteins and low density lipoproteins compete for the same binding site, the low-density-lipoprotein-receptor [4]. This could be explained by the common contents of apolipoprotein B-100 in both particles. To exclude this possibility by contamination of chylomicrons, lymph was obtained from the mesenteric duct and chylomicron remnants were prepared in vitro by incubation in postheparin plasma free of very low density lipoproteins. The resultant remnants were shown to contain apolipoprotein B-48 but no B-100. Earlier it was shown that apolipoprotein-E-containing liposomes bind to the hepatic low-density-lipoprotein-receptor [4]. Thus it seemed reasonable to assume, that also chylomicron remnants which are rich in apolipoprotein E would bind to this receptor, unless apolipoprotein B-48 prevents this binding. In this case specific binding should be restricted to the apolipoprotein-E-receptor. To exclude this possibility and to provide evidence for the binding to the low-density-lipoprotein-receptor, competition studies had to be performed with low density lipoproteins which were free of apolipoprotein E. In agreement with the hypothesis that chylomicrons and their remnants by virtue of their content in apolipoprotein E and low density lipoproteins due to apolipoprotein B-100 share the low-density-lipoprotein-receptor as a common binding site, low density lipoproteins efficiently competed for the binding of chylomicron remnants as well as for that of serum chylomicrons to hepatic membranes.

Studies in humans homozygous for familial hypercholesterilemia and in Watanabe heritable hyperlipidemic rabbits have demonstrated an undisturbed chylomicron remnant removal under conditions where low-density-lipoprotein-receptors are grossly or completely absent [6]. Thus, there have to exist alternative removal mechanisms as the well characterized apolipoprotein-E-receptor [5]. As in research by others, it has not been possible to demonstrate this binding site with a membrane assay in vitro for unknown reasons [6]. But this may explain the mentioned discrepancies between the findings in vitro versus in vivo. Therefore experiments in live animals or with perfused organs are needed to be able to further assess the significance of the low-density-lipoprotein-receptor for the chylomicron remnant removal.

References

1. Windler E, Preyer S, Greten H (1985) Correlation between the content in lysophosphatidylcholine and the C-apolipoproteins of human triglyceride-rich lipoproteins. Eur J Clin Invest 15
2. Windler E, Chao Y-s, Havel RJ (1979) Determinants of hepatic uptake of triglyceride-rich lipoproteins and their remnants in the rat. J Biol Chem 255: 5475-5480

3. Windler E, Chao YS, Havel RJ (1980) Regulation of the hepatic uptake of triglyceride-rich lipoproteins in the rat. J Biol Chem 255: 8303-8307
4. Windler E, Kovanen PT, Chao YS, Brown MS, Havel RJ, Goldstein JL (1980) The estradiol-stimulated lipoprotein receptor of rat liver. J Biol Chem 254: 10464-10471
5. Hui DY, Innerarity TL, Milne RW, Marcel YL, Mahley RW (1984) Binding of chylomicron remnants and ß-very low density lipoproteins to hepatic and extrahepatic lipoprotein receptors. J Biol Chem 259: 15060-15068
6. Kita T, Goldstein JL, Brown MS, Watanabe Y, Hornick CA, Havel RJ (1982) Hepatic uptake of chylomicron remnants in WHHL rabbits: A mechanism genetically distinct from the low density lipoprotein receptor. Proc Natl Acad Sci USA 79: 3623-3627
7. Därr WH, Greten H (1982) In vitro modulation of the distribution of normal human plasma high density lipoprotein subfractions through the lecithin: cholesterol transferase reaction. Biochim Biophys Acta 710: 128-133

Metabolism of Human Triglyceride-rich Lipoprotein Remnants

C. J. PACKARD, A. MUNRO, R. J. CLEGG, R. JAMES, D. POMETTA, and J. SHEPHERD

Department of Pathological Biochemistry, Royal Infirmary, Glasgow, UK and Division of Diabetology, Hospital Cantonal, Geneva, Switzerland

The liver is believed to play an important role in clearing from the plasma metabolic end products (or "remnants") generated during the lipolysis of triglyceride-rich lipoproteins [1]. We have recently undertaken a series of studies designed to examine the genesis and removal of such remnants following administration of radiolabeled very low density lipoproteins (VLDL) to normal and hyperlipoproteinaemic subjects. In a typical experiment large, triglyceride-rich VLDL of Sf 100-400 were isolated from fasting plasma, radioiodinated with ^{125}I, and reinjected into the bloodstream of the donor. Thereafter at timed intervals, VLDL of Sf 100-400, intermediate lipoproteins of Sf 12-100 and LDL of Sf 0-12 fractions were prepared and the radioactivity and protein present in their apolipoprotein B (apo B) measured following its precipitation with 1, 1, 3, 3 tetramethylurea and delipidation with chloroform/methanol [2]. Normal subjects transferred Sf 100-400 apo B rapidly into the Sf 12-100 remnant density range ($t^{1}/_{2}$ for Sf 100-400 VLDL apo B was 1.1 hours). From there, the apo B decayed more slowly (mean residence time of about 0.8 days), with most of the radioactivity being cleared directly from the circulation and little appearing in LDL of Sf 0-12 [3]. This indicated that this material made a minimal contribution to the production of LDL in the intravascular compartment. On the other hand, when smaller VLDL particles of Sf 20-100 were labelled with radioiodine and their metabolism was studied in normal subjects, a high proportion of the apo B radioactivity was transferred into the LDL range indicating that the LDL precursor lipoproteins were probably secreted into the Sf 20-100 density range.

Comparative catabolic rates for large VLDL and its remnant in normal, type III, type IV and FH homozygous subjects are presented in the Table 1 below:

Table 1

Subject Group	Fractional catabolic rate (pools/d)	
	Sf 100-400 VLDL apo B	Sf 12-100 remnant apo B
Normal (n = 4)	14.9 ± 2.1	1.29 ± 0.23
type IV (n = 5)	7.0 ± 2.9	1.38 ± 0.62
type IV on bezafibrate	31.2 ± 21.6	0.98 ± 0.38
type III (2)	11.5, 16.1	0.60, 0.60
FH homozygote (1)	10.8	0.4

Receptor-Mediated Uptake
in the Liver
Edited by H. Greten, E. Windler, U. Beisiegel
© Springer-Verlag Berlin Heidelberg 1986

The type III and FH homozygous subjects converted their large VLDL to remnants at an approximately normal rate, but the process was 50% slower in the type IV individuals. It could be promoted in the latter by the administration of bezafibrate [4] which presumably activated the lipoprotein lipase responsible for this initial conversion. Subsequent removal of these Sf 12-100 remnants occurred at a normal rate and did not change during bezafibrate therapy. Intermediate lipoprotein catabolism was slower, however, in the type III and FH homozygous subjects who lack functional apolipoprotein E and LDL (or "B/E") receptors respectively. These findings suggest that remnant removal from the plasma depends on the interaction between the particle and a receptor on cell membranes. To test this hypothesis in control subjects we isolated large VLDL of Sf 100-400 and divided it into two aliquots one of which was labelled with ^{125}I, the other with [131]I. The latter was modified with 1, 2 cyclohexanedione as previously described [5] and each subject received an injection of ^{125}I-labelled native and ^{131}I-labelled 1, 2 cyclohexanedione (CHD) treated Sf 100-400 VLDL. B protein in both tracers transferred into the SF 12-100 remnant density interval at the same rate but thereafter their metabolism diverged. The CHD treated material had a clearance rate from the Sf 12-100 range that was half that of the untreated lipoprotein (ie the FCR of CHD modified VLDL in the Sf 12-100 lipoprotein was 0.63 + 0.07 pools/day, n = 4).

There is now a substantial body of evidence that indicates that the LDL (or "B/E") receptor plays an active role in VLDL as well as LDL metabolism. In situations, such as those described above and elsewhere [6, 7] where the interaction of ligand with receptor is blocked the catabolism of apolipoprotein B in intermediate density lipoproteins is retarded. Since the site of remnant catabolism is believed to be the liver then it appears that hepatic receptors are important in controlling the plasma levels of not only LDL but also VLDL remnants and their primary function may be to clear these potentially atherogenic lipoproteins from the bloodstream.

Acknowledgements. This study was supported by grants from the Medical Research Council (G 8111558SA) and Scottish Home and Health Department (HERT 673). Miss Joyce Pollock provided excellent secretarial assistance.

References

1. Havel RJ, Goldstein JL, Brown MS (1980). Lipoproteins and lipid transport. In: Metabolic Control and Disease, 8th ed., edited by Bondy PK and Rosenberg LE, Saunders Co. Philadelphia PA pp 393-494
2. Packard CJ, Shepherd J, Joerns S, Gotto AM, Taunton OD (1980). Apolipoprotein B metabolism in Normal, type IV and type V hyperlipoproteinaemic subjects. Metabolism 29: 213-222
3. Packard CJ, Munro A, Lorimer AR, Gotto AM, Shepherd J (1984) Metabolism of apolipoprotein B in large triglyceride-rich lipoproteins of normal and hypertriglyceridemic subjects. J Clin Invest 74: 2178-2192

4. Shepherd J, Packard CJ, Stewart JM, Atmeh RF, Clark RS, Boag DE, Carr K, Lorimer AR, Ballantyne D, Morgan HG, Lawrie TDV (1984) Apolipoprotein A and B (Sf 100-400) metabolism during bezafibrate therapy in hypertriglyceridemic subjects. J Clin Invest 74: 2164-2177
5. Shepherd J, Bicker S, Lorimer AR, Packard CJ (1979) Receptor-mediated low density lipoprotein catabolism in man. J Lipid Res 20: 999-1006
6. Kita T, Brown MS, Bilheimer DW, Goldstein JL (1982) Delayed clearance of very low density and intermediate density lipoproteins with enhanced conversion to low density lipoproteins in WHHL rabbits. Proc Natl Acad Sci USA 79: 5693-5697
7. Soutar AK, Myant NB, Thompson GR (1982) The metabolism of very low density and intermediate density lipoproteins in patients with familial hypercholesterolemia. Atherosclerosis 43: 217-231

Suppression of Apoprotein-E Receptor by LP-X

A. K. WALLI and D. SEIDEL

Abt. Klinische Chemie, Zentrum Innere Medizin der Universität Göttingen, 3400 Göttingen, Federal Republic of Germany

Cholestasis brings about numerous changes in hepatic lipoprotein metabolism. The most pronounced alterations are hypercholesterolemia, hyperlipidemia and appearance of a unique lipoprotein, lipoprotein-X, in plasma. This lipoprotein is characterized by a high content of phospholipids and unesterified cholesterol with a small amount of protein. About 60% of the protein is albumin which is in the core of the vesicle. Apo-C forms the surface apoprotein, whereas apo-B and apo-E are absent. Lipoprotein-X is formed when bile lipids reflux into the plasma [1-4]. Even though LP-X is rich in cholesterol, it is surprising that cholesterol circulating in the form of LP-X does not exert feed-back control through HMG-CoA reductase on hepatic cholesterol synthesis during cholestasis. Despite the high cholesterol content of LP-X, its infusion has no significant effect on hepatic cholesterol biosynthesis in normal rats or in rats with a bile fistula [5], in contrast to the inhibitory effect of LDL. As a result of a disturbance in cholesterol homeostasis, hepatic cholesterol synthesis is increased in cholestasis [6]. Its role as a possible causative factor for cholestatic hypercholesterolemia has gained interest in recent years [7].

When ^{125}I-LP-X is injected into rats it rapidly disappears from the circulation showing a biphasic decay curve. Analysis of the plasma decay curve yielded a mean biological half life of 15.5 min as calculated from the fast component of the curve, and biological half life of 9.5 hours corresponding to a mean fractional catabolic rate of 1.782 days, as calculated from the slow component of the curve [7]. Measurement of radioactivity in various organs of rats showed that on a weight basis, spleen takes up several fold more LP-X than liver (Fig. 1). The mean biological half life of ^{125}I-LP-X in various tissues of rat was calculated so that it could be compared to the slow component of the plasma decay curve. The values obtained showed that spleen had $t_{1/2}$ of 51.6 h compared to 18.3 h for liver.

These data show that LP-X in vivo is mainly removed by the reticuloendothelial system, primarily by spleen. Even though on a weight basis (cpm/g) liver takes up only a fraction of ^{125}I-LP-X taken up by the spleen, on the basis of total tissue weight, the amount of LP-X removed by the liver is significant. Liver tissue consists of parenchymal and non-parenchymal cells which may have different relative rates of uptake of LP-X. Measurement of the distribution of ^{125}I radioactivity in isolated livers that were perfused with ^{125}I-LP-X or perfused livers that were isolated from rats, that were injected with ^{125}I-LP-X before cell isolation, showed that non-parenchymal cells took up 8-10 fold more LP-X than parenchymal cells [7].

Receptor-Mediated Uptake
in the Liver
Edited by H. Greten, E. Windler, U. Beisiegel
© Springer-Verlag Berlin Heidelberg 1986

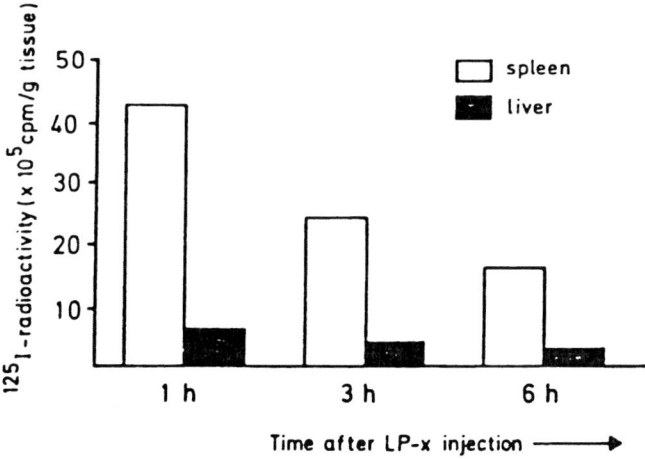

Fig. 1. Comparison of ^{125}I-activity in liver and spleen of rats after intravenous injection of ^{125}I-LP-X

The role of reticuloendothelial cells in removal of LP-X is further confirmed by the uptake of this lipoprotein in various cell systems in vitro (Table 1). Incubation of parenchymal liver cells, non-parenchymal liver cells, human lymphocyte suspensions or fibroblast cultures with LP-X reveals that non-parenchymal cells bind more LP-X than parenchymal cells or fibroblasts, while lymphocytes take up 20 fold more LP-X than do hepatocytes. LP-X is not taken up by specific binding to a receptor. Incubation of cells in the presence of increasing amounts of unlabeled LP-X showed no displacement of ^{125}I-LP-X uptake. Even in the presence of over 50-fold excess of unlabeled LP-X, no displacement was noted. Thus LP-X uptake even though concentration dependent, is not saturable and is non-specific (Fig. 2).

When these observations are considered together with the data from the in vivo experiments, it is evident that LP-X is mainly taken up by the cells of the reticuloendothelial system both in vivo and in vitro. During cholestasis, even though the levels of unesterified cholesterol are high, most of this is transported by LP-X. Since LP-X is not taken up significantly by hepatic parenchymal cells it cannot exert a feed-back control on hepatic cholesterol synthesis.

Table 1. Uptake of [125]-I-LP-X by isolated parenchymal and non-parenchymal cells, suspensions of human lymphocytes and monolayer cultures of human skin fibroblasts

Concentration of LP-X in the medium (µg LP-X protein/ml)	Uptake ng LP-X protein/mg cell protein			
	parenchymal cells	non-parenchymal cells	fibroblasts	lymphocytes
5 µg	24	75	34	324
10 µg	41	158	66	791
15 µg	58	229	91	1158

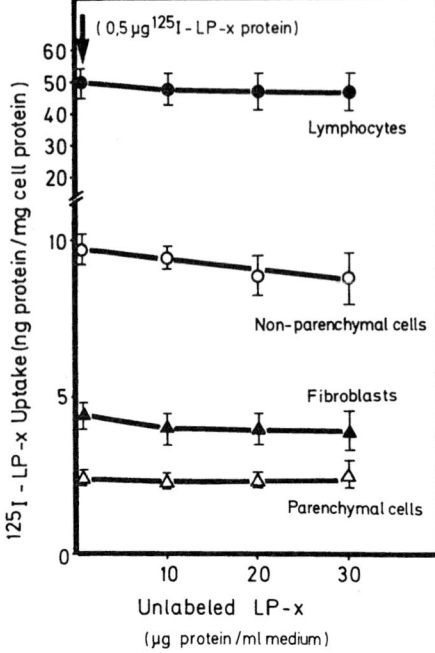

Fig. 2. Failure of increasing concentrations of unlabeled LP-X to suppress the uptake of ^{125}I-LP-X in isolated cell in suspension or culture. ^{125}I-LP-X was added to medium to give a LP-X protein concentration of 0.5 µg/ml

From these observations one might conclude that LP-X acts primarily on reticuloendothelial cells. However, since enhanced hepatic cholesterogenesis, coupled with increased activity of hepatic HMG-CoA reductase, is a feature of cholestasis, the effects of LP-X on this enzyme as well as lipoprotein uptake were investigated [6, 8].

Hepatic cholesterogenesis is closely related to the activity of HMG-CoA reductase activity [8]. In cholestasis enhanced cholesterogenesis is accompanied by the elevated activity of the enzyme despite the elevated levels of unesterified cholesterol, the reasons for which are unclear. Bile acids do not appear to directly affect hepatic cholesterol synthesis but biliary lipids which reflux into plasma need to be considered. Bile contains a protein lipid complex which is capable of inhibiting HMG-CoA reductase in isolated microsomes [9]. In contrast to this, the total lipoprotein fraction and particularly that fraction isolated in d<1.063 g/ml from cholestatic rat serum, which was not characterized, increased the activity of HMG-CoA reductase by several fold [10]. The density fraction d<1.063 g/ml in both cholestatic serum and bile contains LP-X or its precursor. This indirectly suggests that LP-X may affect the activity of HMG-CoA reductase. In order to verify this, isolated livers from rats were perfused in the absence or presence of either LDL or LP-X (Fig. 3). LP-X increased the activity of HMG-CoA reductase by over 2 fold when compared with control or livers perfused with LDL.

This contrasts with the data obtained in lymphocytes. LP-X inhibited the activity of the reductase in lymphoycte suspensions. The degree of the inhibition of the enzyme is similar for LDL and LP-X (Fig. 4). The data obtained from these incu-

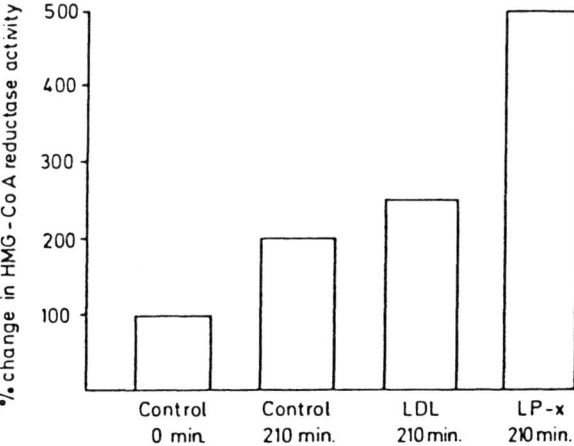

Fig. 3. Effect of LP-X and LDL on the activity of HMG-CoA reductase in isolated perfused rat livers

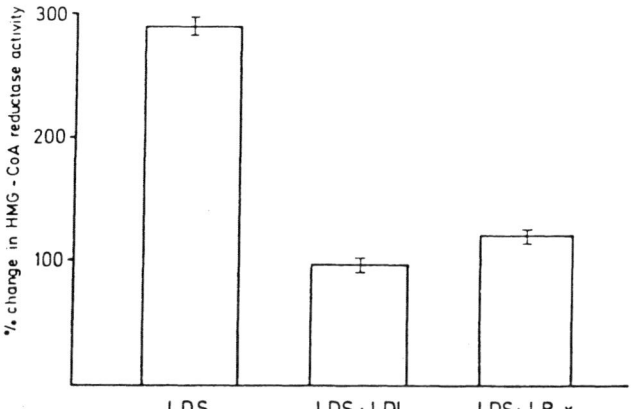

Fig. 4. Effect of LP-X and LDL on the activity of HMG-CoA reductase in lymphocytes from human blood. Lymphocytes were incubated for 48 h in 10% lipoprotein deficient serum (LDS). LP-X or LDL (125 μg cholesterol/ml medium) was added to culture dishes. The reductase activity was measured 24 h later in lymphocytes

bation experiments are in agreement with these measurements performed in lymphocytes from cholestatic patients who were LP-X positive. The enzyme activity was significantly lower as compared to that measured in control subjects (11.5 compared to 55 pmole/mg protein/h).

LP-X is capable of suppressing the HMG-CoA reductase in isolated hepatic microsomes in a concentration dependent manner. The presence of small amounts of bile acids that are present in LP-X were not responsible for the inhibition of the activity of the reductase. Incubation of isolated microsomes with even 10 fold higher concentration of bile salts that are present in LP-X caused no inhibition of the enzyme [7, 11].

It thus becomes evident that when no barriers for LP-X uptake exist, its cholesterol moiety is capable of inhibiting the reductase activity. This may be due to delivery of cholesterol from LP-X to microsomes. The activation of the reductase in perfused livers or in cells which do not take up LP-X may be due to its physicochemical properties. LP-X is rich in phospholipids, the molar ratio of phospholipids to cholesterol being about 1. Phospholipid vesicles are known to promote efflux of cholesterol from a variety of cells and increase the activity of the reductase [12-16]. On the basis of our data and from earlier observations, we suggest that LP-X in the circulation causes an efflux of cholesterol from cells which do not readily take it up. In contrast, LP-X suppresses the activity of the reductase in cell types such as lymphocytes in vitro or lymphocytes isolated from cholestatic patients where LP-X is taken up and delivers its cholesterol to cells thereby suppressing the activity of HMG-CoA reductase.

Normally chylomicron remnants are rapidly removed from the circulation by the liver and are most effective in suppressing hepatic cholesterogenesis [17, 18]. Should the disturbance in chylomicron remnant removal be a causative factor for enhanced hepatic cholesterol synthesis during cholestastis, it would then be expected that their uptake is impaired. Surprisingly, LP-X causes a marked inhibition of remnant uptake by isolated perfused liver and isolated hepatocytes, even though it is devoid of apo-B and apo-E and shows a poor uptake by hepatocytes (Fig. 5). Analysis of data from Lineweaver-Burk plots show that whereas K_m for remnant uptake in normal cells is 4.55 μmol protein/ml, it is increased to 10.00 μmol protein/ml in the presence of LP-X. On the other hand, the V_{max} remains essentially unchanged. (105 Vs 97 n mol protein/mg cell protein) (Fig. 6). This suggests a competitive type of inhibition in the presence of LP-X.

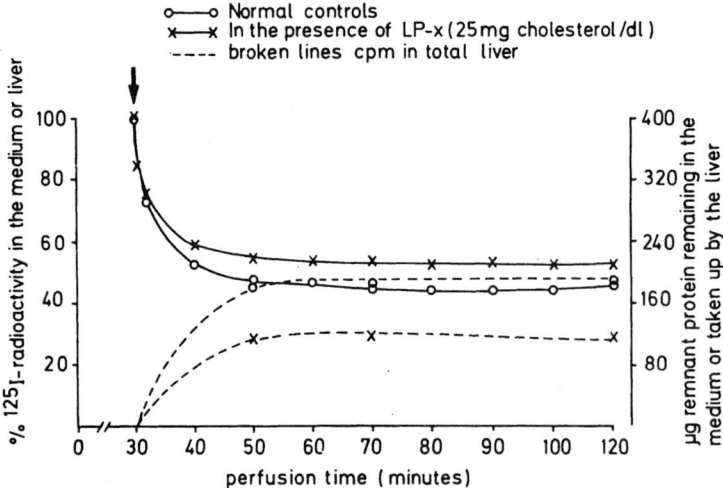

Fig. 5. Effect of LP-X on the ^{125}I-labeled chylomicron remnants in isolated perfused livers

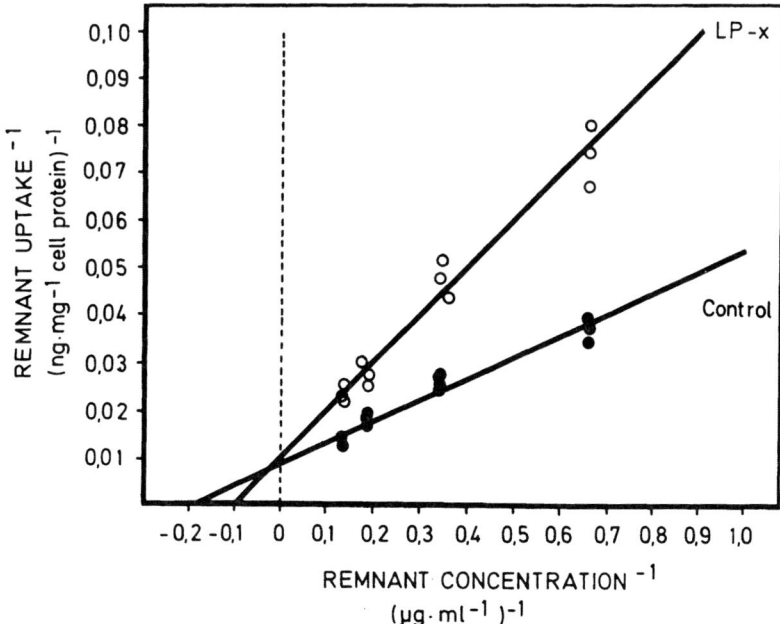

Fig. 6. Lineweaver-Burk Plot of ^{125}I-labeled chylomicron remnant uptake by isolated hepatocytes in the presence and absence of LP-X

A parallel finding is a marked hypertriglyceridemia, which is often noted in cholestatic patients, and may indicate accumulation of remnant-like particles [19].

Plasma LDL is catabolized by a variety of cells in culture after specific binding to high affinity receptors [20]. However, in normal rats only a small amount of circulating LDL is reported to be taken up by liver suggesting that this organ does not usually possess a large number of LDL receptors. Administration of ethinyl estradiol results in the expression of specific binding sites for LDL on the hepatic plasma membranes [21]. Similarly, livers of estrogen treated rats bind and degrade human LDL as well as rat LDL in amounts which are several fold higher than found in normal livers [22].

In contrast to direct effects of LP-X on remnant uptake, the degradation of LDL by perfused livers from rats treated with ethinyl estradiol is unchanged in the presence of LP-X [7]. Similarly, no effect of LP-X was noted on in high affinity binding and degradation of LDL in fibroblasts, which possess apo B-E receptors for LDL binding.

In order to understand the relevance of these in vitro systems to the situation in vivo, we perfused livers from cholestatic rats which had LP-X in their serum. Such livers degraded twice as much ^{125}I LDL as normal livers. These data strongly suggest that, whereas LP-X leads to inhibition of chylomicron remnant uptake, it increases hepatic LDL receptor activity. The supply of LDL cholesterol during cholestasis may not be sufficient to counteract the enhanced hepatic cholesterol synthesis, even in a situation of increased LDL receptor activity. A similar situa-

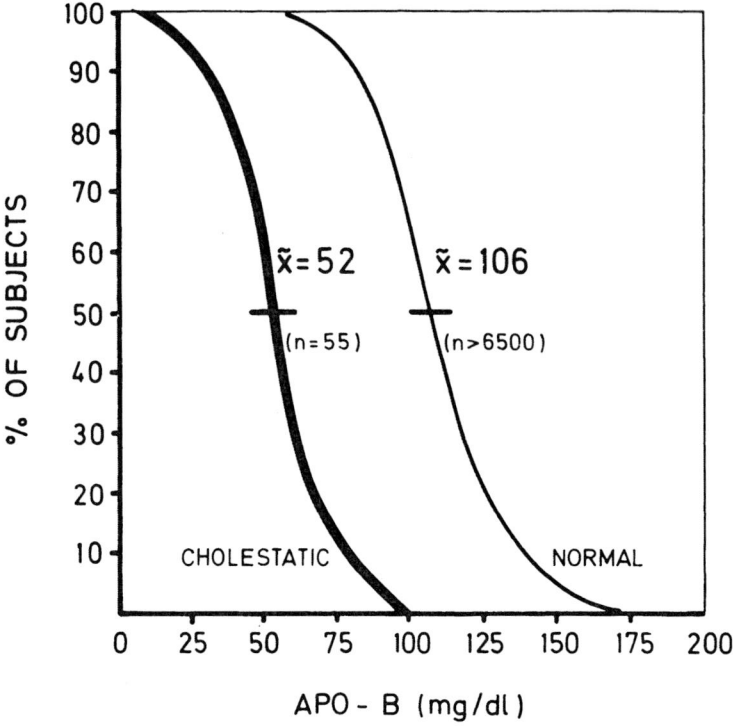

Fig. 7. Distribution of apo-B in plasma of normal and cholestatic patients

tion is observed in patients with cholestasis. The median apo-B concentration in serum of cholestatic patients is nearly reduced to half of that found in normal subjects, reflecting a reduced LDL concentration (Fig. 7).

From these results the role of LP-X in bringing about cholestatic hypercholesterolemia can be summarized as follows:

1. LP-X does not deliver its cholesterol to hepatocytes. Instead, it causes efflux of cellular cholesterol, which leads to activation of hepatic HMG-CoA reductase activity.
2. LP-X inhibits the receptor mediated uptake of chylomicron remnants by liver, thereby rendering this class of lipoproteins unable to regulate hepatic cholesterogenesis.
3. Its presence in vivo (in cholestasis) activates apo B-E receptor activity, but the availability of lipoproteins, which are removed by this receptor, may not be sufficient to suppress the enhanced hepatic cholesterogenesis of cholestasis.
4. These observations are of particular interest with respect to receptor activity. Although LP-X is devoid of apo-B and apo-E, yet it appears to affect apo-E receptor directly and apo B-E receptor indirectly.

In conclusion it is tempting to postulate that an interplay of these two receptors is important for maintaining the cholesterol homeostasis.

References

1. Seidel D, Alaupovic P, Furmann RH (1969) A lipoprotein characterizing obstructive jaundice. I. Method for quantitative separation and identification of lipoproteins in jaundiced subjects. J Clin Invest 48: 1211-1223
2. Seidel D, Alaupovic P, Furman RH, McConathy WJ (1970) A lipoprotein characterizing obstructive jaundice. II. Isolation and partial characterization of protein moieties of low density lipoproteins. J Clin Invest 49: 2396-2407
3. Seidel D, Büff HU, Fauser U, Bleyl U (1976) On the metabolism of lipoprotein-X (LP-X). Clin Chim Acta 66: 195-207
4. Manzato E, Fellin R, Baggio G, Neubeck W, Seidel D (1976) Formation of lipoprotein-X: its relationship to bile compounds. J Clin Invest 57: 1248-1260
5. Liersch M, Baggio G, Heuck CC, Seidel D (1977) Effect of lipoprotein-X on hepatic cholesterol synthesis. Atherosclerosis 26: 505-514
6. Fredrickson DJ, Loud AV, Hinkelmann BT, Schneider HS, Frantz ID (1954) The effect of ligation of common bile duct on cholesterol synthesis in rat. J Exp Med 99: 43-53
7. Walli AK, Seidel D (1984) Role of lipoprotein-X in the pathogenesis of cholestatic hypercholesterolemia. Uptake of lipoprotein-X and its effect on 3-hydroxy-3-methylglutaryl coenzyme A reductase and chylomicron remnant removal in human fibroblasts, lymphocytes, and in the rat. J Clin Invest 74: 867-879
8. Rodwell VW, Nordstrom JL, Mitschelen JJ (1976) Regulation of HMG-CoA reductase. In: Advances in Lipid Research. R Paoletti, D Kritschevsky editors, Academic Press, London 14: 1-74.
9. McNamara DJ, Rodwell VW (1975) Regulation of 3-hydroxy-3-methyl glutaryl coenzyme A reductase. In vitro inhibition by a protein present in bile. Arch Biochem 168: 378-385
10. Barak AJ, Sorrell MF, Tuma JD (1979) Effect of serum lipoproteins of bile obstructed rats on 3-hydroxy-3-methyl glutaryl coenzyme A reductase activity in perfused rat liver. Lipids 14: 883-887
11. Seidel D, Walli AK (1983) Liver in metabolic diseases. Bianchi et al. editors. MTP Press Limited Lancaster England p 81-95
12. Griffin E, Breckenridge WC, Kukis A, Bryan MH, Angel A (1979) Appearance and characterization of lipoprotein-X during continuous intralipid infusions in the neonate. J Clin Invest 64: 1703-1712
13. Cooper RA, Arner EC, Wiley JS, Shattil SJ (1975) Modification of red cell membrane structure by cholesterol rich lipid dispersions. A model for the primary spur cell defect. J Clin Invest 55: 115-126
14. Edwards PA (1975) Effect of plasma lipoproteins and lecithin: cholesterol dispersions on the activity of 3-hydroxy-3-methyl glutaryl coenzyme A reductase in isolated rat hepatocytes. Biochem Biophys Acta 409: 39-50
15. Stein O, Stein Y (1973) The removal of cholesterol from Landschütz Ascites cells by high density lipoproteins. Biochem Biophys Acta 326: 232-244
16. Stein O, Vanderhoeck J, Stein Y (1976) Cholesterol content and sterol synthesis in human skin fibroblasts and rat aortic smooth muscle cells exposed to lipoprotein depleted serum and high density apolipoprotein/phospholipid mixtures. Biochim Biophys Acta 431: 347-358
17. Sherill BC, Dietschy JM (1977) Characterization of sinusoidal transport process responsible for uptake of chylomicrons by liver. J Biol Chem 253: 1895-1867
18. Cooper AD, Erickson SK, Nutik R, Shrewsbury MA (1982) Characterization of chylomicron remnant binding to rat liver membranes. J Lipid Res 23: 42-52
19. Müller P, Fellin R, Lamprecht J, Agostini B, Wieland H, Rost W, Seidel D (1974) Hypertriglyceridemia secondary to liver disease. Europ J Clin Invest 4: 419-428
20. Goldstein JL, Brown MS (1977) The low-density lipoprotein pathway and its relation to atherosclerosis. Ann Rev Biochem 46: 897-930
21. Kovanen PT, Brown MS, Goldstein JL (1979) Increased binding of low-density lipoproteins to liver membranes from rats treated with 17 α-Ethinyl estradiol. J Biol Chem 254: 11367-11373
22. Chao YS, Windler E, Chen G, Havel JR (1979) Hepatic catabolism of rat and human lipoproteins in rats treated with α-Ethinyl estradiol. J Biol Chem 254: 11360-11366

A Novel Mechanism by which High Density Lipoprotein Selectively Delivers Cholesterol Esters to the Liver

RAY C. PITTMAN and DANIEL STEINBERG

Division of Endocrinology and Metabolism, Department of Medicine, University of California, San Diego, La Jolla, CA 92093

One of the most dramatic developments in the epidemiologic investigation of coronary heart disease risk factors during the last decade has been the mushrooming evidence that a high level of HDL decreases while a low level of HDL increases the risk of clinical disease. A seminal paper by Miller and Miller in 1975 [1] focused attention on this problem by pointing out the several risk factors for coronary heart disease that were associated with low levels of plasma HDL. Despite the high level of interest in this problem and the many studies that have been done, we still do not know exactly how this HDL-coronary heart disease relationship works. By all odds the most widely accepted hypothesis is that HDL serves the function of removing cholesterol from peripheral tissues and carrying it to the liver for reutilization or excretion in the bile [2]. Many studies in cell culture show that HDL is capable of acting as an acceptor of cholesterol from cells overloaded with it [3-8]. On the other hand, delipidated serum is also able to facilitate the removal of cholesterol from cholesterol-loaded cells in culture [9]. More direct evidence is needed before the role of HDL in reverse cholesterol transport can be considered established.

Recent work by Oram and his colleagues has described a saturable binding of HDL to human cells in culture [10, 11]. This binding activity is increased by loading the cells with cholesterol, and it is postulated to mediate the efflux of cholesterol to HDL. Such efflux to HDL, coupled with the action of lecithin-cholesterol acyltransferase and the eventual hepatic uptake of the resulting cholesterol ester (either in HDL or in another lipoprotein to which it has transferred) comprises an attractive hypothetical system for reverse cholesterol transport. However, to date the evidence quantifying the extent to which such a system actually functions in vivo is scanty. If excess cholesterol is taken from extrahepatic cells by HDL for removal to the liver, then there must also be a mechanism for uptake by that organ. Indeed saturable binding of HDL to liver membranes and hepatocytes has been described [12-14]. But how this binding relates to cholesterol uptake is not clear.

Over the last several years we have carried out a series of studies of HDL metabolism that allowed us for the first time to quantify, tissue by tissue, the fate of HDL apoprotein and cholesterol esters fluxing through the plasma pool. These studies have disclosed a mechanism that could play an important role in reverse cholesterol transport, namely the direct uptake of HDL cholesterol esters by liver parenchymal cells in excess of the uptake of HDL apoproteins.

Receptor-Mediated Uptake
in the Liver
Edited by H. Greten, E. Windler, U. Beisiegel
© Springer-Verlag Berlin Heidelberg 1986

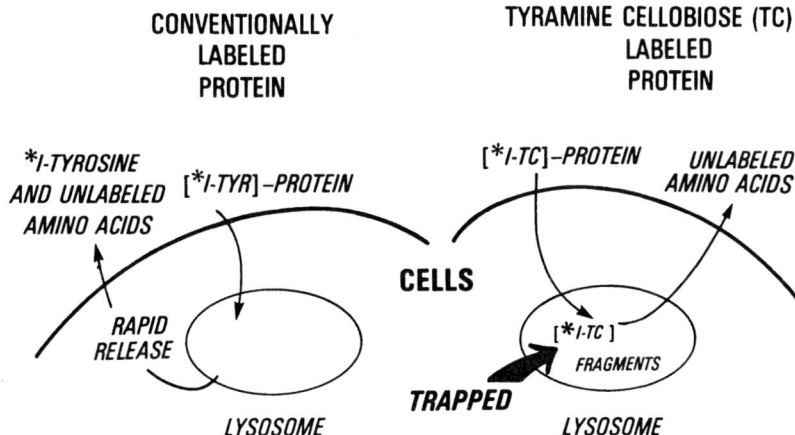

Fig. 1. Principle of the "trapped label" approach to quantifying the sites of protein degradation *in vivo*

Our studies began with the realization that, because of the mobility of the apoprotein and lipid components of HDL, the fates of these components might be independently determined. To trace HDL apoproteins we used the "trapped ligand" approach developed in this laboratory [15, 16] for determining the sites of irreversible degradation of plasma proteins *in vivo* (Fig. 1). We then added another dimension by simultaneously incorporating cholesteryl ethers into the HDL particles as markers of cholesterol esters [17, 18], a method developed by Stein, Halperin and Stein [19, 20]. In our early studies [17] we incorporated cholesteryl ether into HDL by a partial delipidation-reconstitution method [21], and later by the action of plasma cholesterol ester transfer protein [22, 23]. As shown in Fig. 1, iodinated tyramine cellobiose (^{125}I-TC) is covalently attached to apo A-I. On uptake and catabolism of the labeled apo A-I, the ^{125}I-TC ligand remains unhydrolyzed. Due to its size and chemical nature it remains trapped in the cell and thus serves as a cumulative marker of total apo A-I uptake. Similarly, as shown in Fig. 2, the [^{3}H]cholesteryl-oleyl ether incorporated into HDL enters the cell in parallel with HDL cholesterol esters; because it is not hydrolyzed and cannot cross membranes, it too remains trapped in the cell as a cumulative marker of uptake. We have shown [17, 18, 24], using biologically labeled HDL for comparison, that the metabolism of these two tracer molecules faithfully reflects that of their counterpart moieties in native HDL *in vitro,* as discussed in more detail below. Studies *in vivo* have been carried out as well, comparing plasma decay kinetics of the two types of preparations [17, 24].

The main problem facing the experimenter when trying to understand the metabolism of HDL is the speed with which its components can exchange. Essentially all of the apoproteins of HDL can exchange with apoproteins in chylomicrons and VLDL; in most species, including the rabbit, the cholesterol esters of HDL exchange very rapidly with cholesterol esters and/or triglycerides of other lipoprotein

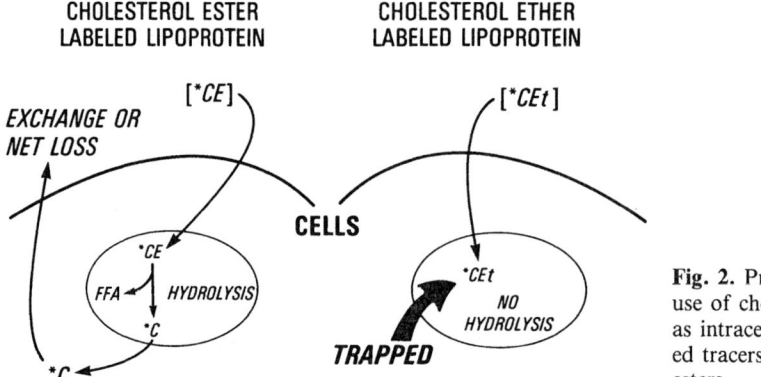

Fig. 2. Principle of the use of cholesteryl ethers as intracellularly trapped tracers of cholesterol esters

fractions. These considerations led us to use the rat in our initial studies, recognizing of course the possibly important differences between HDL metabolism in the rat and in man. In contrast to man and some other animals, rats have very low LDL levels [25], high HDL levels, and appear to depend primarily on HDL rather than LDL for delivery of cholesterol to extrahepatic tissues, at least to steroidogenic tissues [26]. In the fasted rat, virtually all plasma apo A-1 is in the HDL fraction [27, 28] and plasma cholesterol ester exchange is not evident [29]. However, we assume that the rat also must have some provision for return of cholesterol from the periphery to the liver and that such a mechanism will be at least qualitatively like that of other mammals.

Fig. 3 shows the tissue distribution of both [3H]cholesteryl ether and 125I-TC 24 h after injection of doubly labeled HDL. That this label distribution closely approximates the true mass flux of the tracee under the conditions of these experiments is supported on both experimental and theoretical grounds [30]. The data show that the liver accounts for approximately two-thirds of total HDL cholesteryl ether clearance. What fraction of the total reverse cholesterol transport this accounts for is uncertain because the total cholesterol "burden" that must be returned to the liver from the periphery is not known with certainty. All that can be said at this time is that the predominance of the liver in uptake of the cholesteryl ether tracer is compatible with an important role for HDL in reverse cholesterol ester transport in the rat.

We can see from Fig. 3 that the liver makes a smaller contribution to overall apo A-I catabolism than it does to cholesteryl ether uptake, and conversely that kidney is very active in apo A-I uptake but shows almost no cholesteryl ether uptake. As shown elsewhere [24], this uptake by kidney is probably due to glomerular filtration and tubular reabsorption of free apo A-I, explaining the dissociation of apo A-I uptake from cholesteryl ether uptake. Curiously, the preferential uptake of cholesteryl ether by the liver and the preferential uptake of apo A-I by the kidney approximately balance each other. Consequently the plasma fractional catabolic rates of the two components are similar as shown in Fig. 4.

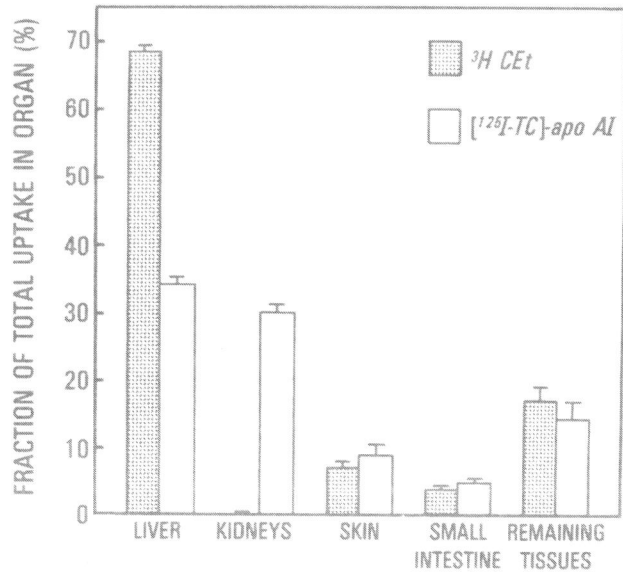

Fig. 3. Contribution of individual tissues of rat to overall uptake of apo A-1 and cholesterol esters of HDL, determined using HDL labeled with ^{125}I-TC-apo A-1 and [^{3}H]CEt (cholesterol ester)

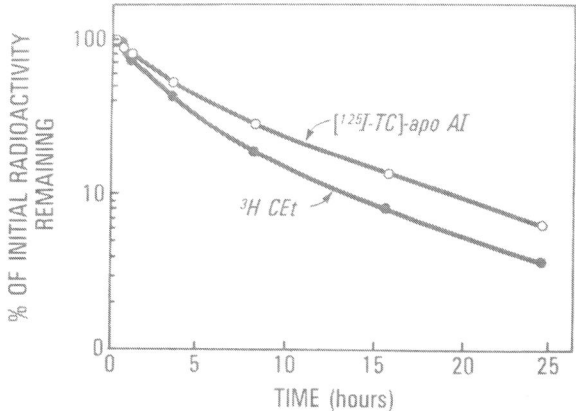

Fig. 4. Plasma decay of doubly labeled HDL in rats

The uptake of HDL cholesteryl ethers by the liver in excess of apo A-I can be seen more directly when the same data are presented in terms of a fractional rate for uptake of the two HDL components per unit weight of tissue (Fig. 5). For every HDL particle equivalent of apo A-I taken up, the liver takes up almost 2 particle equivalents of cholesteryl ether. The steroidogenic tissues display higher absolute rates of uptake of both tracers, but disproportionately higher rates for cholesteryl ether. However, all of the other tissues examined take up the two labels at about equal rates *in vivo*.

The unexpected finding that liver and steroidogenic tissues can selectively take up HDL cholesterol esters without concomitant uptake of apo A-I *in vivo* could have had rather trivial explanations. For example, it might reflect exchange of apo

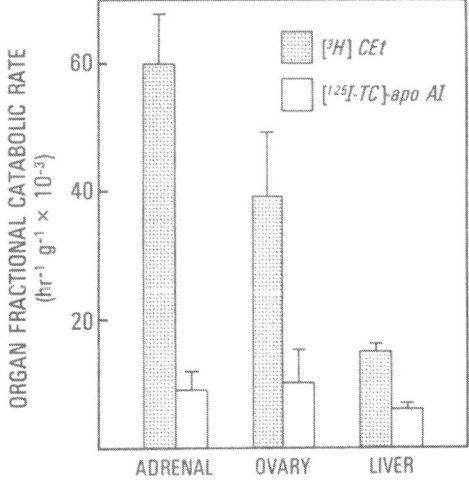

Fig. 5. Fractional rate of uptake of HDL-associated apo A-1 and cholesterol esters by selected tissues of the rat. Data are expressed as the fraction of the plasma pool of HDL taken up per hour per gram of tissue

A-I without parallel exchange of cholesteryl ether to other more rapidly cleared lipoprotein particles (e.g. to VLDL or a more rapidly cleared subfraction of HDL). To help rule out such possibilities, the selective uptake process was studied *in vitro* in the absence of any other lipoproteins. The preferential uptake of cholesteryl ether by primary cultures of rat hepatocytes and adrenal cells was even greater than that observed *in vivo* (Fig. 6). This uptake in the absence of other li-

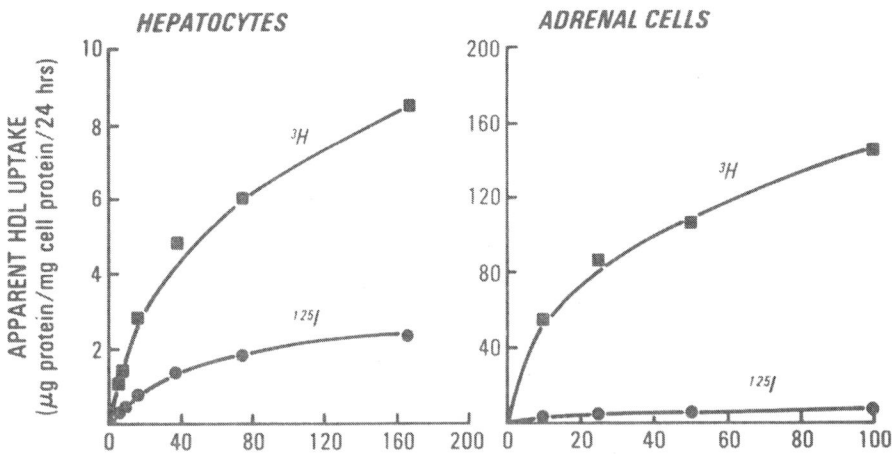

Fig. 6. Uptake of HDL labeled with ^{125}I-TC-apo A-1 and [^{3}H]CEt by primary cultures of rat hepatocytes and adrenal cells. Cultures were incubated with the indicated concentrations of ^{3}H, ^{125}I-HDL for 24 h at 37° C. Cells were then exhaustively washed, "chased" with 100 μg/ml native HDL, and finally treated with trypsin to remove remaining cell-bound ^{125}I, ^{3}H-HDL. Cells were then analyzed for ^{3}H, ^{125}I and protein content. Data are expressed as the amount of HDL protein that would deliver the indicated amounts of label if uptake were of whole particles

poproteins or apoproteins added an important element of substantiation to our *in vivo* results.

The significance of the preferential uptake rests squarely on the assumption that the metabolism of the reconstituted labeled HDL mirrors that of native HDL. This assumption was best supported by a direct comparison of reconstituted HDL with *biologically labeled* HDL, as shown in Fig. 7. In this experiment the uptake of our usual HDL preparation labeled with both [^{3}H]cholesteryl ether and ^{125}I-TC-apo A-I was compared to that of HDL biologically labeled in the cholesterol ester moiety by feeding a donor rat [^{3}H] cholesterol and then labeling the apo A-I moiety by exchange. Results are shown here for hepatocytes but similar results were obtained for adrenal cells. We can see that the uptake of both the lipid and apoprotein labels of the two preparations was quite similar. Absolute rates of uptake were almost identical. The uptake of the lipid was in both cases much higher than that of the apoprotein, and to a comparable extent in both cases whether using biologically labeled HDL or reconstituted HDL. The uptake of both the lipid and apoprotein label was inhibited by added native HDL, and to much the same extent in the two preparations. Thus, hepatocytes take up both the labeled components

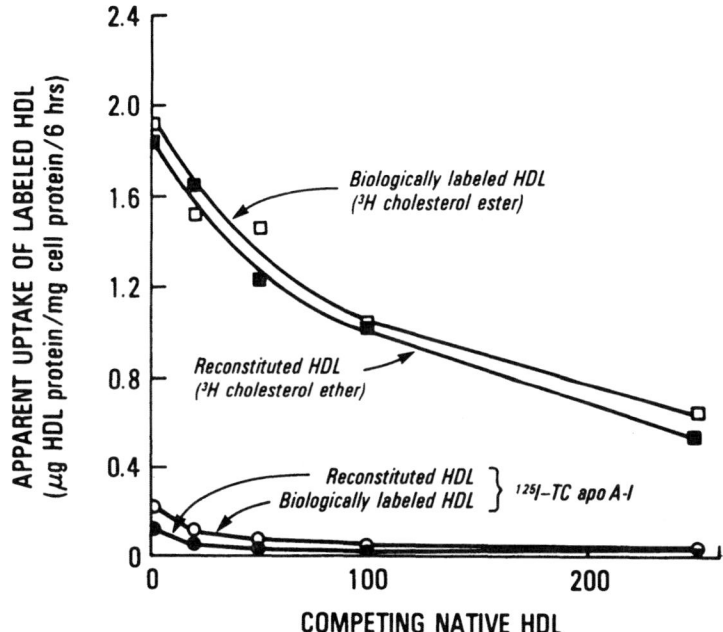

Fig. 7. Competition by native HDL for uptake of doubly labeled HDL by primary cultures of rat hepatocytes. HDL was labeled in two ways: 1. (closed symbols) [^{3}H]CEt was incorporated by partial delipidation-reconstitution and then ^{125}I-TC-apo A-1 was incorporated by exchange; 2. (open symbols) label was incorporated into the cholesterol ester moiety by [^{3}H]cholesterol feeding, HDL isolation, biological screening to remove free cholesterol and reisolation of HDL, and then the particle was labeled in the apo A-1 moiety by exchange of ^{125}I-TC-apo A-1. Cultures were incubated with 10 μg/ml of the labeled preparations for 6 h at 37° in the presence of the indicated amounts of HDL. Apo A-1 label uptake is shown in circles and lipid label uptake in squares

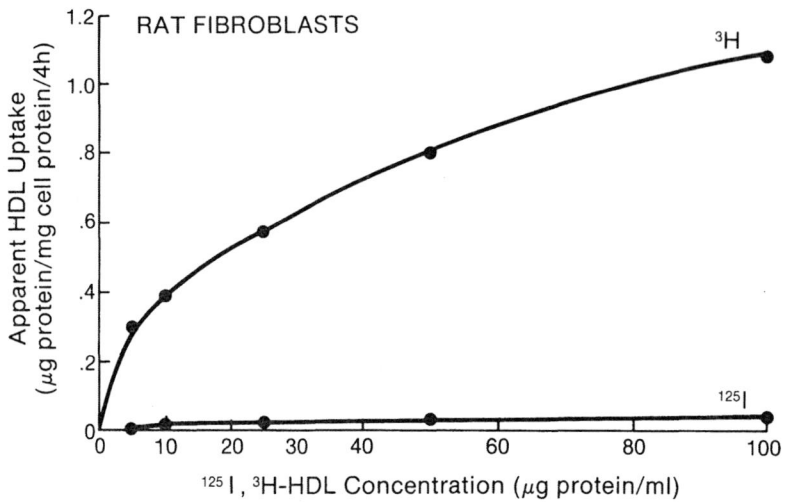

Fig. 8. Uptake of doubly labeled HDL by cultured rat fibroblasts. Conditions were as indicated for Figure 6, except incubation time was 6 h

in HDL by saturable processes, at rates similar to those for biologically labeled HDL, and in processes competed for comparably by native HDL.

The preferential uptake of the cholesteryl ether label from doubly labeled HDL is not confined to the rat, nor is it confined to hepatocytes and steroidogenic cells, at least in cell culture. Thus, as shown in Fig. 8, rat fibroblasts also preferentially take up cholesteryl ethers from HDL by a saturable mechanism evidently similar to that of adrenal cells and hepatocytes. As shown in Fig. 9, both cultured human fibroblasts and a human hepatoma line also take up the cholesteryl ether label preferentially. In all these cases the preferential uptake is inhibited by native HDL.

If the preferential uptake is observed in a broad range of cells in culture, then why do we observe it only in the liver and in steroidogenic tissues in the intact rat? Several possibilities can be considered. It may relate to:
a) down-regulation of the pathway for preferential uptake *in vivo;*
b) differences between HDL in the extravascular spaces and HDL in the plasma (liver and adrenal cells have direct access to plasma HDL through fenestrated endothelium);
c) the involvement of other pathways for HDL uptake *in vivo* that are not readily observed *in vitro* (e.g., the involvement of apo E, as discussed below).

The mechanism of the preferential uptake of HDL cholesterol esters is not clear. An early hypothesis was that *in vitro* it represented uptake of a subclass of particles rich in apo E and poor in apo A-I. Since only a small fraction of the medium HDL is taken up *in vitro,* even a rather minor contamination by such particles could explain the results. The preferential uptake observed *in vivo,* where we studied the uptake of *all* labeled HDL, cannot be faulted in this way. However, there might have been exchange of the abundant plasma apo E into our labeled HDL

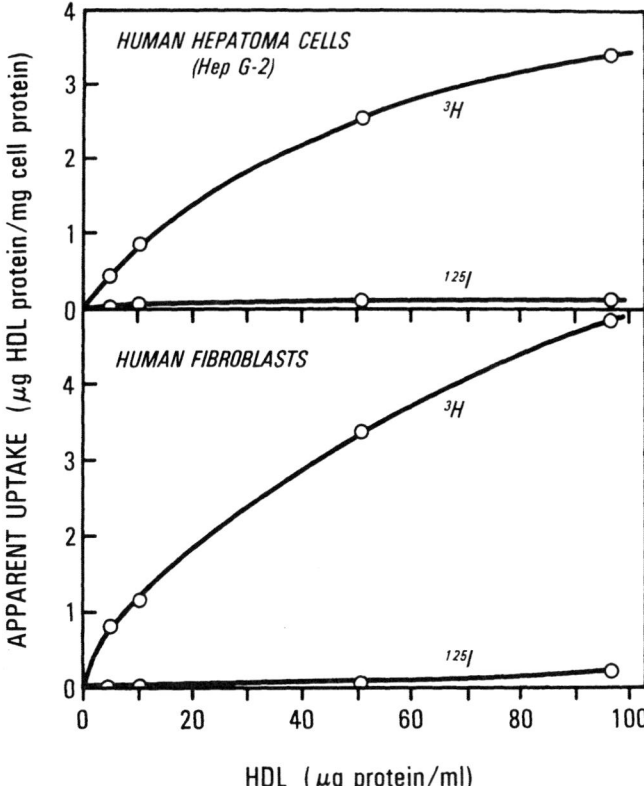

Fig. 9. Uptake of doubly labeled HDL by cultured human cells. Conditions were as indicated for Fig. 8

particles, displacing labeled apo A-I. As a result, cholesterol esters might now be taken up in particles enriched in apo E and poor in apo A-I via an apo E receptor; such preferential uptake would be observed in tissues rich in apo E receptors such as the liver [31]. A similar mechanism has been proposed by Mahley and co-workers [32] to contribute to reverse cholesterol transport. In this scenario, HDL particles become progressively enriched in both cholesterol esters and apo E, to be eventually cleared by hepatic apo E receptors. However, as shown in Fig. 10, blockade of apo E receptor recognition by reductive methylation [33] did not significantly reduce the preferential uptake of cholesteryl ethers by rat adrenal cells. Again, removal of apo E-containing particles by heparin-sepharose affinity chromatography [34] failed to reduce preferential uptake. Thus recognition of apo E in our doubly labeled preparation does not appear to be required for the preferential uptake. However, this does not rule out an important role for apo E in HDL clearance *in vivo* by exchange [35] onto labeled particles as outlined above. Because apo E mediates the uptake of the holo-particle, such a mechanism might explain the apparent lesser importance of the pathway for preferential uptake *in vivo* than *in vitro* if the added apo E does not displace apo A-1.

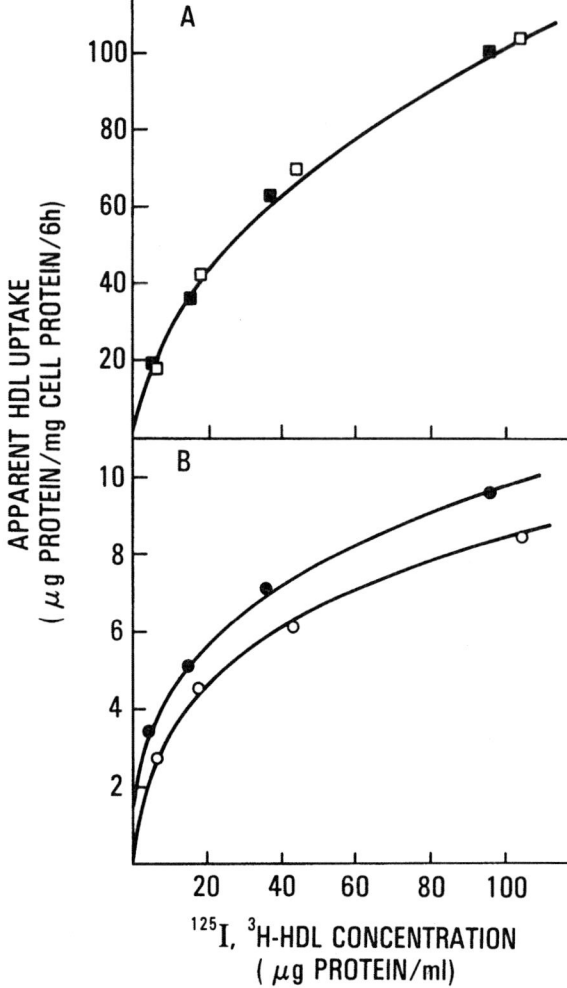

Fig. 10. Effect of reductive methylation on uptake of doubly labeled HDL by primary rat adrenal cultures. Conditions were as indicated for Figure 8. Closed symbols represent control ^{125}I, ^{3}H-HDL, and open symbols represent reductively methylated ^{125}I, ^{3}H-HDL. Panel A represents [^{3}H]CEt uptake and panel B represents ^{125}I-TC-apo A-1 uptake

The studies thus far described do not rule out the possibility that, rather than apo E in the HDL preparation itself, apo E secreted by the cultured cells during the incubation is involved in the preferential uptake. It is known that apo E is produced, at least to some extent, by many and perhaps all human and rat cell types [36-38]. The possibility of involvement of such apo E in the preferential uptake *in vitro* was tested in experiments in which heparin, which inhibits binding of both apo E and apo B to their receptors [39, 40], was added to cultured cells during HDL uptake. A subclone of Y-1 mouse adrenal tumor cells was used in these experiments because they take up LDL by the B/E receptor and also display a high rate of preferential uptake of HDL cholesterol esters. As shown in Table 1, there was little effect of heparin on HDL uptake at heparin levels that drastically in-

Table 1. Effect of heparin (10 mg/ml) on lipoprotein uptake by Y-1 mouse adrenal tumor cells (Percent of uptake in the absence of heparin)

Lipoprotein	Label	
	^{3}H Cholesteryl ether	^{125}I-Apoprotein
HDL (Apo E-free)	86	69
HDL (Apo E-rich)	65	39
LDL	—	8

hibited LDL uptake, indicating that interaction with the B/E receptor was not requisite for the preferential cholesteryl ether uptake. These experiments also indicate that the involvement of lipoprotein lipase, as proposed by the Stein laboratory [41-43] to account for an apparent preferential uptake of cholesterol esters from chylomicrons, was not involved in this case. Levels of heparin well above those that disrupted lipoprotein lipase-cell interaction and prevented preferential cholesterol ester uptake from chylomicrons [43], did not affect the preferential uptake of HDL cholesteryl ether either by rat hepatocytes or by Y-1 adrenal cells.

Precedent suggests the likelihood that the preferential uptake might depend on specific recognition of HDL apoprotein. The obvious candidate for such a role is apo A-I, the prevalent and characteristic apoprotein of HDL. To examine this question we prepared HDL-like particles using sonication procedures developed in the laboratory of Dr. Donald Small. Cholesteryl ether incorporated into such particles was preferentially taken up when particles were made to contain apo A-I. But particles containing either a mixture of apo C's or apo E also yielded some degree of preferential uptake, albeit in every experiment less than was observed with apo A-I particles. It is possible that some degree of apparent preferential uptake is the consequence of heterogeneity in the cosonicated preparations. In any case, the available data are at least consistent with a requirement for apo A-I in the preferential uptake of cholesterol esters.

In considering the mechanisms that might account for preferential uptake of cholesterol esters, we must take into account the fact that in cultured rat adrenal cells the fractional rate of uptake of HDL cholesteryl ether is usually 20 to 50 times the rate of uptake of apo A-I, and in rat hepatocytes it is usually 5-20 times. If the preferential uptake results from endocytosis of particles containing cholesterol esters, then either apo A-I must be almost wholly excluded from those endocytotic vesicles or it must be almost quantitatively returned to the medium. A precedent for such a mechanism is found in the case of the delivery of iron to the liver by transferrin [44-47]. After receptor-mediated uptake of this protein by target cells, the transferrin divests itself of its transported iron in a prelysosomal acidic pool. The apotransferrin is then returned to the cell surface still attached to the receptor; at the cell surface the apotransferrin is released into the medium at neutral pH. Inhibitors of receptor recycling inhibit this process. As shown in Table 2, however, such inhibitors had little effect on the uptake of cholesteryl ethers by either rat hepatocytes or Y-1 mouse adrenal cells, although they did significantly inhibit uptake of the apo A-I component. In contrast, the receptor-mediated uptake of LDL in parallel plates of Y-1 cells was highly inhibited by these agents. This suggests that

Table 2. Effect of metabolic inhibitors on uptake of doubly labeled HDL by G-2 human hepatoma cells

	HDL ^{125}I	Uptake ^{3}H	sucrose pinocytosis	asialofetuin uptake
Control	(100)	(100)	(100)	(100)
Chloroquine, 50 uM	49	69	—	37
Monensin, 50 uM	23	108	—	20
Colchicine, 1 uM	49	78	—	63
Na azide, 5 mM	27	124	33	—

the transferrin model is not applicable, and in fact that a receptor recycling event is not involved. Further "pulse-chase" experiments suggest the same result. Cells were briefly exposed to HDL at 16° C where endocytosis occurs but progression to acidic vesicles and lysosomal fusion does not [48]. On subsequent warming, preferential release of apo A-I was not observed. In fact, the ratio of ^{3}H to ^{125}I uptake at 16° was even greater than at 37°. Thus, we must conclude that HDL cholesterol esters are most likely taken up initially without the particle's complement of apo A-I.

In summary, we have described the selective uptake of HDL cholesterol esters in liver and steroidogenic tissues of the rat *in vivo* and in a wider range of cells in culture. In rats the total uptake of cholesterol ester from HDL is much greater in the liver than in any other tissue and the liver also consistently shows preferential cholesterol ester uptake, albeit less striking than that in the adrenal. These findings support the notion that this pathway may be involved in reverse cholesterol transport as well as in the provision of cholesterol to steroidogenic tissues of rats. The mechanism of the selective uptake does not appear to involve uptake of the holo-particle with recycling of apo A-I to the cell surface, but rather appears to involve the direct uptake of cholesterol ester (and perhaps other HDL components) but with less than equivalent uptake of apo A-I. This could occur by uptake of the particle *per se* minus its complement of apo A-I but our evidence suggests that the selective uptake process does not require endocytotis. We therefore suggest that preferential uptake may involve a "fusion" of HDL to the cell membrane that facilitates entry of cholesterol ester, or the presence in the cell membrane of a hypothetical cholesterol ester transfer protein.

References

1. Miller GJ, Miller NE (1975) Lancet i: 16-19
2. Glomset JA (1968) J Lipid Res 9: 155-167
3. Miller NE (1978) Biochem Biophys Acta 529: 131-137
4. Daniels RJ, Gurtler LS, Parker TS, Steinberg D (1981) J Biol Chem 256: 4978-4983
5. Daerr WH, Gianturco SH, Patsch JR, Smith LC, Gotto AM Jr (1980) Biochim Biophys Acta 619: 287-301
6. Stein O, Vanderhoek J, Stein Y (1976) Biochim Biophys Acta 431: 342-358
7. Innerarity TL, Pitas RE, Mahley RW (1982) Arteriosclerosis 114-124
8. Brown MS, Ho YK and Mahley RW (1980) J Biol Chem 255: 9344-9352

9. Bailey JM (1968) Biochim Biophys Acta 125: 226-236
10. Biesbroeck R, Oram JF, Albers JJ, Bierman EL (1983) J Clin Invest 71: 525-539
11. Oram JF, Brinton EA, Bierman EL (1983) J Clin Invest 72: 1611-1621
12. Bachorik PS, Franklin FA, Virgil DG, Kwiterovich PO Jr (1982) Biochemistry 21: 5674-5684
13. Rifici VA, Eder HA (1984) J Biol Chem 259: 13814-13818
14. Bachorik PS, Franklin FA Jr, Virgil DG, Kwiterovich PO Jr (1984) Arteriosclerosis 5: 142-152
15. Pittman RC, Green SR, Attie AD, Steinberg D (1979) J Biol Chem 254: 6876-6879
16. Pittman RC, Carew TE, Glass CK, Green SR, Taylor CA, Attie AD (1983) Biochem J 212: 791-800
17. Glass CK, Pittman RC, Weinstein DB, Steinberg D (1983) Proc Natl Acad Sci USA 80: 5435-5439
18. Glass C, Pittman RC, Civen M, Steinberg D (1985) J Biol Chem 260: 744-750
19. Stein O, Halperin G, Stein Y (1978) Biochim Biophys Acta 620: 247-260
20. Stein Y, Stein O, Halperin G (1983) Arteriosclerosis 2: 281-289
21. Krieger M, Brown MS, Faust JR, Goldstein JL (1978) J Biol Chem 253: 4093-4101
22. Morton RE, Zilversmith DB (1981) J Biol Chem 258: 11751-11757
23. Son Y-SC, Zilversmith DB (1984) Biochim Biophys Acta 795: 473-480
24. Glass CK, Pittman RC, Keller GA, Steinberg D (1983) J Biol Chem 258: 7161-7167
25. Lasser NL, Roheim PS, Edelstein D, Eder HA (1973) J Lipid Res 14: 1-8
26. Gwynne JT, Strauss JF III (1982) Endocrinol Rev 3: 299-329
27. Swaney JB, Braithwaite F, Eder HA (1973) J Lipid Res 14: 1-8
28. Weisgraber KH, Mahley RW, Assmann G (1977) Atherosclerosis 28: 121-140
29. Barter PJ, Lally JI (1979) Metabolism 28: 230-236
30. Carew TE, Beltz WF (1982) in *Lipoprotein Kinetics and Modeling* (Berman M, Grundy S eds) pp 169-179, Academic Press, New York
31. Sherill BC, Innerarity TL, Mahley RW (1980) J Biol Chem 255: 1804-1807
32. Mahley RW (1982) Med Clin North Am 66: 375-402
33. Weisgraber KH, Mahley RW (1980) J Lipid Res 21: 316-325
34. Biesbroeck R, Oran JF, Albers JJ, Bierman EL (1983) J Clin Invest 71: 525-539
35. Weisgraber KH, Mahley RW, Assman G (1977) Atherosclerosis 28: 121-140
36. Basu SK, Brown MS, Ho YK, Havel RJ, Goldstein JL (1981) Proc Natl Acad Sci USA 78: 7545-7549
37. Blue ML, Williams DL, Zucker S, Khan SA, Blum CB (1983) Proc Natl Acad Sci USA 80: 283-287
38. Driscoll DA, Getz GS (1984) J Lipid Res 25: 1368-1379
39. Goldstein JL, Basu SK, Brunschede GY, Brown MS (1976) Cell 7: 85-95
40. Hui DY, Innerarity TL, Mahley RW (1981) J Biol Chem 256: 5646-5655
41. Chajek-Shaul T, Friedman G, Halperin O, Stein O, Stein Y (1981) Biochim Biophys Acta 666: 156-164
42. Friedman G, Chajek-Shaul T, Stein O, Olivecrona T, Stein Y (1981) Biochim Biophys Acta 666: 154-164
43. Chajek-Shaul T, Friedman G, Stein O, Olivecrona T, Stein Y (1982) Biochim Biophys Acta 712: 200-210
44. Karin M, Minta B (1981) J Biol Chem 256: 3245-3252
45. Van Renswounde J, Bridges KR, Harford JB, Klausner RD (1982) Proc Natl Acad Sci USA 79: 6186-6190
46. Harding C, Heuser J, Stahl P (1983) J Cell Biol 97: 329-339
47. Pan BT, Johnstone R (1984) J Biol Chem 259: 9776-9782
48. Dunn WA, Hubbard AL, Aronson NN (1980) J Biol Chem 255: 5971-5978

Saturable Binding of HDL$_3$ to Human Liver Membranes

F. M. Maggi, S. Marcovina[1], E. Trezzi, G. Maione[2], and A. L. Catapano

[1] Institute of Pharmacology and Pharmacognosy, Via A. Del Sarto 21 Milano
Istituto di Ricerca S. Raffaele, Milano
[2] III Surgical Clinic. Milano, Italy

Introduction

In vitro and in vivo evidences show that the liver of several animal species and humans catabolizes lipoproteins [1]. In particular two different lipoprotein receptors are expressed by the liver; the E and LDL receptors [2, 3]. While the LDL receptor on the liver is probably identical to the well characterized LDL receptor found in peripheral cells [2, 3] the E receptor seems to be peculiar to the liver and probably mediates the catabolism of chylomicron remnants.

The mechanism by which HDL is catabolized, however, are unknown. Experimental evidence, in rats suggest that the HDL cholesteryl ester catabolism is partly uncoupled from that of the protein moiety in the liver, adrenal glands and ovaries [4].

Several groups have demonstrated that HDL binds to specific high affinity sites present on human skin fibroblasts [5] rat adrenals [6], rat testes [7], rat canine and pig liver [8, 9, 10], bovine endothelial cells [11], intestinal cells [12], macrophages [13] and human hepatoma cells [14]. The binding of HDL however does not trigger internalization of the lipoprotein as a whole, it rather modulates the cholesterol homeostasis within the cells [15, 11, 12] probably via exchange of lipids. Many of these experiments however could not differenciate among the binding of HDL either to the B/E or E receptor or to a specific HDL binding site because of the presence of Apo E and B in the HDL preparations used. Recent data by Biesbroek et al. [15] suggest that a binding site, independent from the presence of Apo B or Apo E, exists on human skin fibroblasts cultured in vitro, Bahkornik et al. [16] reported similar results with pig liver hepatocytes. We have also reported on the presence of a binding site for HDL$_3$ Apo E free to human liver membranes [17]. The studies reported here were aimed to better characterize the binding of HDL$_3$ as well as the portion of these lipoproteins responsible for the binding.

Materials and Methods

Liver biopsies were obtained from male patients during surgery, informed consent was obtained. Liver specimens were immediately rinsed in buffer A (150 mM NaCl, 1 mM CaCl$_2$, 10 mM Tris, 1 mM PMSF, pH 8) and frozen at -70° C. The day of the preparation of liver membranes the tissue was thawed and homogenized

Receptor-Mediated Uptake
in the Liver
Edited by H. Greten, E. Windler, U. Beisiegel
© Springer-Verlag Berlin Heidelberg 1986

in buffer A with 3 x 20 s strokes of a politron tissue mincer at 0°C. Liver membranes were prepared as described previously [8, 17]. Immediately before the experiment the membranes were suspended in buffer B (50 mM NaCl, 50 mM $CaCl_2$, 20 mM Tris, pH 8) and sonicated (3 x 15 s with a micro tip at the max setting) at 0°C.

The binding was performed as described by Kovanen et al. [8] in buffer C (25 mM NaCl, 25 mM $CaCl_2$, 50 mM Tris pH 8 containing 2% albumin) with minor modifications [17].

Lipoproteins were isolated by sequential ultracentrifugation from the plasma of normolipemic volunteers [18]. The apoprotein pattern of the HDL was determined by SDS gel electrophoresis. Apo B and Apo E concentrations were determined by radial immunodiffusion using monospecific antisera raised in rabbits against purified Apo B and E. Only trace amounts of Apo E were found in HDL_3 (less than 0.7% of the total protein). Heparin sepharose affinity chromatography of HDL_3 was performed as described by Weisgraber et al. [19]. Apo E was not detectable in the first fraction eluted from the column both by SDS gel electrophoresis and immunodiffusion. Lipoproteins were labeled with ^{125}I by a modification of the McFarlane procedure [20], specific activity of the preparations used was 85-275 cpm (range of 6 different preparations), TCA non precipitable radioactivity was always less than 0.5% of total radioactivity. Protein concentration was determined by the method of Lowry [21] using bovine serum albumin as standard.

Monoclonal antibodies to Apo A-I were raised against purified A-I in mice as described [22], the antibodies reacted against Apo A-I as demonstrated by immunoblotting [23]. In the experiments aimed to verify the effect of these antibodies on HDL binding ^{125}I-HDL_3 were pre-incubated with a 10 fold molar excess of the antibody (vs Apo A-I) for 1 h at room temperature, the binding was performed as described.

Apo A-I Egg PC cholesterol complexes were prepared as described by Pownall et al. [24] in presence of Na Deoxycholate and purified A-I. The stoichiometry of the complexes was 1 mole of Apo A-I vs 100 moles of PC.

Results

The characteristics of the binding of HDL_3 Apo E free to human liver membranes are reported in Fig. 1. The binding of Apo A-I containing particles was very similar to that of whole HDL (data not shown).

Furthermore binding of ^{125}I-HDL_3 was competed by HDL_3 or A-I PL complexes in a very similar fashion thus suggesting identity of the binding site (Fig. 2). Scatchard analysis of the data showed indeed similarity.

Monoclonal antibodies to human Apo A-I showed no inhibition of binding of HDL_3 at molar ratios ranging from 0.03 to 10. Only minor changes of specific binding were found and no dose related effect was evident.

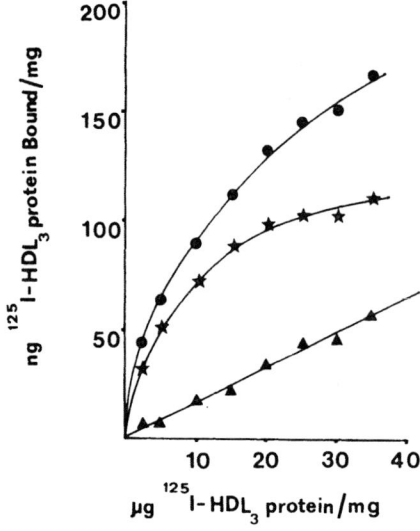

Fig. 1. Binding of HDL_3 Apo E free to human liver membranes ●-● total binding, - non specific binding, △-△ specific binding

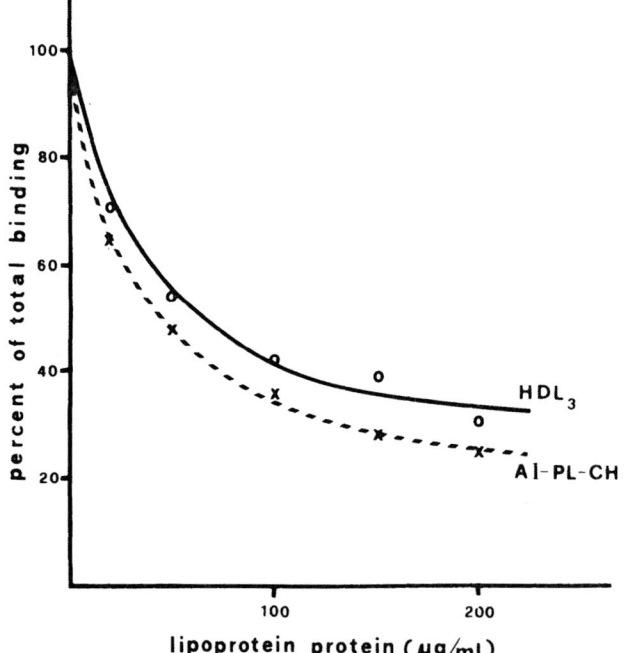

Fig. 2. Competition of HDL ●-● or A-I PL CH complexes for the binding of ^{125}I HDL_3 Apo E free

Discussion

Aim of this work was to identify the component (s) of HDL responsible for the binding of HDL_3 Apo E free to human liver membranes. Brinton et al. suggested that the binding site of fibroblasts has a broad specificity [25]. Similar data were obtained by Backorick et al. [16] for the binding of HDL to pig hepatocytes.

Our previous data showed that LDL could compete for the binding of ^{125}I HDL$_3$ but less efficiently than HDL$_3$ [17]. The data on the ability of the A-I PL complexes to compete with HDL$_3$ for binding indicate that this complex behaves like mature HDL therefore suggesting that either A-I or a lipid component could be the ligand for the binding site. This is in agreement with the suggestions made by Rifici and Eder on rat hepatocytes that A-I is the determinant for binding [26].

The studies performed using monoclonal antibodies however do not allow a clear answer since neither antibodies was effective in inhibiting the binding of HDL$_3$.

Our finding can be interpreted in several ways:

1. monoclonal antibodies bind to epitopes on Apo A-I which are distinct from the areas involved in the binding.
2. Apo A-II or C peptides may be responsible for the binding of HDL$_3$.
3. The binding is lipid mediated and requires the presence of apoproteins only to obtain clusters of lipids on the lipoprotein surface.

The latter interpretation would be in agreement with data by Tabas and Tall [27] who have suggested that no specific receptor exists on peripheral cells to bind HDL.

Further work is in progress in order to better understand the role of this binding site for HDL$_3$ in the human liver.

Summary

We have shown that human HDL$_3$ Apo E free bind to human liver membranes. This binding is saturable, specific and temperature sensitive. Furthermore it is Ca^{++} independent, and pronase treatment of the membranes does not affect its properties. Here we show that Apo A-I, Egg PC, cholesterol complexes bind to liver membranes as well as HDL, however two monoclonal antibodies raised against Apo A-I are unable to inhibit the binding of HDL$_3$ to human liver membranes.

These data suggest that binding of LDL to human liver membranes may not depend upon Apo A-I.

Acknowledgements. This work was supported in part by a MPI to ALC and CNR grant PF malattie degenerative to SM and ALC. The authors wish to thank Miss Silvana Magnani for typing the manuscript.

References

1. Brown MS, Kovanen PT, Goldstein J (1981) Science 212: 628-635
2. Hui DY, Innerarity TL, Mahley RW (1981) J Biol Chem 256: 5646-5655
3. Mahley RW, Hui DY, Innerarity TL, Weisgraber KH (1981) J Clin Invest 68: 1197-1206
4. Glass C, Pittman RC, Weinstein DB, Steinberg D (1983) Proc Natl Acad Sci USA 80: 5435-5439
5. Miller NE, Weinstein DE, Steinberg D (1977) J Lipid Res 18: 439-450

6. Kovanen PT, Schneider WJ, Hillman GM, Goldstein JL, Brown MS (1977) J Biol Chem 254: 5498-5505
7. Chen YDI, Kraemer FB, Reaven GM (1980) J Biol Chem 255: 9162-9167
8. Kovanen PT, Brown MS, Goldstein JL (1979) J Biol Chem 254: 11367-11373
9. Bachorik PS; Kwiterovich PO, Coone JC (1978) Biochemistry 17: 5287-5299
10. Hui DY, Innerarity TL, Mahley RW (1981) J Biol Chem 256: 5646-5655
11. Tauber JP, Coldminz D, Gospodarowicz D (1981) Eur J Biochem 119: 327-339
12. Suzuki N, Fidge N, Nestel P, Yin J (1983) J Lipid Res 24: 253-264
13. Assmann G personal communications
14. Dashti N, Wolfrauber G, Alaupovic P (1985) Biochim Biophys Acta 833: 100-110
15. Biesbroeck R, Oram JF, Albers JJ, Bierman EL (1983) J Clin Invest 71: 515-539
16. Backorik PS, Franklin FA, Virgil DA, Kwiterovich PO Jr (1982) Biochemistry 21: 5625-5684
17. Trezzi E, Maione G, Catapano AL (1984) IRCS Med Sci 12: 472-473
18. Havel RJ, Eder HA, Bragdon JM (1966) J Clin Invest 34: 1345-1354
19. Weisgraber KH, Mahley RW (1980) J Lipid Res 21: 316-325
20. Bilheimer DW, Eisenberg S, Levy RI (1982) Biochim Biophys Acta 260: 212-224
21. Lowry OH, Rosebrough NJ, Farr AL, Randall RJ (1951) J Biol Chem 193: 265-275
22. Galfre G, Howe SC, Milstein C, Butcher GW (1979) Nature 266: 550-552
23. Roma P, Marcovina S, Catapano AL manuscript in preparation
24. Pownall HJ, Winkle WB (1982) Biochim Biophys Acta 713: 494-503
25. Brinton EA, Oram JF, Chen CH, Albers JJ, Bierman EL (1984) Arteriosclerosis 4, 536a
26. Rifici VA, Eder HA (1984) J Biol Chem 259: 13814-13818
27. Tabas I, Tall AR (1984) J Biol Chem 259: 13897-13902

Subcellular Dissection and Characterization of Plasma Lipoprotein Secretory (Golgi) and Endocytic (Multivesicular Bodies) Compartments of Rat Hepatocytes

R. L. HAMILTON

With colleagues R. J. Havel, C.A. Hornick, E. Jost-Vu, J. Belcher, E. Spaziani, and G.H. Enders

Cardiovascular Research Institute and the Departments of Anatomy and Medicine, University of California, San Francisco

Background

Virtually 100% of chylomicron remnants are taken up by liver and degraded within lysosomes in hepatic parenchymal cells [1]. Most (>50-95%) remnants of very low density lipoproteins (VLDL) and most (ca. 50-70%) low density lipoproteins (LDL) are also catabolized by the same metabolic pathway in liver cells [1-3], although remnants of chylomicrons may bind initially to a different receptor than LDL (1 and Mahley, this volume). This enormous traffic of incoming lipoprotein particles is unique to liver and is related to two specialized structures also unique to liver. The first is the sieve plate structure of the sinusoidal lining in which the endothelial cell cytoplasm is perforated by numerous pores averaging about 100-120 nm in diameter, sufficiently large to permit most remnants entry into the space of Disse from plasma and easy access to receptors on hepatocyte microvilli [4].

The second special structure, related to this immense flow of endocytosed lipoprotein particles, is that of the hepatocyte multivesicular body (MVB) compartment which differs from MVBs of most other cells (see Fig. 1 and legend). The MVB compartment in hepatocytes is so completely filled with endocytosed remnants of both chylomicrons and VLDL that the characteristic internal bilayer vesicles (50-80 nm) are very difficult to visualize (see Fig. 2 and 3). And, because MVBs are typically located so close to the Golgi apparatus, they frequently have been identified incorrectly as secretory vesicles originating from this organelle which contains nascent VLDL of about the same size and staining properties of the remnant particles within MVBs. Because hepatocyte MVBs are about the same size as Golgi secretory vesicles, contain lipoproteins of similar size and staining properties, and are located in the same subcellular region of the hepatocyte, it is very difficult to distinguish these metabolically opposite compartments by routine electron microscopic methods. Moreover, the characteristic feature of MVBs is the presence of several internal bilayer vesicles which are very difficult to visualize in hepatocyte MVBs for two reasons:

This work was supported by the National Institutes of Health Grant HL-14237 Arteriosclerosis SCOR

Receptor-Mediated Uptake
in the Liver
Edited by H. Greten, E. Windler, U. Beisiegel
© Springer Verlag Berlin Heidelberg 1986

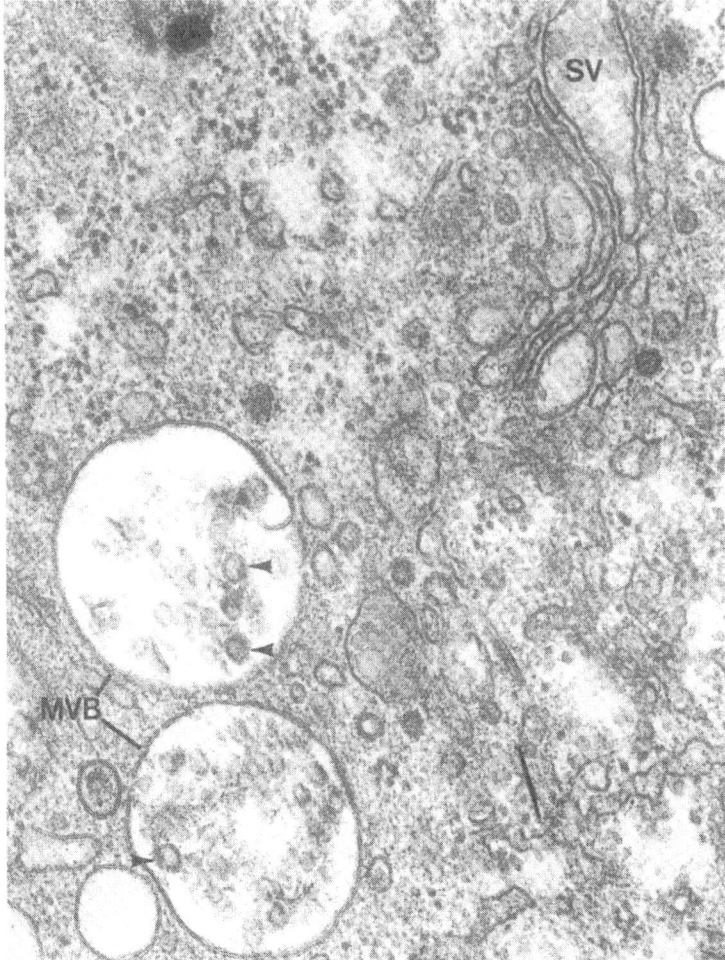

Fig. 1. X 45,000. Golgi/MVB area of hepatocyte from a rat liver perfused for 4 h with medium containing only red blood cells and buffer. Because the perfusion medium completely lacked remnants of chylomicrons, remnants of VLDL, and LDL, the endocyte compartment of MVBs look much like those of most other cell types which take up comparatively few lipoproteins, i. e., the latter MVBs contain much space permitting the bilayer vesicles to be seen clearly (arrowheads), together with a few lipoproteins and precipitated protein. Note the nearby Golgi secretory vesicles (SV) containing nascent VLDL

1. in contrast to MVBs in most other tissues, whose vesicles are often surrounded by space which makes them stand out (Fig. 1), the remnants in hepatocyte MVBs completely fill the internal compartment, often compressing the bilayer vesicles, thereby decreasing the contrast between the lipoprotein particles and the bilayer vesicles (Fig. 3);
2. the very rich lipid environment within hepatocyte MVBs may inhibit the deposition of heavy metals which stain the vesicle bilayers.

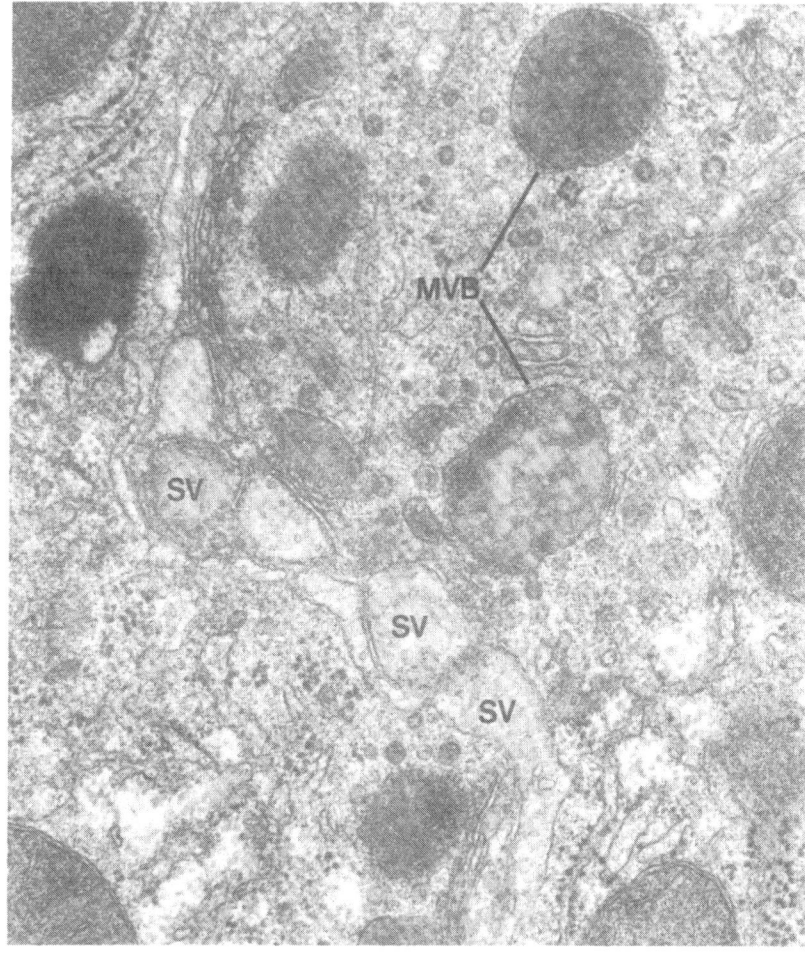

Fig. 2. X 45,000. Golgi/MVB area of hepatocyte of a chylomicron injected rat (30 min), illustrating close similarity of Golgi secretory vesicles (SV) and MVBs, which often makes it difficult to impossible to distinguish these two metabolically opposite compartments

We have found that an intense block staining procedure (2% uranyl acetate at 37°C for 48 h) causes hepatocyte MVBs to become more electron dense than the nearby Golgi secretory vesicles (Fig. 2 and 3). This stain also enhances the contrast of the bilayer vesicles of 50-80 nm (Fig. 3 and 4, top). There are other morphologic features that are sometimes present which can aid in the distinction between hepatocyte MVBs and Golgi secretory vesicles. Careful inspection reveals that MVB content lipoprotein particles are more heterogeneous in size and in staining properties than are Golgi nascent VLDL. Like MVBs in other cells, hepatocyte MVBs sometimes have a staight segment of limiting membrane which is often thickened by a (clathrin?) coating (Fig. 3). They sometimes have a smooth membranous tu-

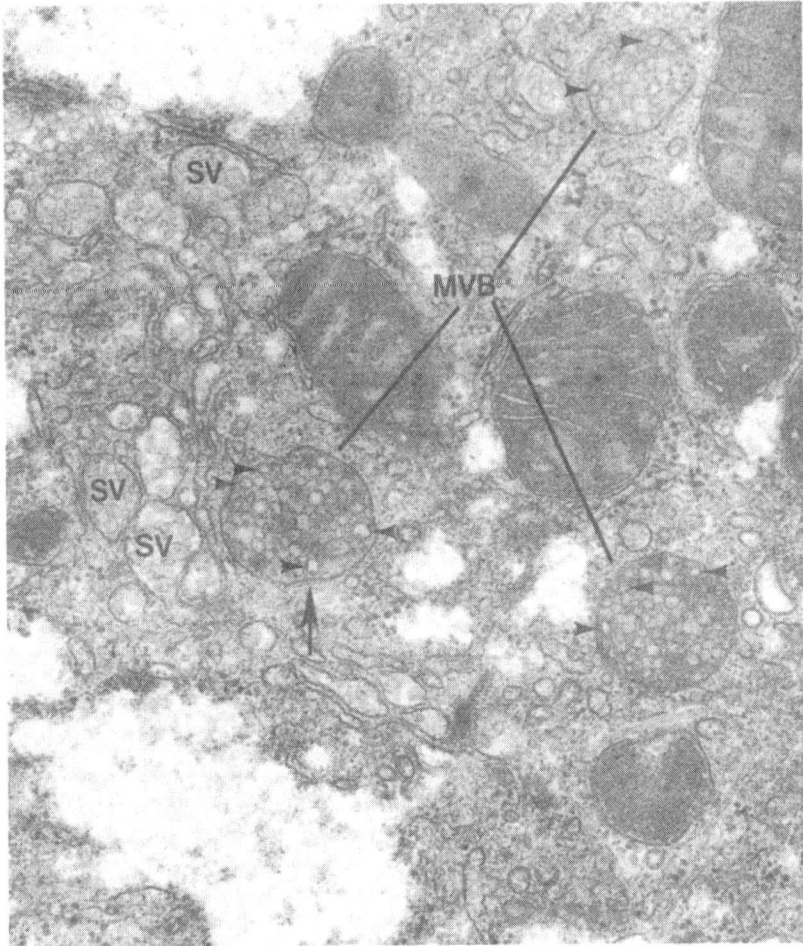

Fig. 3. X 35,000. Golgi/MVB area of hepatocyte of estradiol-treated rat illustrating differences in size and staining properties between MVBs and Golgi secretory vesicles (SV). The internal bilayer vesicles (arrowheads), heterogeneity of content lipoproteins, and increased electron density aid in the identification of MVBs. A straight membrane segment with a plaque is also sometimes present on these MVBs (arrow)

bular appendage and sometimes the surface membrane is indented, suggestive of an endocytic event that could give rise to the content bilayer vesicles. These features are always absent from Golgi secretory vesicles (Fig. 1-3).

MVB Isolation

The MVB compartment in hepatocytes became a focus of great interest to our research group because:

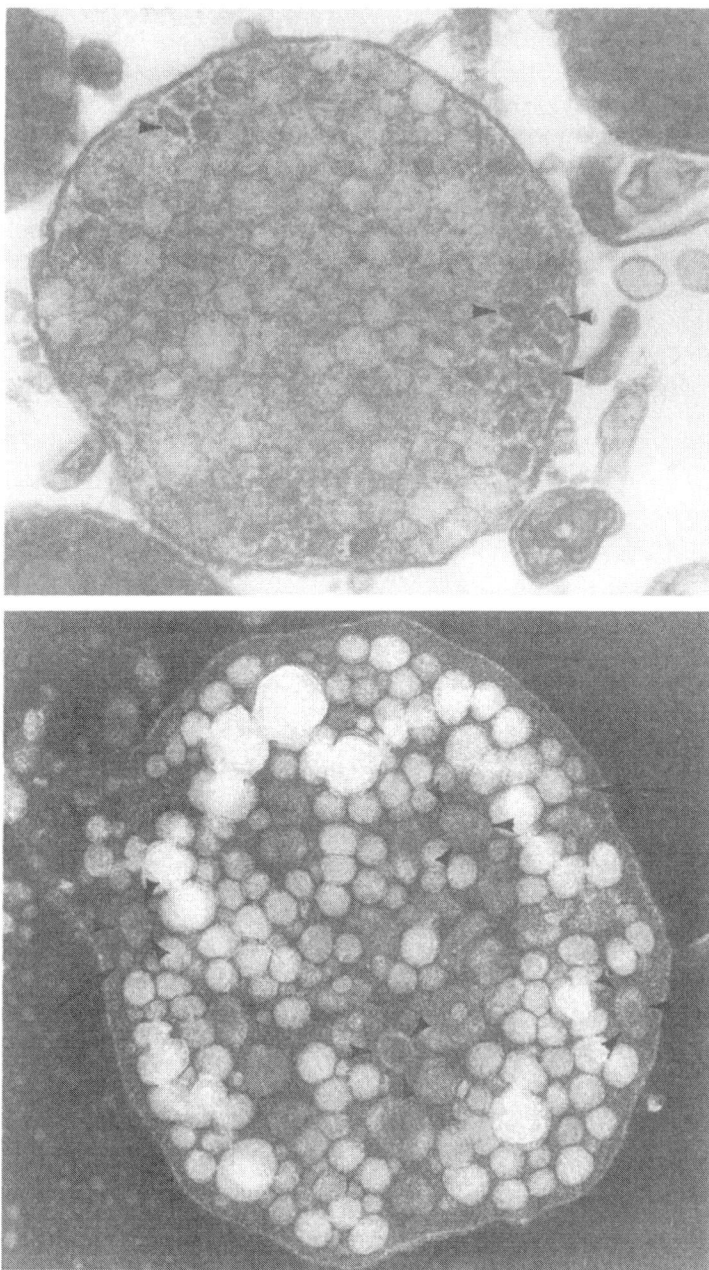

Fig. 4. X 65,000. Higher magnifications of isolated MVBs to illustrate clearly their content internal bilayer vesicles and remnant lipoproteins. *Top:* thin section of one intensely stained MVB showing internal bilayer vesicles (arrowheads) amongst remnants. *Bottom:* negative stain of one isolated MVB showing numerous content remnants together with collapsed internal bilayer vesicles (arrowheads) and some injected ^{125}I-LDL (arrows)

1. a large fraction (12-35%) of autoradiographic silver grains accumulated over this organelle soon (10-35 min) after intravenous injection of ^{125}I-labeled lipoproteins [5, 7];
2. estradiol-treated rats not only have 10-20-fold increased LDL-receptors in their livers and greatly increased LDL uptake, but their hepatocyte MVBs are larger and more numerous (Fig. 3) than in control livers [5, 7];
3. chloroquine increases the amount of ^{125}I radioautographic grains fivefold in further enlarged MVBs in these estradiol-treated rats, strongly supporting the hypothesis that MVBs are a prelysosomal compartment [7].

In addition, the literature indicated that a procedure to isolate MVBs was not available. We reasoned that because of the great similarity in size and content lipoproteins of hepatocyte MVBs and Golgi secretory vesicles, separation of these two organelles by standard centrifugal techniques might be difficult, a prediction borne out by preliminary experiments indicating that these two structures tend to co-isolate.

Therefore, we took advantage of the properties of livers of estradiol-treated rats:

a) greatly enhanced uptake of ^{125}I-LDL to intensely label the MVB compartment 10-15 min after intravenous injection (prior to any detectable degradation by lysosomal enzymes) [5]; and
b) substantially enlarged MVB size (2-3-fold) over that of Golgi secretory vesicles, which are smaller in livers of estradiol-treated rats (Fig. 3).

Because of the similarities between Golgi secretory vesicles and MVBs, we differentially labeled nascent VLDL triglycerides by intravenous injection of ^{3}H-palmitate at 10 min before liver homogenization, to preclude secretion of newly synthesized triglycerides. In addition, we homogenized one-half of the livers with a Polytron apparatus to isolate "intact" Golgi fractions from the same livers used for tracking ^{125}I-LDL in MVBs. By following the ^{125}I through a series of centrifugal steps including a Percoll gradient and a sucrose cushion, an isolation procedure was worked out with a ^{125}I-LDL purification of about 100-fold over that of the original homogenate [8].

Properties of Isolated MVBs

In thin sections, the bulk of the MVB pellet contains large vesicles of 0.4-0.75 μm diameter (0.55 μm average) with variable electron density of contents. Distinctive features are two types of appendages: one is a large double bilayer membranous appendage that often is nearly as large as the MVB from which it extends. The second appendage is a small finger-like projection. Each MVB usually has several electron dense structures, seen at low magnification, which are identifiable at higher magnifications as 50-70 nm bilayer vesicles (Fig. 4, top). Occasionally, the limiting membrane has an indentation suggestive of an endocytic event [8]. In negatively stained fractions, isolated MVBs have the same diameter when the limiting membrane remains intact, but the contents are obscured. Rupture of the limiting membrane permits stain to enter, revealing the following contents: numerous remnant particles, from 10-30 distincive internal bilayer vesicles which are collapsed

(Fig. 4, bottom), some smaller LDL-sized particles (presumably ^{125}I-LDL that was injected), and sometimes a few discoidal structures [8].

The differential labeling of the endocytic and secretory components shows that a large fraction of injected ^{125}I-LDL (12% of homogenate) was recovered in the MVB pellet whereas the amount of ^{3}H-palmitate in the MVB content remnants was miniscule, indicating the absence of Golgi contamination. Golgi VLDL contained a large amount of ^{3}H-palmitate, but they also contained a significant amount of [125]I (1.6% of homogenate), indicative of MVB contamination. This was confirmed morphologically. Much of this contamination can be eliminated by the simple procedure of diluting the "intact Golgi rug" fraction 10-12-fold with distilled water rather than a smaller volume of saline just prior to the final pelleting spin of 5,000 rpm for 20 min. This further dilution with water apparently permitted MVBs that were entrained in the Golgi tubular meshwork to be set free, so that only the "intact" Golgi compartment was pelleted by low speed sedimentation.

The MVB content lipoproteins had a higher proportion of cholesteryl esters, free cholesterol, and protein than Golgi content lipoproteins, consistent with the fact that they are remnants of chylomicrons and VLDL. In addition, the MVB membranes had threefold higher ratio of free cholesterol to phospholipid, the same as that of plasma membranes from which they are probably derived during the endocytic process. Whereas almost one-half of homogenate galactosyltransferase was recovered in "intact" Golgi fractions, only a trace of this Golgi marker enzyme activity was found in MVB pellets [8].

The Birth of Secondary Lysosomes

The postulated prelysosomal nature of MVBs was tested directly by chemical assay of arylsulfatase activity and by cytochemical studies for the lysosomal enzyme activities of arylsulfatase and acid phosphatase. Chemical measurements showed that less than 0.1% of the total homogenate arylsulfatase was present in MVB pellets [8]. However, cytochemical assays showed that about 10-15% of isolated MVBs in highly purified MVB pellets were reactive for the lysosomal enzymes tested [9]. In partially purified MVB fractions only, we identified small (ca. 70-120 nm), round, and intensely stained vesicles as putative primary lysosomes, often apparently fusing with an individual MVB. Reaction product for acid phosphatase with cerium (rather than lead) as capturing ion appeared as uniform precipitates surrounding endocytosed remnants within the few positively stained MVBs. Arylsulfatase reaction product appeared as a distinct arc or plaque just inside the MVB limiting membrane, often in continuity with intense reaction product of a 70-120 nm primary lysosome fusing with the MVB membrane. In isolated "intact" Golgi fractions these intensely stained primary lysosomes were also occasionally found beside a Golgi stack [9].

We conclude that in hepatocytes, MVBs represent the last or immediate prelysosomal compartment of the endocytic pathway of catabolism of macromolecules which give birth to secondary lysosomes in the Golgi region of the cell by direct fusion with primary lysosomes arising from closely adjacent Golgi compartments [9].

Contamination of Golgi fractions with MVBs

While these studies on the isolation of MVBs were in progress, a report was published on the properties of nascent plasma lipoproteins from hepatocyte Golgi fractions isolated by a different procedure [10, 11]. In that study, the content lipoproteins were more like endocytosed remnants than nascent VLDL and more than 50% of the content lipoproteins were recovered in the LDL and HDL density range [11]. Moreover, the morphology of the Golgi fractions (GF_{1+2}) obtained by this procedure [10, 12] shared many of the properties that we observed in our MVB fraction:
a) large, double bilayer membranous appendages,
b) heterogeneity of content particles,
c) variable degrees of content electron density,
d) small electron densities reminiscent of bilayer vesicles, and
e) positive reaction for acid phosphatase [13].

To test the hypothesis that the GF_{1+2} fraction contains MVBs, we labeled LDL with ^{125}I and chylomicrons with ^3H-cholesterol and, in the same animals receiving these injected ligands, we differentially labeled nascent VLDL triglycerides. Homogenized livers were divided equally and Golgi fractions (GF_{1+2}) and "intact" Golgi fractions [8] were obtained from the same livers. In GF_{1+2} fractions the ratio of endocytosed labeled lipoproteins to that of newly synthesized lipoproteins was about equal, whereas in "intact" Golgi fractions the ratio of newly synthesized triglycerides to endocytosed label was from 20 to 60-fold greater. Electron microscopic examination of GF_{1+2} fractions confirmed the presence of many MVBs mixed with Golgi secretory vesicles [14]. By a different biochemical approach, another group of investigators has shown recently that GF_{1+2} fractions contain a large amount of injected ^{125}I-labeled insulin within endocytic lipoprotein-filled structures [15].

Conclusions

1. Hepatocyte MVBs, unlike MVBs in most other cells, are closely similar to Golgi secretory vesicles in morphology, size, and content lipoproteins. Thus, because of their juxtaposition to Golgi compartments, hepatocyte MVBs are often mistaken for Golgi secretory vesicles.
2. Because of their similarity of size and contents, MVBs co-isolate with Golgi secretory vesicles from normal rat livers during standard centrifugal isolation methods.
3. MVBs can, however, be isolated in highly pure form from livers of ethinyl estradiol-treated rats.
4. These isolated MVBs are characterized by:
   a) internal bilayer vesicles
   b) several membranous appendages
   c) heterogeneity of content particles
   d) content remnant-like lipoproteins
   e) high free cholesterol to phospholipid content of limiting membrane

f) absence of galactosyltransferase

g) presence of LDL receptors and a proton pump (Havel, this volume)

5. MVBs are the immediate prelysosomal compartment of endocytosis because they give birth to secondary lysosomes by fusion with Golgi derived primary lysosomes in the Golgi/lysosomal region of the hepatocyte.

6. MVBs substantially contaminate Golgi GF_{1+2} fractions of hepatocytes [14, 15] obtained by the most commonly used Golgi isolation technique [12].

"Intact" Golgi fractions contain some MVBs [8], but the extent of contamination is comparatively much less [14]. Therefore, we recommend that Golgi fractions obtained by any of the different isolation procedures be analyzed for extent of MVB (endosome) contamination.

References

1. Havel RJ (1985) Annu Rev Physiol Palo Alto CA: Annual Reviews Inc, in press
2. Havel RJ (1984) J Lipid Res 25: 1570
3. Pittman RC, Steinberg D (1984) J Lipid Res 25: 1577
4. DeZanger R, Wisse E (1982) In: Sinusoidal Liver Cells (Knook DL, Wisse E, eds) Amsterdam: Elsevier, pp 69-79
5. Chao YS, Jones AL, Hradek GT, Windler EET, Havel RJ (1981) Proc Natl Acad Sci USA 78: 597
6. Jones AL, Hradek GT, Hornick CA, Renaud G, Windler EET, Havel RJ (1984) J Lipid Res 25: 1151
7. Hornick CA, Jones AL, Renaud G, Hradek GT, Havel RJ (1984) Am J Physiol 24: G187
8. Hornick CA, Hamilton RL, Spaziani E, Enders GH, Havel RJ (1985) J Cell Biol 100: 1558
9. Jost-Vu E, Hamilton RL, Hornick CA, Belcher JD, Havel RJ Submitted manuscript
10. Howell KE, Palade GE (1982) J Cell Biol 92: 822
11. Howell KE, Palade GE (1982) J Cell Biol 92: 833
12. Ehrenreich JH, Bergeron JJM, Sickevitz P, Palade GE (1973) J Cell Biol 59: 45
13. Farquhar MG, Bergeron JJM, Palade DF (1974) J Cell Biol 60: 81
14. Hamilton RL, Hornick CA, Havel RY Unpublished data
15. Kay DG, Khan MN, Posner BI, Bergeron JJM (1984) Biochem Biophys Res Comm 123: 1144

Immunoelectron Microscopy on Receptor and Ligand Sorting Sites

H. J. GEUZE

Laboratory of Cell Biology, Medical Faculty, University of Utrecht, Nic Beetsstraat 22, 3511 HG Utrecht, The Netherlands

While several methods are available for characterizing ligand localization (e. g. labeling with radioactive or electrondense tracers), receptor molecules themselves can only be localized in situ by immunocytochemical means. The increasing need for precise subcellular detection has coincided with recent developments of powerful immunoelectron microscope techniques. Of these we have chosen a method which relies on ultrathin cryosections and labeling with colloidal gold particles [1]. Double-labeling can easily be achieved using gold preparations of different sizes [2]. Immuno double-labeling is of special value when different receptors and ligands are studied simultaneously. Using this method we have directly compared the endocytotic pathways of the receptors for asialoglycoproteins (ASGP-R), mannose 6-phosphate residues on lysosomal enzymes (MP-R) and polymeric IgA (IgA-R) in liver parenchymal cells and hepatoma cells (Hep G2). ASGP-R is exclusively present in liver cells and mediates the endocytosis of ASGP-ligand from the blood. The uptake in coated vesicles is followed by a rapid transfer through an acidic prelysosomal compartment to lysosomes. The low pH facilitates uncoupling of receptors and ligands. Next, receptors recirculate to the plasma membrane via an as yet unknown pathway. The MP-R on the other hand, binds to its ligand somewhere intracellularly but like ASGP-R makes use of an acidic prelysosomal compartment for ligand uncoupling. In addition, in many cell types surface MP-R is engaged in the internalization of exogenous ligand. Both ASGP-R and M-R target their ligands to lysosomes and recycle for many rounds of ligand delivery. The IgA-R provides for an example of yet another receptor pathway, because it does not involve receptor uncoupling and recycling. The IgA-R with its covalently bound ligand is transported across the cell in a process called transcytosis. We felt that a precise description of the intracellular distributions would help in understanding the cell biological differences in receptor-ligand trafficking. We have used immunocytochemistry to address questions like: What are the precise intracellular routes taken by each receptor system? Does each of these receptors utilize the same transport vesicles and compartments? Where in the cell are these compartments localized and what are their structural features? Where does receptor-ligand uncoupling occur? Where do recycling receptors segregate from those which undergo degradative down regulation or transcytosis? Does a receptor for endogenous ligand such as MP-R make use of the same compartments as a receptor which directs exogenous ligands, such as ASGP-R?

Receptor-Mediated Uptake
in the Liver
Edited by H. Greten, E. Windler, U. Beisiegel
© Springer-Verlag Berlin Heidelberg 1986

We found ASGP-R, MP-R and IgA-R present in liver cells, but only the first two in Hep G2 cells. All three receptors were found in the Golgi complex, along the entire plasma membrane, in coated pits and vesicles and in a system of pleiomorphic vesicles. At the cell surface the receptors were randomly distributed as were all three in coated pits and vesicles regardless of whether little or an overdose of one of the ligands (ASGP) was administered to the cells. We also found ASGP-ligand and IgA in the same coated pits, indicating that in liver cells pits do not segregate ligands destined for lysosomal degradation from ligands which by-pass the lysosomes. Quantitation of label for the three receptors was consistent with nonselective internalization. We concluded that the smooth surfaced sinusoidal plasma membrane and the coated membrane area are quantitatively similar with respect to their composition of these three receptors. However, coated pits and vesicles may contain greater receptor density, i.e. molecules per unit length of membrane, than the plasma membrane [5]. Double-labeling of ASGP-R and ligand led to the identification of the intracellular pleiomorphic vesicles as the compartment of uncoupling receptors and ligands (CURL). CURL appeared to be composed of anastomosing tubules and some vesicles. Most of the receptors were found in the tubules whereas ASGP-ligand was mainly confined to the detaching vesicles [3]. These CURL vesicles (in literature also termed endosomes and receptosomes), including those with internal vesicles (multivesicular bodies) were shown to accumulate the lysosomotropic amine primaquine, and thus provide for the acidic environment needed for receptor-ligand uncoupling [4]. In CURL we also found segregation between IgA-R and the two others. CURL appeared to contain IgA-R enriched microdomains. Internalized IgA and IgA-R were found to be transferred from these tubulor microdomains to detaching vesicles which appeared to mediate transcytosis of receptor and ligand to the bile pole of liver cells [5]. Thus, in addition to receptor-ligand uncoupling CURL is clearly involved in receptor sorting.

All three receptors were present in the Golgi complex. For ASG-R, the Golgi pool of receptors amounted to 30% of the intracellular receptors. In addition, all three receptors are glycoproteins which pass through the Golgi during biosynthesis. Thus, in order to address the possible nature of the receptors in Golgi complexes we had to distinguish between possible recycling receptors and those in transit from their site of synthesis to the plasma membrane. Since inhibition of protein synthesis does not interfere with transport kinetics, we have used cycloheximide to deplete newly synthesized receptors from the cells. Using quantitative immunogold double-labeling and morphometry in rat liver parenchymal cells, we found that 2 h and 4 h after *in vivo* administration of cycloheximide the densities of ASGP-R and MP-R in the membranes of the Golgi complex were unaltered as compared with untreated liver. Similarly, no effect was found on receptor occurrence in coated pits, coates vesicles and CURL. As expected, other classes of proteins such as secretory proteins (e.g. albumin), structural cell surface enzymes (e.g. 5'-nucleotidase) and transcytosed ligand (e.g. IgA) and receptor (e.g. IgA-R) were not present in Golgi complexes or other intracellular compartments following treatment with cycloheximide. These observations are consistent with an involvement of the Golgi complex and CURL pools of ASGP-R and MP-R in receptor trafficking and recycling. Surprisingly, the Golgi complex of Hep G2 cells is most likely not involved in receptor recycling to a major degree. The proportion of the

Golgi receptor in Hep G2 cells (i.e. a few percent) is consistent with that expected solely from those receptor molecules in synthetic transit through the Golgi (transit time 1 h from RER to cell surface) when one considers the slow turnover (lifetime 80 h) of ASGP-R and MP-R.

Hep G2 cells enabled a more precise localization of lysosomal enzymes in relation to the MP-R and secretory protein. Because of discrepancies in literature with respect to Golgi sidedness of MP-R, we directly compared the localization of MP-R and galactosyl transferase. Preliminary observations show that MP-R is predominantly located in CURL and in a trans-Golgi reticulum (TGR) of smooth surfaced and coated membranes. In Golgi and TGR lysosomal enzymes, MP-R and albumin co-distribute, but in CURL only enzymes and MP-R were found. Treatment of the cells with primaquine resulted in an accumulation of MP-R and ASGP-R in CURL and TGR. The data obtained thus far lead us to conclude that MP-R assisted lysosomal enzyme delivery, involves TGR, and to a lesser extent, CURL.

References

1. Slot JW, Geuze HJ (1983) In: Immunocytochemistry. AC Cuello eds IBRO, Wiley and Sons Chichester UK pp 323-346
2. Geuze HJ et al (1981) Cell Biol 89: 653
3. Geuze et al (1983) Cell 32: 277
4. Schwartz et al (1985) EMBO J in press
5. Geuze et al (1984) Cell 37: 195

The Epidermal Growth Factor Receptor; Studies in Cultured Hepatocytes and During Liver Regeneration

H. Shelton Earp, Joyce Blaisdell, R. A. Rubin, and Qixiong Lin

Cancer Research Center, Department of Medicine, School of Medicine University of North Carolina, Chapel Hill, NC 27514 and Qingdao Medical College, Qingdao, China

Introduction

Epidermal growth factor is a mitogen for a broad range of cell types [1]. Infusion of EGF in intact rats induces hepatic DNA synthesis [2]; similar results are seen when EGF is incubated with primary cultures of rat hepatcoytes [3]. To determine whether EGF plays a role in the physiologic regulation of growth we have begun a series of studies of EGF-EGF receptor interaction during the course of liver regeneration and in primary cultures of hepatocytes. EGF transduces its signal by binding to a 170,000 molecular weight transmembrane glycoprotein. The binding of EGF leads to receptor clustering and internalization [4, 5]. The EGF receptor contains a ligand stimulated protein kinase activity located on the cytoplasmic side. This intrinsic kinase phosphorylates tyrosine residues, an enzymatic activity analogous to other growth factor receptors and oncogene products [6]. The binding of EGF activates the tyrosine kinase activity in vitro [6, 7]. However, the nature and localization of the critical substrates is unknown.

We have previously shown that EGF receptor number decreases in a time dependent manner following partial hepatectomy [8]. A 50% fall in receptor number is seen by 24 hours post-operatively. This is prior to first wave of mitosis in periportal hepatocytes. The decrease in receptor number during regeneration may occur by one of the following mechanisms:
1. A ligand-directed increase in the rate of receptor internalization. The ligand may be EGF itself or an EGF-like molecule such as TGF alpha.
2. An alteration in the extracellular and intracellular distribution of the EGF receptor triggered by a humoral component of the regenerative signal.
3. An alteration in the metabolic fate of the internalized EGF receptor; for example, a switch from receptor recycling to receptor degradation.
4. A decrease in EGF receptor synthesis that fails to replace constitutively degraded receptor.

These mechanisms are not mutually exclusive, and the decrease in receptor number during liver regeneration may be due to a combination of the above factors.

Whether the EGF receptor is recycled or degraded after ligand-directed internalization may depend upon the cell type. In mouse 3T3 cells, receptor labeled with ^{125}I-EGF appeared to be degraded after internalization [9]. Similar conclusions were reached when A431 cells prelabeled with heavy amino acids were studied after EGF binding [10]. More recent studies using human fibroblasts and an antibody

Receptor-Mediated Uptake
in the Liver
Edited by H. Greten, E. Windler, U. Beisiegel
© Springer-Verlag Berlin Heidelberg 1986

to the EGF receptor again showed rapid receptor degradation, i.e. loss of ^{35}S prelabeled receptor upon addition of EGF [11]. However, careful studies of the perfusion of rat liver with ^{125}I-EGF indicated that EGF was internalized to an extent that exceeds by 3-4 fold the number of receptors available on the surface. The data has been reasonably interpreted as showing receptor recycling in the hepatocyte [12]. The following studies were performed to examine these problems.

Methods

^{125}I-EGF Binding

EGF was iodinated with chloramine T to a specific activity of 1-2 X 10^6 CPM per ng EGF. Microsomal membrane fractions were made and the ^{125}I-EGF binding reaction carried out as previously described [8]. Purified rat liver hepatocytes were prepared by collagenase perfusion. Cells were cultured on plastic 35 mm dishes, the medium (Waymouth) was changed at 4 h and the incubation continued overnight. Binding studies were performed by incubating hepatocytes with ^{125}I-EGF (400,000 cpm) at 0° for 2 hours. Non-specific binding was assessed using a 1,000 fold excess of native EGF [13]. ^{125}I-EGF was chemically cross linked to membranes using disuccinimidyl suberate by the method of Pilch and Czech [14]. Eight percent SDS polyacrylamide gel electrophoresis was performed and dried gels were assessed by autoradiography.

Phosphorylation

Membranes were incubated with 20 mM Pipes, 30 mM Mg 2^+ and 1 μM ATP containing 5 μCi [γ ^{32} P]-ATP per assay. The reaction was performed with or without 1-10 ug/ml EGF [15]. Membrane solubilization was achieved by incubation in 1% Triton X 100 and 10% glycerol for 1 hour at 0° C. The residue was pelleted at 105,000 x g. Solubilized preparations were incubated with 10 ug/ml EGF for 40 min at 21° prior to the onset of a 0° 1 min phosphorylation that was begun by the addition of ATP.

Immunoprecipitation

An antiserum (799) was raised to rat liver EGF receptor purified by the method of Cohen [7] using an EGF-Affigel affinity column. The antiserum specifically immunoprecipitates both phosphorylated p170 from membranes and ^{35}S-labeled p170 from rat liver, cultured hepatocytes and hepatic cells. (Unpublished results)

Primary cultures were plated in Waymouth media in 1% fetal calf serum and 0.1 μM insulin for 3 hours. The medium was changed to MEM with 2% of the normal concentration methionine and 50 μCi of ^{35}S-labeled methionine and incubated for 12 to 16 hours. The medium was changed again to one containing 2 times the normal methionine concentration without [35]S. Unlabeled EGF at the indicated concentration was added. At the end of the incubation hepatocytes were washed and then solubilized in 1% NP40 containing Tris HCL pH 8.5, 150 mM NaCl and the protease inhibitors PMSF and leupeptin. The solubilized material was scraped and the residue pelleted in a microfuge. The samples were preincubated with pansorbin and normal rabbit serum for 10 min, recentrifuged and the supernatant incubated with 5 μl of antiserum (799 or normal rabbit serum) for 30 min at room temperature. Pansorbin was added for 45 min and the immunoprecipitates were washed with 0.5% NP40-0.5 MNaCl, 0.5% NP 40-0.15 MNaCl and 0.1% NP40. The pellets were resuspended in SDS containing sample buffer, boiled and run on 6% polyacrylamide gels. Fluorography was performed after treating the gels with 1 M Na salicylate.

Results

Our previous studies had shown a time-dependent decrease in EGF receptor binding during liver regeneration. Scatchard analysis of plasma membranes prepared from sham operated and partially hepatectomized rats indicated that the decrease in EGF binding was due to decrease in EGF receptor number [8]. In order to determine whether there had been any alteration in the molecular form of the EGF receptor, ^{125}I EGF was crosslinked to membranes from sham operated and regenerating liver. Fig. 1 shows that the molecular size of the EGF receptor was not changed during the process of liver regeneration; there is simply less available for ^{125}I EGF to bind to. Quantitation of the crosslinked ^{125}I-EGF showed a 60-70% drop in EGF receptor 36 hours following partial hepatectomy, in agreement with binding studies.

We demonstrated that EGF-directed EGF receptor autophosphorylation also fell during the course of liver regeneration [15]. Since this activity represents an intrinsic phosphorylation of tyrosine residues in the terminal part of the cytoplasmic domain, it supported the hypothesis that there were fewer EGF receptors in regeneration membranes. The phosphorylation experiment was repeated in solubilized membrane fractions to rule out the possibility that receptors were shifted to a masked compartment in regenerating rat liver (so called cryptic receptors). The solubilized membranes were preincubated for 40 min with 10 μg/ml of EGF. This vast excess of EGF was used to rule out any alterations in affinity that might have occured during solubilization or as a consequence of regeneration. Phosphorylation under these conditions again showed 60-70% loss of EGF receptor at 36 hours.

In order to understand the biosynthesis and fate of the EGF receptor in a controlled situation, these parameters were studied in primary cultures of hepatocytes. We initially showed by binding criteria that dexamethasone (1-100 ng/ml) and hydrocortisone (.1-50 μM) increased EGF receptor number in primary cultures of hepatocytes. The increase in binding was detectable by 4 to 8 hours and was maximal (70-100% increase) within 24 hours [13]. In order to show that this effect was dependent upon protein and RNA synthesis, the cells were incubated with or without 50 μM hydrocortisone for 18 hours in the presence of increasing concentrations of cycloheximide and actinomycin D. These inhibitors produced an unexpected re-

Fig. 1. ^{125}I-EGF crosslinked to liver membranes prepared from sham-operated (S) and partially hepatectomized rats (R). The major band is p170

sult, emphasizing the need to be cautious in interpreting results of receptor synthesis done with inhibitors. Cycloheximide (Fig. 2) and actinomycin D (Fig. 3) produced dose dependent increases in ^{125}I-EGF binding in the control cultures (incubated with 0.1 μM insulin). Cycloheximide and actinomycin D inhibited the rise in EGF binding seen with glucocorticoid but at higher doses the binding began to rise again. Scatchard analysis of cells treated with cycloheximide at 0.5 μg/ml for 18 hours indicated the increase in ^{125}I-EGF binding was not due to an increase in receptor number but rather an increase in receptor affinity (data not shown). Direct assessment of receptor biosynthesis has recently been analyzed by immunoprecipitating p170 labeled with ^{35}S-methionine in the presence or absence of 0.5 ug/ml of cycloheximide for 18 hours. Cycloheximide abolished EGF receptor synthesis, showing that the inhibitor does block protein and p170 synthesis and yet still raised ^{125}I-EGF binding.

In order to determine the fate of the EGF receptor after internalization, experiments were performed using primary cultures. Cultured hepatocytes were incubated with native EGF for 2-4 h at 37°. The surface bound EGF was washed and ^{125}I-EGF used to assess remaining surface receptors. Greater than 10 ng/ml decreased EGF surface receptor number by 60-80% at 4 h. A similar result was reported by Moriarity and Savage [16].

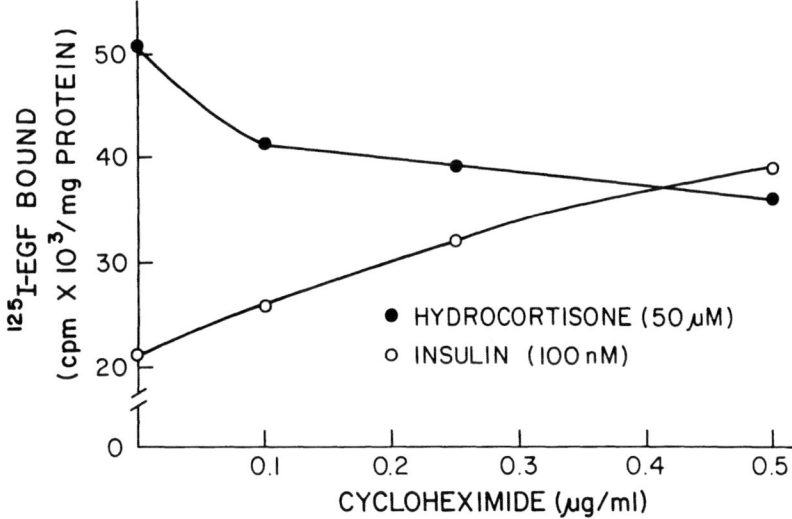

Fig. 2. ^{125}I-EGF Bound: Primary cultures of rat hepatocytes incubated overnight with the indicated agents

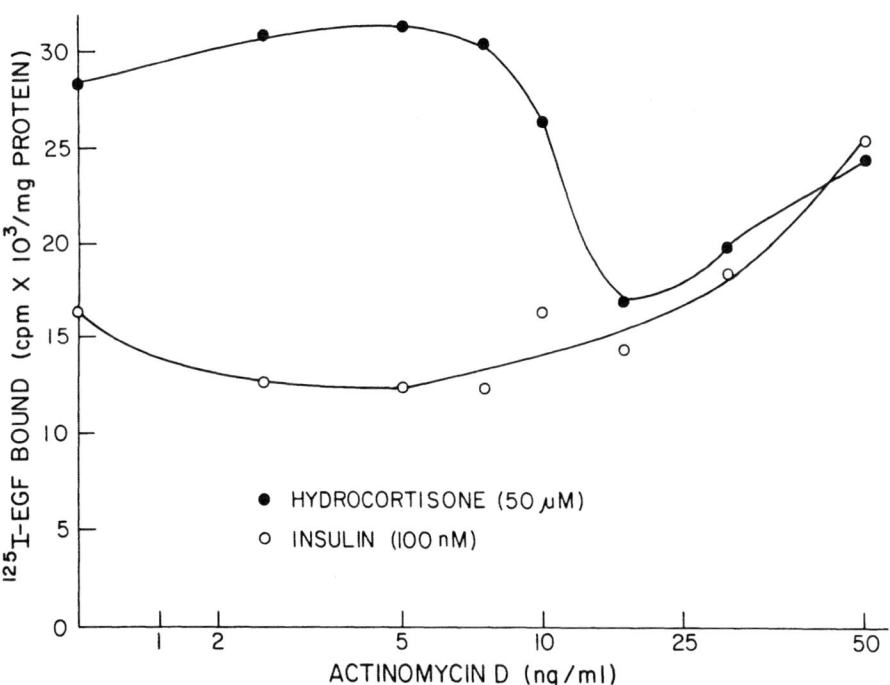

Fig. 3. ^{125}I-EGF Bound: Primary hepatocyte cultures were incubated with the indicated concentration of ActD for 18 h

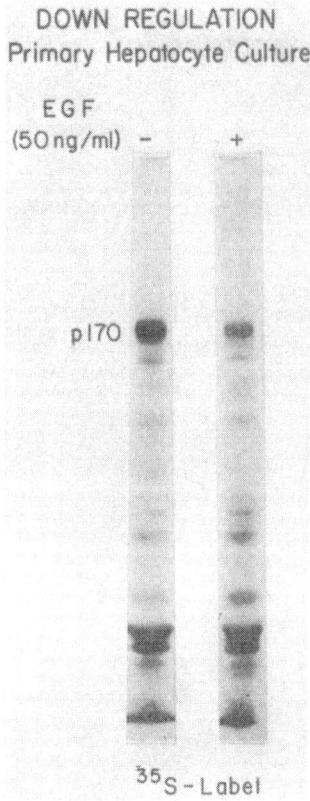

DOWN REGULATION
Primary Hepatocyte Culture

EGF
(50 ng/ml)   −   +

p170

^{35}S − Label

Fig. 4. Immunoprecipitation of ^{35}S labeled p170 by EGF

To study the fate of the internalized receptor, hepatocyte cultures were incubated overnight in ^{35}S-methionine containing media. After a 16 h incubation, the labeling was stopped with the addition of medium containing 2 times normal methionine concentration. The cells were then treated with or without added (50 ng/ml) EGF. Immunoprecipitation after 4 hours showed a significant loss of ^{35}S-prelabeled EGF receptor. Densitometry of the autoradiogram showed a 60% loss of p170 (Fig. 4). Thus, internalization in the primary culture resulted in loss of pre-labeled receptor.

Discussion

The down regulation of the EGF receptor during an in vivo growth response following partial hepatectomy has been demonstrated. The decrease in EGF receptor number has been assessed by ^{125}I-EGF binding studies [8]. ^{125}I-EGF crosslinking to the receptor indicates that the molecular size of the receptor is not changed during regeneration. Studies of EGF directed EGF receptor autophosphorylation come to the same conclusion [15]. There is less receptor present during the course of regeneration. Phosphorylation of detergent solubilized membranes showed that regenerating membrane vesicles to not sequester receptor in any cryptic form.

The explanation for the growth related loss of growth factor receptor has not been determined. The simplified explanation is that a mitogenic peptide has bound to, internalized, and promoted degradation of the receptor. If this is so, it would appear that EGF or EGF like substances are true physiologic regulators of cell growth. Since no laboratory has convincingly demonstrated an increase in plasma EGF during regeneration, the explanation may be more complex.

Certain transformed cells can secrete a polypeptide factor referred to as TGF α that binds to the EGF receptor [17]. The mRNA for one form of TGFα has been demonstrated in normal rat liver [18]. It is possible that the humoral signal that mediates regeneration increases the secretion of TGFα which binds to and internalizes the EGF receptor. This would be a form of autocrine stimulation [18] and would explain the lack of increased EGF-like activity in the systemic circulation.

An additional aspect of EGF receptor metabolism in the liver must also be taken into account. Unlike cultured fibroblasts and carcinoma cells [9, 11], the EGF receptor in the perfused liver may be recycled [12]. The lack of receptor degradation would mean that the loss of receptor observed during regeneration may require an additional level of control. In primary cultures of hepatocytes, EGF can promote significant receptor degradation within 4 h (Fig. 4). The extent of degradation for exceeds that seen in the perfused liver [12]. The results do not preclude recycling in the cultured hepatocytes; they only indicate that degradation is more likely under these conditions. Our present interpretation is that the extent of EGF receptor degradation or recycling may be a regulated process in the hepatocyte. The signal that governs regeneration may shift the metabolism of the receptor toward the

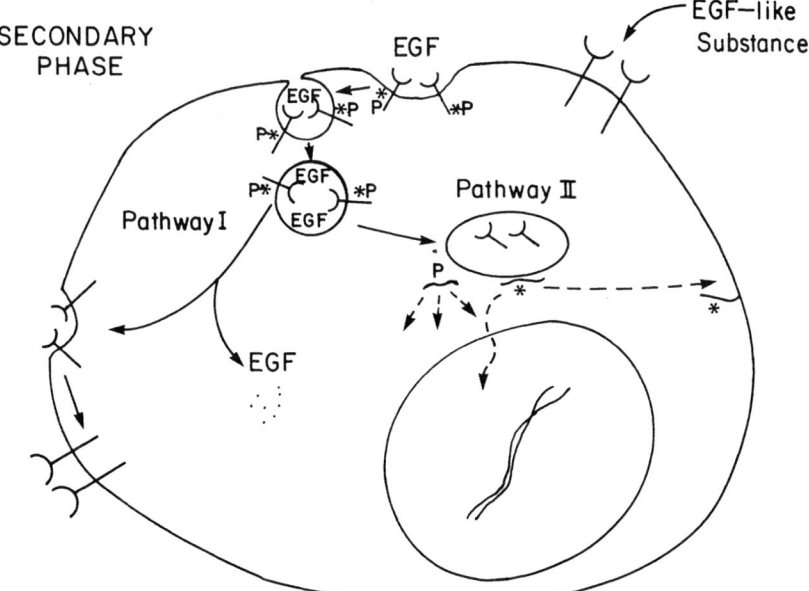

Fig. 5. Potential pathways of the EGF receptor after ligand directed internalization

pathway II shown in Fig. 5. This would lead to lysosomal degradation. The shift to the lysosome may result in the generation of an internal signal important for triggering hepatocyte growth. Alternatively since other experiments indicate that mitogenesis requires extracellular EGF for 6-8 h [1] the clearance of receptor from the surface may play another role in the complex process by which this normally quiescent tissue renews itself.

References

1. Carpenter G, Cohen S (1979) Annu Rev Biochem 48: 193-216
2. Bucher NLR, Patel U, Cohen S (1978) Adv Enzymol Reg 16: 205-213
3. Richman RA, Claus TH, Pilkis SJ, Friedman DL (1976) Proc Natl Acad Sci USA 79: 776-780
4. Adamson ED, Rees AR (1981) Molecular and Cellular Biochemistry 34: 129-152
5. Schlessinger J, Schreiber AB, Levi A, Lax I, Libermann T, Yarden Y (1983) CRC Critical Reviews in Biochemistry Vol 14, 2: 93-111
6. Carpenter G (1984) Cell 37: 357-58
7. Cohen S, Ushiro H, Stoscheck C, Chinkers M (1982) J Biol Chem 257: 1523-1531
8. Earp HS, O'Keefe EJ (1981) J Clin Invest 67: 1580-1583
9. Das M, Fox CF (1978) Proc Natl Sci USA 75: 2644-2648
10. Krupp MN, Connolly DT, Lane MD (1982) J Biol Chem 257: 11489-11496
11. Stoscheck CM, Carpenter G (1984) J Cell Biology 98: 1048-1053
12. Dunn WA, Hubbard AL (1984) J Cell Biology 98: 2148-2159
13. Lin Q, Blaisdell J, O'Keefe E, Earp HS (1984) J Cellular Physiology 119: 267-272
14. Pilch PF, Czech MP (1979) J Biol Chem 254: 3375-3381
15. Rubin RA, O'Keefe EJ, Earp HS (1982) Proc Natl Acad Sci USA 79: 776-780
16. Moriarity DM, Savage CR Jr (1980) Arch Biochem Biophys 203: 506-518
17. De Larco JE, Todaro GJ (1978) Proc Natl Acad Sci USA 75: 4001-4005
18. Lee DC, Rose TM, Webb NR, Todaro GJ (1985) Nature 313: 489-491
19. Sporn MB, Roberts AB (1985) Nature 313: 745-747

Insulin Interaction with Target Cells Morpho-Functional Aspects

Jean-Louis Carpentier[1], Phillip Gorden[2], and Lelio Orci[1]

[1] Institute of Histology and Embryology, University of Geneva Medical Center, Geneva, Switzerland
[2] Diabetes Branch, National Institutes of Arthritis, Diabetes and Digestive and Kidney Diseases, National Institutes of Health, Bethesda, Maryland 20205, USA

Introduction

When a polypeptide such as insulin binds to a specific receptor on a target cell several events are initiated. First a biological signal is generated, the nature of which depends on the cell. For instance, in adipose and muscle cells, glucose transport is controlled by insulin but in hepatocytes glucose transport is unaffected and instead intracellular enzyme activation and other actions are stimulated. Following the hormone-receptor interaction, other events occur that are remarkably common among different cell types including both target and non-target cells. These events include degradation of the ligand and regulation of the receptor. Both of these actions are receptor mediated and depend on the formation of the hormone-receptor complex.

In the present review we will explore how direct visual probes of the insulin-receptor interaction have extended our concepts of:
a) the nature of the cell surface binding;
b) the subsequent fate of the ligand, and the receptor, and
c) the possible relevance of these processes to insulin degradation and receptor regulation.

Cell surface events

There are three features of the cell surface, discernable morphologically, that have been studied in detail. For many cells that bind insulin, the surface is covered with numerous microvilli; this is true for example for cultured human lymphocytes and freshly isolated rat hepatocytes. In these two cell types, microvilli constitute ~55% of the cell surface [1, 2]. These microvilli are variable in length, contain abundant cytoskeletal structures, increased density of intramembrane particles and are largely devoid of cytoplasmic organelles [1].

Small segments of the plasma membrane are decorated with a cytoplasmic bristle coat made up predominantly of the protein clathrin [3] and at least two other minor proteins [4]. These coated segments predominate in invaginated portions of the membrane and are referred to as coated pits [5]. Though their occur in essentially all cells, their importance with respect to receptor mediated endocytosis was

Receptor-Mediated Uptake
in the Liver
Edited by H. Greten, E. Windler, U. Beisiegel
© Springer-Verlag Berlin Heidelberg 1986

first recognized by Anderson et al., who found that the internalization of low density lipoprotein occurred essentially exclusively by way of coated pits [5].

The remainder of the surface of most cells is comprised of a smooth surface which can be pitted by small uncoated invaginations.

When ^{125}I-insulin is incubated with freshly isolated rat hepatocytes, autoradiographic grains localize initially and preferentially to the microvillous surface of the cell [2]. Preferential localization also occur to coated pits [2]. With time there is a redistribution of the labeled material to the non-villous portion of the membrane more precisely to coated regions. Studies using both autoradiography to localize ^{125}I-labeled ligands [6] and video-intensification microscopy to detect fluorescently labeled ligands have shown that the ligand-receptor complex is mobile in the plane of the membrane [7, 8]. These observations suggest that the hormone-receptor complex moves in the plane of the membrane from the villous surface to the non-villous and coated surface. These data are also consistant with the idea that the

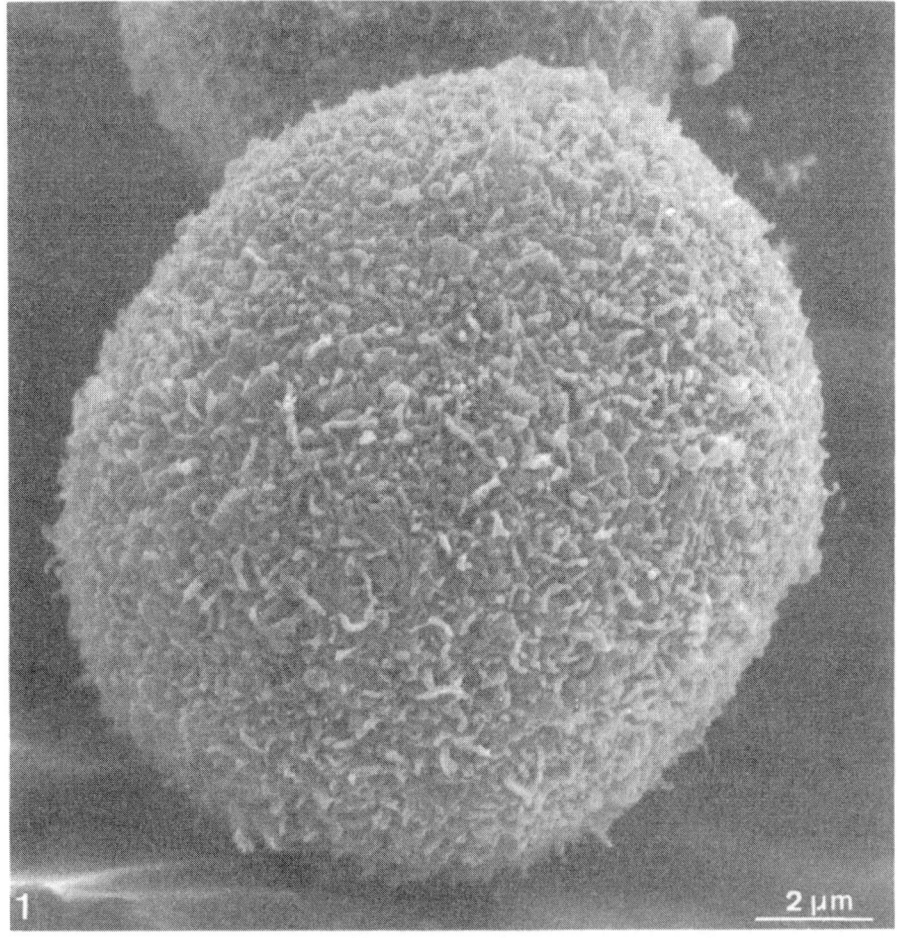

Fig. 1. General view of a freshly isolated rat hepatocyte seen at the scanning microscope. The surface of the cell is filled with microvillosities and cytoplasmic projections. X 9.000

affinity for insulin may be higher in receptor in the non-villous portions of the membrane that in receptor in the villous regions. This is emphasized by the finding of a correlation between slowed dissociation of ^{125}I-insulin from the plasma membrane of cells and concentration of the ligand in coated pits on the non-villous surface of these cells [2].

Internalization of the insulin-receptor complex

Coated pits represent a preferential pathway for the internalization of many ligands. This also appears to be true for polypeptide hormones but there is no evidence that this is an exclusive mechanism as appears to be the case for low density lipoproteins.

Coated pits are exposed to the external environment of the cell thus the ligand either binds initially to receptors in these structures or the complex moves into coated pits by lateral mobility. The neck of the coated pit then fuses and subsequently fissions from the membrane surface to form a coated vesicle. These vesicles have been demonstrated morphologically by serial sections which have verified that they are closed vesicular structures [9, 10, 11]. The lifetime of the coated vesicle is short i.e. 1-2 minutes or less and by some unknown mechanism, the coat is shed from the membrane-limited vesicle. Recent studies suggest that clathrin in coated vesicles is initially acted upon by a 70.000 M.W. polypeptide containing ATPase activity [12, 13].

Following association with coated vesicles, the next structure with which the insulin associate is a larger clear non-coated vesicle or endosome [14]. These structures have been shown to have important functional properties. Maxfield and associates have shown that the endosome has a protein pump in its limiting membrane capable of acidifying the internal milieu of the vesicle [15]. This acidic environment could be ideal to promote dissociation of ligand from receptor, thus allowing the ligand to be sequestered and processed separately from the receptor.

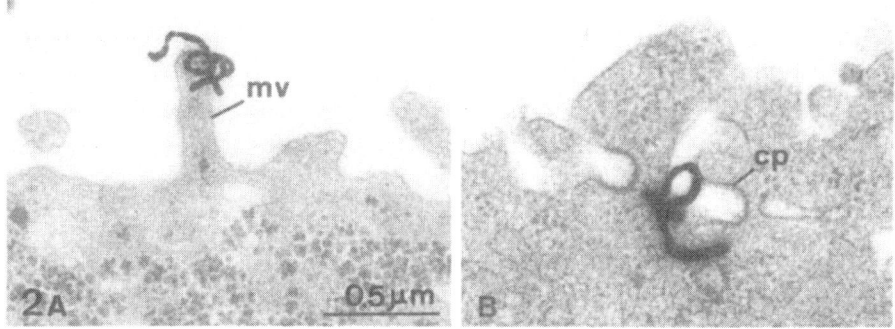

Fig. 2. Periphery of freshly isolated rat hepatocytes incubated for short periods of time (2 minutes) (A) or longer periods of time (60 minutes) at 20° C in the presence of ^{125}I-insulin. Following 2 minutes of incubation the labeled material is frequently associated with microvilli (mV) why at longer incubation time ^{125}I-insulin concentrates in coated pits (cp). x 36.000

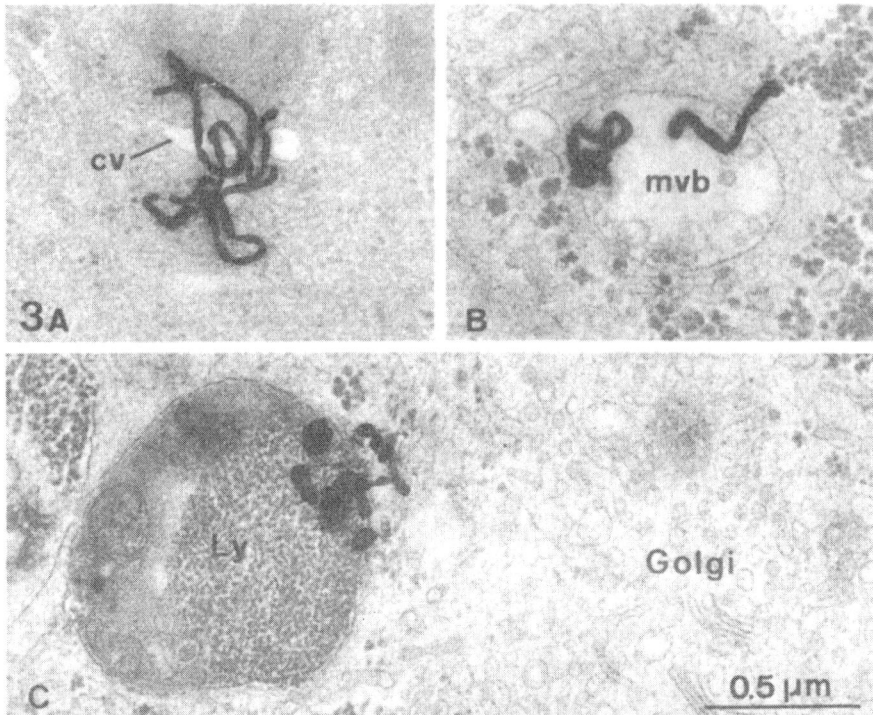

Fig. 3. Representative examples of intracellular structures with which a preferential association of the labeled material is observed. The hepatocytes were incubated for 2 hours at 15° C with ^{125}I-photoreactive insulin, exposed to UV, washed and further incubated in the absence of labeled ligand for 0 minutes (**a** and **b**) or 30 minutes (**c**) at 37° C. X 42.000

The next structure seen is the multivesicular body. This organelle is larger than the clear endosome and is further characterized by occasional or many small vesicles and by a plaque bearing a fuzzy coat. The biogenesis of these structures is unclear: whether they exist de novo or are formed by the fusion of endosomes and other vesicles remains to be established. The multivesicular body appears to be an intermediate in a continous process: the next structure visualized is, therefore, the lysosome [14, 16]. Though the lysosome has distinctive morphologic features, strictly speaking it can be identified only by cytochemical techniques that reveal biologically active enzymes. Unfortunately, these techniques may be relatively insensitive unless rigorously applied and multiple enzymes are sought. Thus it is most appropriate to call structures like multivesicular bodies which have been considered a form of lysosome as "lysosome-like". Finally, ambiguity of nomenclature is avoided if one considers the endosome, multivesicular body and lysosome as a continuum involved in processing of ligands, their receptors or both.

Insulin receptor recycling

Using a photoreactive insulin analogue that can be covalently coupled to the insulin receptor by exposition to U.V. light we have shown both biochemically and morphologically that the insulin receptor is internalized together with the hormone in both freshly isolated rat hepatocytes and hepatocytes in primary culture [17, 18]. These observations have also been supported by biochemical experiments [19, 20]. It has further been shown morphologically that following its internalization the receptor may be recycled back to the plasma membrane [21, 22].

The fate of the receptor following internalization may be the same or different from the ligand. That is, an uncoupling step may take place following initial endocytosis. With respect to polypeptide hormone the nature of this uncoupling remains obscur. As mentioned above the endosome fulfill most of the characteristics required to promote this uncoupling. Moreover, in other systems, the endosomal compartment have been shown to participate in the uncoupling and in the sorting. For instance, when the asialoglycoprotein receptor was tagged by an antibody specific for the receptor and the ligand separately tagged by an antibody against the

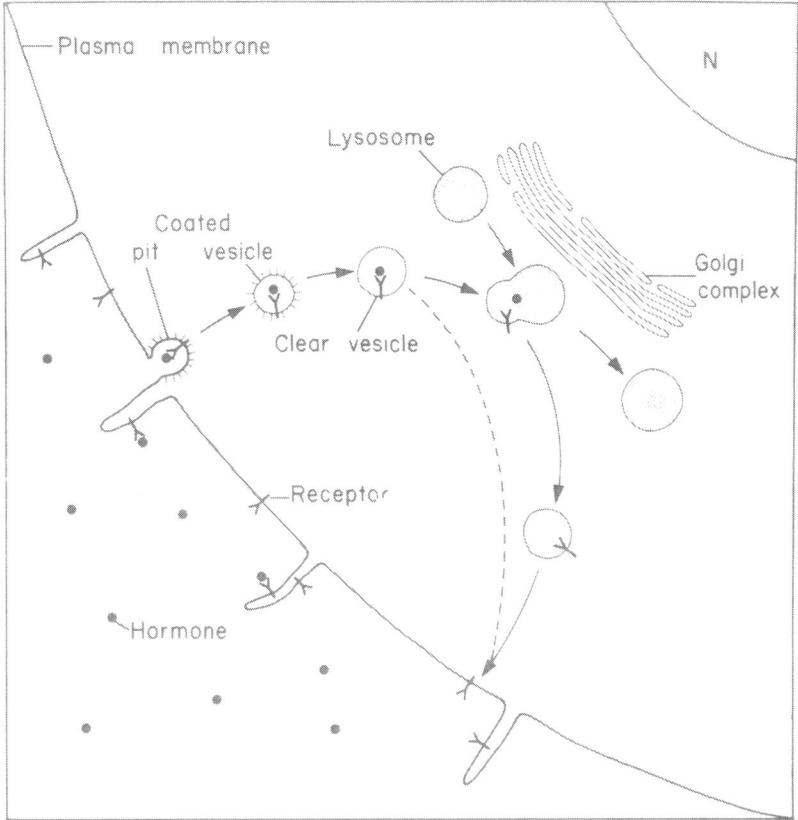

Fig. 4. Schematic drawing illustrating the main morphologic events underlying binding, internalization and recycling of the insulin receptor in a target cell. Reproduced from [32] with permission

ligand, separation of the cellular distribution of the two compartments was visualized morphologically using protein A coupled to colloidal gold particles of different sizes [22]. According to this analysis the ligand appeared destined for the lysosome whereas the receptor entered a tubulovesicular compartment thought to be involved in returning the receptor to the plasma membrane. Supporting the key role played by an acidic compartment in the recycling of insulin receptors back to the cell surface is the observation that acidotropic drugs such as NH_4Cl, or monensine inhibit the recycling process [22, 24].

Separation of ligand and receptor is not, however, required for recycling since in the case of the ^{125}I-photoreactive insulin analogue covalently coupled to the insulin-receptor recycling of the insulin analogue-receptor complex is occurring. In this case, however, recycling proceeds at a slow rate and via lysosomes [24] in the same type of vesicles as described for endocytosis per se.

Functional implications of receptor mediated endocytosis and recycling

Different polypeptide hormones transduce an intracellular signal in different ways following their binding to cell surface receptors. Some polypeptide hormones, such as glucagon, activate adenylate cyclase by a complex coupling mechanism. Other among which insulin, EGF and other growth factors work through an as yet obscure mechanism possibly in part involving receptor autophosphorylation. Yet all of these and other polypeptide hormones undergo a very similar pattern of endocytosis. It is possible that intracellular transport of phosphoprotein subscribes some functions, but the nature of this putative function is unknown. Thus, the

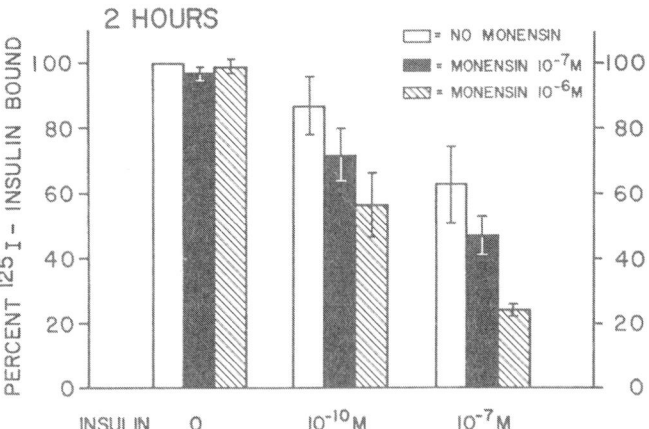

Fig. 5. Effect of monensin and insulin on the down-regulation of insulin receptors on U-937 monocytes. Cultured cells were preincubated in the absence or presence of monensin (10^{-6} or 10^{-7} M) plus or minus unlabeled insulin (10^{-7} or 10^{-10} M) for 2 hours at $37°$ C. The cells were washed and incubated with ^{125}I-insulin with or without excess unlabeled insulin (100 μg/ml): the specific ^{125}I-insulin bound was determined after 90 minutes at $20°$ C. Results are expressed per cent of ^{125}I-insulin specifically bound following a preincubation in the absence of monensin and unlabeled insulin. Data shown are representative of three different experiments. The height of the bar is the mean and the vertical line represents S.E.M. Reproduced from [22] with permission

possible role of endocytosis in polypeptide hormone i. e. insulin action, if any, is obscure.

If cell surface binding activates hormones action, then there must be a regulatory mechanism to terminate that action. For instance, insulin degradation has been shown to be receptor linked [25]. Thus, internalization may be an important mechanism for removing the hormone from the cell surface and initiating its degradation. It is likely that this receptor mediated degradation of insulin is primarily lysosomal: this is supported by the lysosomal localization of the hormone and by the inhibition of insulin degradation by lysosomotropic agents such as chloroquine, ammonium chloride and other similar compounds [26]. Our current thinking is therefore that insulin degradation occurs at least in part through a lysosomal mechanism related to receptor mediated endocytosis of the hormone.

Another general feature or consequence of insulin binding to receptor is insulin induced receptor regulation [27]. Since both insulin and its receptor are internalized, it is clear that endocytosis is an important mechanism of modulating cell surface receptor concentration. Further, it is clear that there is no simple relationship between insulin receptor complexes internalization and insulin receptor regulation. This lack of straightforward relationship between insulin receptor downregulation and internalization relates to recycling. We have pointed out that at some steps in the endocytotic pathway the ligand and the receptor may become uncoupled and each may have a different fate. Thus, the receptor may be recycled, may be degraded, or some combination of these events may take place. In the U-937 human monocyte cell line, small concentrations of insulin induce the loss of cell surface receptors. These receptors are in part recovered in soluble extracts of the cell. Thus, in this case, receptors appear to be internalized and in part recovered intact intracellularly and in part degraded. Monensin, which inhibits recycling, augments down regulation. Monensin, however, does not affect that fraction of receptors destined for degradation. Thus, monensin affects only the recycling component of the receptor. In other cell types where the rate of internalization is low, such as in the IM-9 lymphocytes, monensin has essentially no effect [22].

Hormone and receptor internalization also provide a mechanism for understanding receptor regulation in clinical states. Non-target cells like peripheral blood monocytes have insulin receptors which are regulated in an analogous fashion to hepatocyte receptors. Monocytes and hepatocytes exposed to the same concentration of insulin would, therefore, regulate their receptors in an analogous fashion by way of receptor mediated endocytosis [28].

Further evidence that receptor mediated endocytosis is a regulated process comes from studies in hypoinsulinemic states. If it is true that endocytosis is a mechanism to remove the ligand from the cell surface and terminate its signal, it might be expected that in hypoinsulinemic states this process would be impaired. We have recently found that in streptozotocin induced diabetes in the rat, a hypoinsulinemic state, the internalization of ^{125}I-insulin is impaired. By contrast, the internalization of ^{125}I-glucagon is either normal or increased [29]. Further in insulinopenic type I diabetes of man, ^{125}I-insulin internalization is markedly inhibited [30].

Acknowledgements. This work was supported by grant 3.660.83 from the Swiss National Science Foundation.

References

1. Carpentier JL, Van Obberghen E, Gorden P, Orci L (1981) Surface redistribution of ^{125}I-insulin in cultured human lymphocytes. J Cell Biol 91: 17-25
2. Carpentier JL, Fehlmann M, Van Obberghen E, Gorden P, Orci L Redistribution of ^{125}I-insulin on the surface of rat hepatocytes as a function of dissociation time. Diabetes, in press.
3. Pearse BMF, Clathrin: (1976) a unique protein associated with intracellular transfer of membrane by coated vesicles. Proc Natl Acad Sci USA 73: 1255-1259
4. Woods JW, Woodward MP, Roth TF (1978) Common features of coated vesicles from dissimilar tissues: composition and structure. J Cell Sci 30: 87-97
5. Anderson RGW, Brown MS, Goldstein JL (1977) Role of the coated endocytotic vesicle in the uptake of receptor-bound low density lipoprotein in human fibroblasts. Cell 10: 351-364
6. Barazzone P, Carpentier JL, Gorden P, Van Obberghen E, Orci L (1980) Polar redistribution of [125]Iodine labeled insulin on the plasma membrane of cultured human lymphocytes. Nature 286: 401-403
7. Schlessinger J, Shechter Y, Willingham MC, Pastan I (1978) Direct visualization of binding, aggregation and internalization of insulin and epidermal growth factor on living fibroblastic cells. Proc Natl Acad Sci USA 75: 2654-2663
8. Schlessinger J, Van Obberghen E, Kahn CR (1980) Insulin and antibodies against insulin receptor cap on the membrane of cultured human lymphocytes. Nature 286: 729-731
9. Fan JY, Carpentier JL, Gorden P, Van Obberghen E, Blackett NM, Grunfeld C, Orci L (1982) Receptor-mediated endocytosis of insulin: the role of microvilli, coated pits and coated vesicles. Proc Natl Acad Sci USA 79: 7788-7791
10. Petersen OW, Van Deurs B (1983) Serial-selection analysis of coated pits and vesicles involved in adsorptive pinocytosis in cultured fibroblasts. J Cell Biol 96: 277
11. Van Deurs B (1983) Do coated pinocytic vesicles exist? TIBS 8: 400-401
12. Schlossman DM, Schmid SL, Braell WA, Rothman JE (1984) An enzyme that removes clathrin coats: purification of an uncoating ATPase. J Cell Biol 99: 723-733
13. Braell WA, Schlossman DM, Schmid SL, Rothman JE (1984) Dissociation of clathrin coats coupled to the hydrolysis of ATP: role of an uncoating ATPase. J Cell Biol 99: 734-741
14. Fan JY, Carpentier JL, Van Obberghen E, Blackett NM, Grunfeld C, Gorden P, Orci L (1983) The interaction of ^{125}I-insulin with cultured 3T3-L1 adipocytes: quantitative analysis by the hypothetical grain method. J Histochem Cytochem 31: 859-870
15. Tycko B, Mayfield FR (1982) Rapid acidification of endocytic vesicles containing α_2-macroglobulin. Cell 28: 643-651
16. Carpentier JL, Gorden P, Freychet P, Le Cam A, Orci L (1979) Lysosomal association of internalized ^{125}I-insulin in isolated rat hepatocytes: direct demonstration by quantitative electron microscopic autoradiography. J Clin Invest 63: 1249-1261
17. Fehlmann M, Carpentier JL, Le Cam A, Thamm P, Saunders D, Brandenburg D, Orci L, Freychet P (1982) Biochemical and morphological evidence that the insulin receptor is internalized with insulin in hepatocytes. J Cell Biol 93: 82-87
18. Gorden P, Carpentier JL, Moule ML, Yip CC, Orci L (1982) Direct demonstration of insulin receptor internalization: a quantitative electron microscopic study of covalently bound ^{125}I-photoreactive insulin incubated with isolated hepatocytes. Diabetes 31: 659-662
19. Marshall S, Green A, Olefsky JM (1981) Evidence for recycling of insulin receptors in isolated rat adipocytes. J Biol Chem 256: 11464-11470
20. Hedo JA, Simpson IA (1984) Internalization of insulin receptors in the isolated rat adipose cell. J Biol Chem 259: 11083-11084
21. Fehlmann M, Carpentier JL, Van Obberghen E, Freychet P, Thamm P, Saunders D, Brandenburg D, Orci L (1982) Internalized insulin receptors are recycled to the cell surface in rat hepatocytes. Proc Natl Acad Sci USA 79: 5921-5925
22. Carpentier JL, Dayer JM, Lang U, Silverman R, Gorden P, Orci L (1984) Down regulation and recycling of insulin receptors: effect of monensin on IM-9 lymphocytes and U-937 monocyte-like cells. J Biol Chem 259: 14190-14195
23. Geuze HJ, Slot JW, Strous GJAM, Lodish HF, Schwartz AL (1983) Intracellular site of asialoglycoproteins receptor-ligand uncoupling: double-label immunoelectron microscopy during receptor-mediated endocytosis. Cell 32: 277-287

24. Carpentier JL, Fehlmann M, Van Obberghen E, Gazzano H, Freychet P, Brandenburg D, Orci L (1983) Intracellular pathway of the insulin receptor during internalization and recycling. J Cell Biol 97: 409a

25. Terris S, Steiner DF (1975) Binding and degradation of ^{125}I-insulin by rat hepatocytes. J Biol Chem 250: 8389-8398

26. Gorden P, Freychet P, Carpentier JL, Canivet B, Orci L (1982) Receptor-linked degradation of ^{125}I-insulin is mediated by internalization in isolated rat hepatocytes. Yale J Biol Med 55: 101-112

27. Gavin III JR, Roth J, Neville Jr DM, De Meyts P, Buell DN (1974) Insulin-dependent regulation of insulin receptor concentrations: a direct demonstration in cell culture. Proc Natl Acad Sci USA 71: 84-88

28. Grunberger G, Robert A, Carpentier JL, Dayer JM, Roth A, Stevenson HL, Orci L, Gorden P Human circulating monocytes internalize ^{125}I-insulin in a similar fashion to rat hepatocytes: relevance to receptor regulation in target and non-target tissues. J Lab Clin Med, in press

29. Carpentier JL, Robert A, Van Obberghen E, Freychet P, Gorden P, Orci L (1985) Inhibition of receptor-mediated endocytosis of ^{125}I-insulin into isolated hepatocytes of streptozotocin-treated diabetic rats: evidence for a regulated step in hypoinsulinemia. Abstracts of the Endocrine Society # 22

30. Carpentier JL, Grunberger G, Robert A, Orci L, Gorden P (1985) Regulation of receptor-mediated endocytosis of ^{125}I-insulin in hypoinsulinemic states: differential response in insulin dependent type I diabetes versus non-insulin dependent diabetes. Diabetes 34: Suppl I 7A

31. Carpentier JL, Fehlmann M, Van Obberghen E, Gorden P, Orci L (1984) Morphological aspects and physiological relevance of insulin receptor internalization and recycling. In: Endocrinology, Labrie F, Proulx L (eds.) Elsevier Publishers B.V. pp 349-353

The Regulation and Dynamics of the Transferrin Receptor

A.M. WEISSMAN, K.K. RAO, T. ROUAULT, R.D. KLAUSNER, and J.B. HARFORD

Cell Biology and Metabolism Branch National Institute of Child Health and Human Development, National Institutes of Health Bethesda, Maryland 20205

Introduction

A wide variety of substances that would otherwise be excluded from cells gain entry *via* receptor-mediated endocytosis [1, 2]. Binding of ligands to their specific plasma membrane receptors is followed by internalization involving specialized regions of the membrane termed coated pits [2, 3]. While the pathways that are traversed subsequently by diverse ligands exhibit striking similarities, there are distinctive features that separate endocytic systems into several groups. The endocytosis of low density lipoproteins (LDL) by fibroblasts [4] and of asialoglycoproteins (ASGP) by hepatocytes [5] are representatives of systems in which ligands are catabolized in lysosomes and receptors are reutilized. Constant numbers of receptors are maintained during extended continuous endocytosis of ligand molecules. In other systems, such as those mediating uptake of insulin [6] or epidermal growth factor (EGF) [7], both the ligand and its receptor are degraded in lysosomes. These systems exhibit "down-regulation" in that ligands enhance receptor degradation. As a result of a reduction in the number of receptors, the target cells exhibit lowered responsiveness to the continued presence of these ligands.

In contrast to either of these situations, neither transferrin (Tf) nor the transferrin receptors (TfR) are destroyed as a part of the so-called transferrin cycle involved in cellular iron uptake [8, 9]. Diferric Tf enters the cell bound to the TfR, iron is unloaded intracellularly, and both the apoprotein ligand and the receptor are returned intact to the cell exterior (Fig. 1). An acidic (pH 5 to pH 6) endocytic compartment is instrumental in release of iron from Tf within the cell [10]. The acidic endosome is apparently utilized in different endocytic systems to acheive different ends. For example, in hepatocytes, the same (or similar) organelle is employed for dissociation of ASGP from their receptors [11].

Recently, we have been engaged in examination of the regulation of TfR biosynthesis in K562 cells, a human erythroleukemia cell line, as well as in studies involving perturbations of the dynamics of the Tf/TfR pathway in these cells. It is not our intent here to review extensively the literature related to these areas but to summarize briefly recent findings from our laboratory. We have come to appreciate the complexity of receptor regulation and movement and hope that this chapter will convey this to the reader.

Receptor-Mediated Uptake
in the Liver
Edited by H. Greten, E. Windler, U. Beisiegel
© Springer-Verlag Berlin Heidelberg 1986

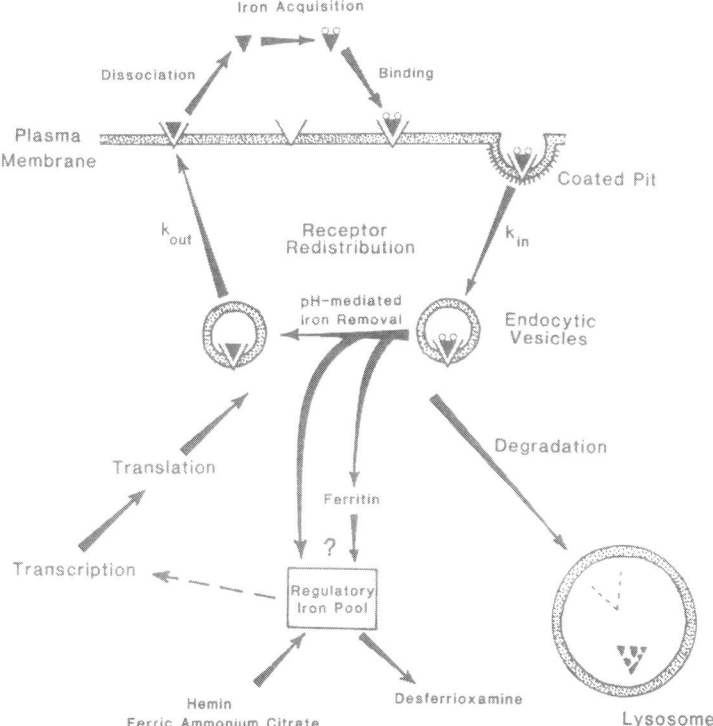

Fig. 1. Schematic diagram of the transferrin cycle. Iron (○) bound to transferrin (▼) enters cells associated with the transferrin receptor (V). Iron is removed in an endocytic compartment of low pH, and the receptor-apotransferrin complex returns to the cell surface where apotransferrin dissociates. For the most part, iron entering the cell via transferrin cycle is found associated with cytoplasmic ferritin. Biosynthesis of the transferrin receptor is regulated at the transcriptional level by a chelatable pool of intracellular iron. Hemin and iron salts are capable of contributing iron to the regulatory pool, and the permeant chelator desferrioxamine can lower the effective size of this pool. The degradation rate of the receptor is unaffected by these manipulations of available iron, but is markedly enhanced by the anti-receptor monoclonal antibody OKT9. In addition, OKT9 treatment influences the distribution of the receptors that are participating in iron uptake

Regulation of transferrin receptor biosynthesis by alterations in cellular iron

Proliferating cells require iron and obtain it via receptor-mediated endocytosis of the iron carrier protein transferrin. Iron, though an essential component of many important cellular processes, is nonetheless a toxic substance. Accordingly, it is important that iron uptake be regulated. A logical site for this regulation is the "port of entry" for iron i. e. the TfR. We have observed that cells regulate the expression of the TfR in response to agents that alter iron availability [12, 13]. When exogenous iron is supplied to K562 cells, the number of TfR decreases and, when iron is removed by the permeant chelator desferrioxamine (Df), there is an increase in

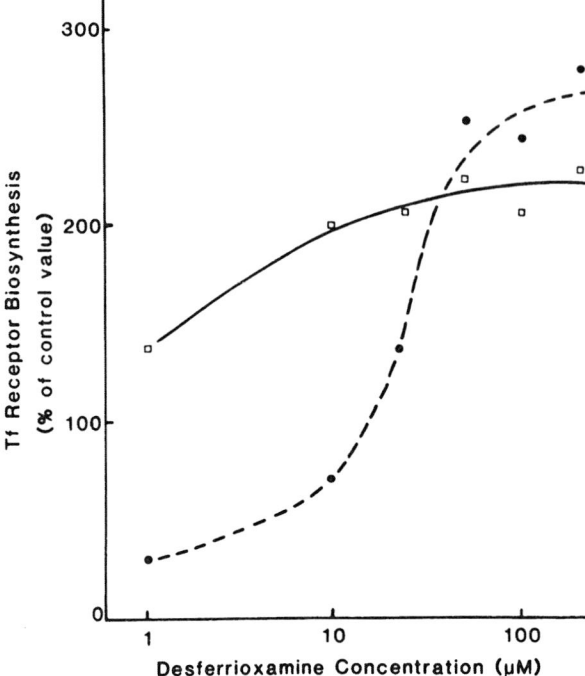

Fig. 2. Regulation of transferrin receptor biosynthesis by chelatable iron. K562 cells were treated for 4 hr with the indicated concentration of desferrioxamine ($\square$—$\square$) or with 50 μM hemin plus desferrioxamine ($\bullet$---$\bullet$). Receptor biosynthesis was measured for a 30 min pulse with [^{35}S]methionine. Quantitation of newly synthesized receptor was achieved by immunoprecipitation, electrophoresis, and densitometry of autoradiographs. Data are expressed as percentages of the value obtained with untreated cells. Additional details may be found in reference 14

receptor number. Iron can be added to the regulatory pool *via* saturating levels of differric Tf or by incubation of cells with ferric ammonium citrate. Recently, we have found that hemin (ferric protoporphyrin IX) is an extremely efficient source of iron capable of depressing TfR expression [14]. All of these iron sources exert their influence on TfR expression by supplying iron to a pool that is accessible to chelation by Df and all act by decreasing the rate of TfR biosynthesis. Conversely, Df itself increases TfR expression by elevating the biosynthetic rate [12-14]. Fig. 2 provides evidence that incubation of K562 cells with increasing concentrations of Df completely abolishes the depression of TfR biosynthesis seen with a fixed concentration of hemin. In an analogous fashion, increasing concentrations of hemin antagonizes completely the increase in TfR biosynthesis seen with a fixed concentration of Df (data not shown). When hemin and Df are added to cells, their composite effect on TfR biosynthesis appears to reflect a direct competition between iron delivery and iron removal.

The alterations of TfR biosynthesis observed when iron availability is experimentally manipulated is a reflection of changes in the levels of cellular mRNA encoding the TfR [13]. This is evidenced by isolation of polyadenylated RNA from cells treated with either Df or an iron supplier such as diferric Tf or hemin. *In vitro* translation experiments revealed a 2.5-fold increase in translatable TfR mRNA in Df-treated cells and a 50% decrease in translatable TfR mRNA in cells treated with diferric Tf. The availability of a cDNA clone for the TfR gene [15] has allowed direct quantitation of mRNA levels in K562 cells after iron provision or iron chelation [16]. The time-dependent increase in the cellular levels of TfR mRNA

Fig. 3. Elevation of transferrin receptor mRNA by treatment with desferrioxamine. K562 cells were treated for the indicated times with 50 uM desferrioxamine before RNA was extracted and mRNA selected by oligo-dT Sepharose. Equivalent amounts of mRNA from each sample were denatured with formaldehyde and immobilized on nitrocellulose. Content of receptor mRNA was assessed by hybridization with [^{32}P]pcDTr1, a cDNA clone of the transferrin receptor [15]. In the lower portion of the figure is shown an autoradiograph of the nitrocellulose after hybridization and washing. In the upper portion of the figure, the autoradiograph has been quantitated by densitometry. Data are expressed as percentages of the value obtained with mRNA from untreated cells. Additional details may be found in reference 16

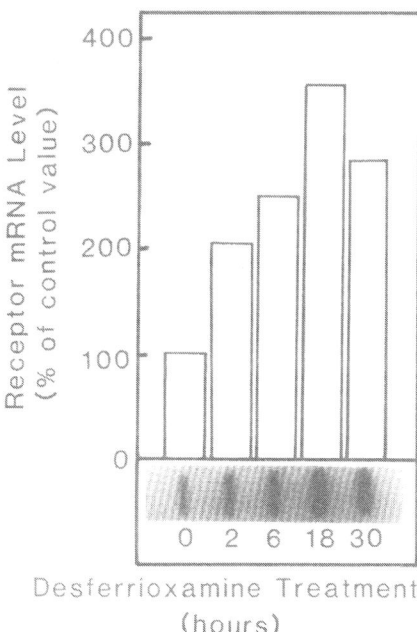

caused by treatment with Df is shown in Fig. 3. Quantitative hybridization with the TfR cDNA clone of Northern blots reveal that the level of the 4.9 kb TfR mRNA in K562 cells is decreased by hemin treatment and increased by treatment with Df. The specificity of these effects was established by demonstrating that neither treatment affected the level of actin mRNA in these cells. When nuclei were isolated from K562 cells after various iron manipulations, it was found that the rate of *in vitro* TfR gene transcription was markedly higher in nuclei from Df-treated cells than in nuclei from cells treated with hemin. Thus, it appears that a chelatable iron pool influences TfR gene expression leading to altered levels of TfR mRNA. In turn, this results in corresponding alterations in TfR biosynthesis and expression in K562 cells. The nature of the transcriptional control of the TfR gene is currently under study. The rapidity with which new steady-state levels of TfR mRNA are reached in either Df-treated or hemin-treated cells is consistent with a very short ($<$ 45 min) half-life for the TfR mRNA. The short mRNA half-life would allow for the rapid modulation of mRNA levels in either direction *via* a corresponding alteration in the rate of transcription.

Receptor redistribution and degradation in response to treatment with an anti-receptor antibody

We have observed that treatment of K562 cells with a monoclonal antibody against the TfR has marked effects on receptor dynamics and the survival of the receptor

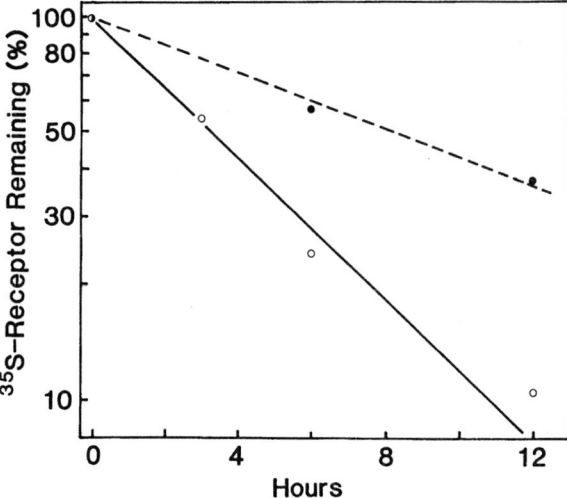

Fig. 4. Enhancement of transferrin receptor degradation by treatment of K562 cells with an anti-receptor antibody. K562 cells were metabolically labeled with [^{35}S]methionine for 2 h. After washing, the cells were divided and 5 ug/ml of OKT9 IgG was added to one-half of the cells. During the subsequent incubation, samples were removed from treated (○) and untreated (●) cells at the indicated times and content of [^{35}S]receptor assessed as described in Fig. 2. Data are expressed as percentages of the value obtained with cells at the time of antibody addition. Additional details may be found in reference 17

[17]. In these studies, we have employed OKT9, a monoclonal antibody that recognizes a determinant distinct from the Tf binding site. This antibody has been used to study the structural features of the TfR [18] and has been instrumental in chromosomal localization [19] and cloning [15] of the TfR gene. When K562 cells are labeled metabolically with [^{35}S]-methionine, the TfR can be quantitated by immunoprecipitation, electrophoresis, and densitometry of autoradiographs. The rate of decrease of radiolabeled TfR during a chase period yields an apparant half-life of approximately 8 h [12, 13, 17]. Inclusions of Df, hemin, ferric ammonium citrate, or the ligand diferric Tf were without effect on the rate of TfR degradation. However, when highly purified OKT9 IgG is included in the chase medium, there is a marked increase in the degradation of radiolabeled TfR (Fig. 4). A similar observation has been made concerning the insulin receptor using antibodies directed against the insulin receptor [20, 21]. Thus, the anti-receptor antibodies mimic the ligand in causing "down-regulation". In the case of the TfR, OKT9 enhances the degradation of a receptor that is not normally "down-regulated".

Treatment of K562 cells with OKT9 also leads to a rapid redistribution of the TfR such that a reduced percentage of the receptors are displayed on the cell surface (Fig. 5, panel A). Receptor redistribution may be caused by altering the internalization rate and/or the externalization rate of the receptor. Antibodies directed against receptors for mannose-6-phosphate [22], insulin [20, 21], and EGF [23] have been shown to cause receptor redistribution. Another monoclonal antibody (B3/25) against the TfR also has this effect in human carcinoma A431 cells [24]. Agents other than antibodies can stimulate TfR redistribution as has been demonstrated by treatment of K562 cells with a tumor-promoting phorbol ester [25].

In addition to the reduction in surface receptors, OKT9 treatment also leads to a less rapid reduction in the number of receptors in what we have termed the "cycling pool" (Fig. 5, panel B). The "cycling pool" is measured by determining the

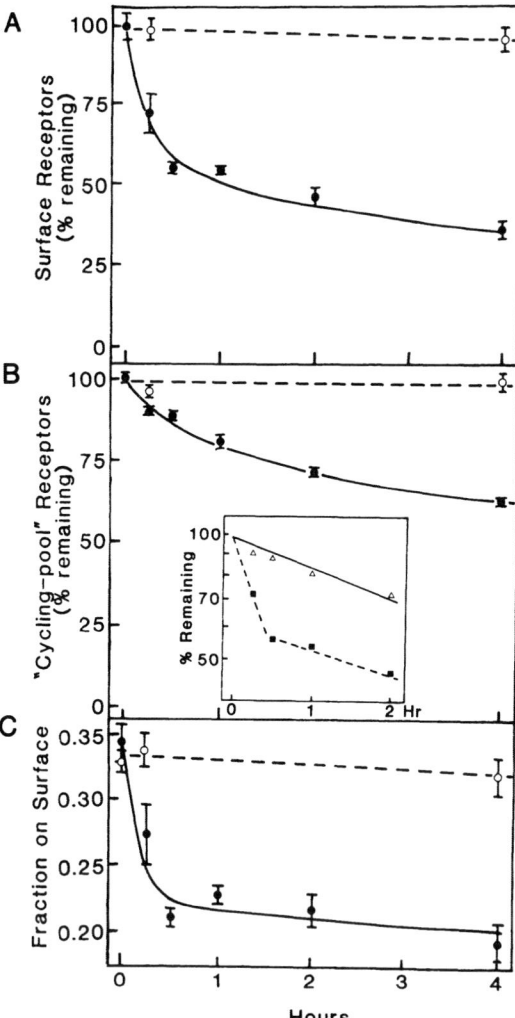

Fig. 5. Effect of OKT9 treatment on the number of cell surface and "cycling pool" transferrin receptors. K562 cells were treated with 1 μg/ml of OKT9 IgG for the indicated times. Portions of the incubations were cooled to 4° C and incubated with [125I]transferrin to determine the number of cell surface transferrin receptors (panel A). Portions of the incubations were incubated with [125I]transferrin at 37° C to determine the maximum amount of ligand that becomes cell-associated (panel B). This latter value is taken as a measure of the transferrin receptors in the "cycling pool" (see text). The ratio of the surface receptors to the receptors in the "cycling pool" is shown in panel C. In each case OKT9-treated cells (●—●) have been compared to cells comparably incubated without OKT9 (○---○). In the inset of panel B, values obtained for surface receptors (■--■) and "cycling pool" receptors (△ — △) in OKT9-treated cells are plotted semilogrithmically. This plot demonstrates that the loss of "cycling pool" receptors appears to be defined by a single exponential function whereas the loss of surface receptors is biphasic. Additional details may be found in reference 17

maximum amount of radioactive ligand that becomes cell-associated when ligand is present at saturating concentrations. This value represents a steady-state between association of diferric Tf and dissociation of apo-Tf (see Fig. 1). Because Tf remains bound to its receptor throughout the Tf cycle and unbound Tf does not accumulate in the cells, this value provides a measure of the receptors that are participating in the cycle. When the number of receptors in the Tf cycle is decreased the rate at which the cells can acquire iron is diminished. Such is the case with OKT9-treated cells [17]. Based on the insights gained from experimental manipulation of available iron (see above), it might be expected that reduction in iron uptake would result in an enhancement of receptor biosynthesis analogous to that

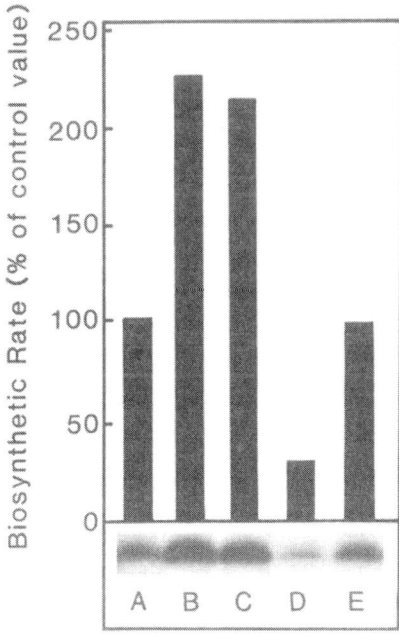

Fig. 6. Effect of OKT9 and transferrin on transferrin receptor biosynthesis. K562 cells were treated for 6 h with no additions (lane A), 5 μg/ml of OKT9 IgG (lane B), 5 μg/ml of B3/25 IgG (lane C), 40 μg/ml human diferic transferrin (lane D), or with OKT9 plus transferrin (lane E). The rate of biosynthesis of the receptor was assessed as described in Fig. 2. In the lower portion of the figure is the autoradiograph of the relevant portion of an SDS-polyacrylamide gel showing the immunoprecipitated, newly-synthesized transferrin receptor. In the upper portion of the Figure, the autoradiograph has been quantitated by densitometry. Data are expressed as percentages of the value obtained with untreated cells. Additional details may be obtained in reference 17

seen when intracellular iron is chelated by Df. Fig. 6 demonstrates that OKT9 treatment enhances the biosynthetic rate of TfR by more than two-fold (lane B). Diferic Tf, which by itself decreases TfR biosynthesis (lane D), abolishes the OKT 9-mediated enhancement resulting in near normal rates of biosynthesis when cells are co-incubated with Tf and OKT9 (lane E). Another anti-TfR monoclonal (B3/25) has as stimulatory effect on TfR biosynthesis (lane C) resembling that of OKT9.

Based solely on the OKT9 effect on TfR degradation, one would predict that a new steady-state of TfR in OKT9-treated cells would be attained that would be less than 50% of that seen in untreated cells. In fact the new steady-state is 70-75% of the control value. This appears to be due to enhanced biosynthesis (caused by iron deprivation) that partially compensates for enhanced degradation (caused by OKT9). When hemin is included as an iron source during treatment with OKT9, a more marked reduction in cellular receptor content results. Presumably, hemin prevents the iron deprivation that stimulates TfR biosynthesis. The net effect of enhanced degradation without enhanced biosynthesis is a more pronounced depletion of cellular TfR.

Although we have observed an enhancement of receptor degradation upon OKT9 treatment, it appears that the majority of TfR with bound OKT9 continues to participate in the Tf cycle. Iron from [^{59}Fe]Tf accumulates linearly in OKT9-treated cells at a rate only 20-30% lower than that seen in untreated cells [17]. The amount of ^{59}Fe that accumulates in either case represents multiple cycles of the TfR in the "cycling pool". Since an insignificant number of new receptors (i.e. without bound OKT9) enter the "cycling pool" in the course of the ^{59}Fe uptake

Table 1. Effect of altering the theoretical recycling efficiency on receptor half-life

Theroetical Recycling Efficiency per Cycle	Resultant Receptor Half-Life
100%	∞
99.1%	16 h
98.2%	8 h
96.5%	4 h
86.6%	1 h
50.0%	12.5 min

The above calculations are based on a first order decay function for the transferrin receptor and the following assumptions:
1. The cycle length is 12.5 min (calculated from experimental data)
2. Receptors must leave the cycling pool to be degraded
3. Receptors that leave the cycling pool are degraded

experiment, this means that the binding of OKT9 does not earmark the TfR for immediate removal and destruction. Rather, it appears that OKT9 binding to the TfR allows recycling yet increases the probability that a receptor will depart the cycle and be degraded. The time required for the Tf cycle is very short (approx. 12.5 min) compared to the normal half-life of the TfR (approx. 8 h). The implication of this disparity is illustrated in Table 1. If departure from the Tf cycle is rate-limiting for receptor degradation, then receptors can recycle with a 98.2% efficiency per cycle and an 8 h half-life for the TfR would result. A relatively small decrase in this recycling efficiency per cycle from 98.2% to 96.5% would cause a 50% reduction in the receptor half-life. In systems that exhibit ligand-mediated "downregulation", it is possible that decreases in recycling efficiency rather than irreversible once-for-all removal of receptors accounts for this phenomenon. Certainly, experiments with these systems would have to be carefully designed if these two possibilities were to be distinguished. Considerable interest exists in the signals for receptor traffic and membrane protein sorting [26]. Our studies with the TfR and OKT9 indicate that, by coupling a rapid pathway (e.g. recycling) with a slower process (e.g. degradation), a significant shift toward the slower process can be achieved through rather subtle changes in the fidelity to the rapid pathway. It is possible that membrane proteins may be sorted and targeted using processes that do not involve absolute once-for-all signals.

Summary and Perspectives

One of the hallmarks of cell biology is the existence of multiple sites of regulation; receptors are no exception. Receptors may be sequestered or made more available through changes in their distribution within the cell. This redistribution makes possible the increase or decrease of ligand binding and responsiveness without altering the total number of receptor molecules present in the cell. This may allow for extremely rapid modulation of receptor function. Alternatively, the cellular content of receptors may be varied by altering receptor biosynthesis and/or degradation.

Finally, receptor function may be controlled by cellular modulation of receptor affinity for ligand or *via* regulation leading from the receptor along signal transducing pathways.

References

1. Steinman RM, Mellman IS, Muller WA, Cohn ZA (1983) J Cell Biol 96: 1-27
2. Goldstein JL, Anderson RGW, Brown MS (1979) Nature (London) 279: 679-685
3. Steer CJ, Klausner RD (1983) Hepatology 3: 437-454
4. Brown MS, Goldstein JL (1979) Proc Natl Acad Sci USA 76: 3330-3337
5. Harford J, Ashwell G (1982) in "The Glycoconjugates" (M Horowitz, ed) Academic Press NY Vol 4: 27-55
6. Kahn CR (1982) J Cell Biol 70: 261-286
7. Schlessinger J, Schreiber A, Levi A, Lax I, Libermann T, Yarden Y (1983) CRC Crit Rev Biochem 14: 93-111
8. Newman R, Schneider C, Sutherland R, Vodinelich L, Greaves M (1982) TIBS 7: 397-401
9. Hanover JA, Dickson RB (1985) in "Receptor-Mediated Endocytosis" (M Willingham, I Pastan, eds) Academic Press NY
10. Rao K, van Renswoude J, Kempf C, Klausner RD (1984) FEBS Lett 160: 213-216
11. Harford J, Wolkoff AW, Ashwell G, Klausner RD (1983) J Cell Biol 96: 1824-1828
12. Mattia E, Rao K, Shipiro DS, Sussmann HH, Klausner RD (1984) J Biol Chem 259: 2689-2692
13. Rao KK, Shapiro D, Mattia E, Bridges K, Klausner RD (1984) Molec Cell Biol 5: 595-600
14. Rouault T, Rao K, Harford J, Mattia E, Klausner RD (submitted to J Biol Chem)
15. Kuhn LC, McClelland A, Ruddle FH (1984) Cell 37: 95-103
16. Rao KK, Harford J, Rouault T, McClelland A, Ruddle FH (submitted to Cell)
17. Weissman A, Klausner RD, Rao KK, Harford J (submitted to J Cell Biol)
18. Schneider C, Sutherland R, Newmann R, Greaves M (1982) J Biol Chem 257: 8516-8522
19. Goodfellow PN, Banting G, Sutherland DR, Greaves MF, Solomon E, Povey S (1982) Somat Cell Genet 8: 197-206
20. Roth RA, Maddux Ba, Cassell DJ (1983) J Biol Chem 258: 12094-12097
21. Taylor SI, Marcus-Samuels B (1984) J Clin Endocrin Metab 58: 182-186
22. von Figura K, Gieselmann U, Hasilik A (1984) EMBO J 3: 1281-1286
23. Gregoriou M, Rees AR (1984) J 3: 929-937
24. Hopkins CR, Trowbridge IS (1983) J Cell Biol 97: 508-521
25. Klausner RD, Harford J, van Renswoude J (1984) Proc Natl Acad Sci USA 81: 3005-3009
26. Farquhar MG (1983) Meth. Enzymol 98: 1-13

Receptor-Mediated Endocytosis of Mannose-Terminated Glycoproteins in Hepatocytes

HELGE TOLLESHAUG[1], RUNE BLOMHOFF[2], HEIDI K. BLOMHOFF[4],
TROND BERG[2], and TERJE B. CHRISTENSEN[3]

[1] Institute for Experimental Medical Research
[2] Institute for Nutrition Research, and
[3] Institute of Biochemistry, University of Oslo
[4] Norsk Hydro's Institute for Cancer Research, The Norwegian Radium Hospital, Oslo, Norway

The parenchymal cells of the liver contain more than 90% of the total hepatic binding capacity for glycoproteins terminating in mannose or N-acetylglucosamine [1, 2]. It was thought that all of this binding capacity was intracellular; mannose-specific uptake of glycoproteins by hepatocytes was suspected [3, 4], but it was not definitely shown to occur until recently [5]. In order to obtain detailed evidence for the receptor-mediated endocytosis of mannose-terminated proteins in hepatocytes, we used a glycoprotein ligand with a high molecular weight: yeast invertase. It contains about 50% mannose by weight in several large polymannose chains which are attached to the peptide via two N-acetylglucosamine residues [6, 7].

Distribution of invertase among liver cell types in the intact rat

Following injection of a trace amount of labelled yeast invertase into rats, 64 ± 13% (S.D., n = 4) of the radioactivity was recovered in the liver after 10-13 min. Of this amount, 38% ended up in the parenchymal cells. An even higher fraction (52%) was found in the endothelial cells. When the recoveries were recomputed to give invertase content per cell, it turned out that each parenchymal cell or Kupffer cell (liver macrophage) contained about the same amount of ligand, while endothelial cells contained 3-4 times more [5]. The recoveries were not corrected for loss of radioactivity due to degradation of invertase during the cell purification procedure.

Uptake of yeast invertase in hepatocytes

[125]I-invertase was added to a suspension of purified rat hepatocytes at 37° C, either the labelled tracer alone or along with unlabelled invertase. The concentrations used ranged between 0.06 and 230 nM. The uptake was clearly saturable (Fig. 1), but a large fraction of the added ligand was taken up even at the highest concentration.

Contamination of the hepatocytes by nonparenchymal cells cannot account for the observed rate of endocytosis of invertase by the hepatocytes. The line of reasoning is this. The number of nonparenchymal cells in the hepatocyte preparation was certainly less than 2% of the total cell number; the uptake of invertase into

Receptor-Mediated Uptake
in the Liver
Edited by H. Greten, E. Windler, U. Beisiegel
© Springer-Verlag Berlin Heidelberg 1986

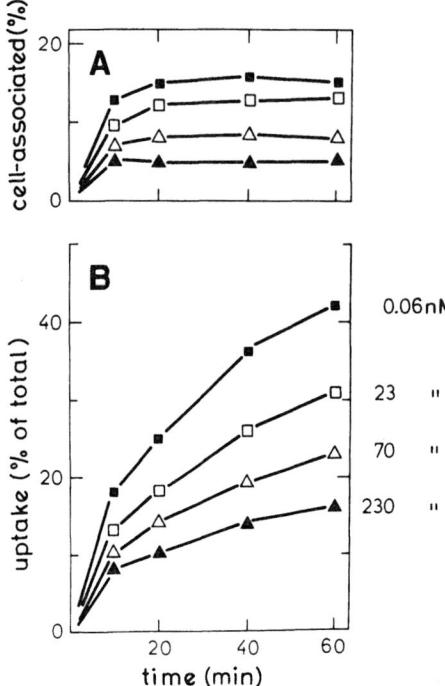

Fig. 1. Endocytosis of ^{125}I-invertase into purified hepatocytes. ■, 0.06 nM; □, 23 nM △, 70 nM; ▲, 230 nM yeast invertase in the initial cell suspension (10 million cells/ml).
Cell-associated radioactivity (upper panel) was determined after centrifuging the cells through oil. Acid-soluble radioactivity was also measured, and the sum of the cell-associated and the acid-soluble radioactivity were added at each time point in order to give total uptake (lower panel)

these two categories of cells proceeded at roughly the same rate (at the same concentrations of ligand) [5]. Consequently, the percentage of ligand molecules which entered nonparenchymal cells was less than 2% in the experiment shown in Fig. 1.

Ten to twenty minutes after the addition of the ligand, the number of cell-associated invertase molecules ceased to increase (Fig. 1). Subsequently, the number of molecules that were broken down equalled the number that entered the cells through receptor-mediated endocytosis. Degradation of invertase continued at the same rate for 90 minutes (not shown) provided the concentration of ligand in the medium was sufficient to support a constant rate of endocytosis. About 0.4% of the intracellular invertase molecules were degraded per minute.

The addition of a 1000-fold molar excess of either asialo-fetuin or asialo-orosomucoid had no effect on the endocytosis of yeast invertase. Treatment of the cell surface with neuraminidase reduced the endocytosis of asialo-fetuin to a small fraction of control values, but there was no effect on the uptake of invertase. However, yeast mannan had a very pronounced inhibitory effect, and so did α-methyl mannoside (Fig. 2) and N-acetyl-glucosamine, even though a high concentration of the inhibitors had to be added. The calcium ion chelator EGTA also inhibited the endocytosis of invertase by hepatocytes (Fig. 2); it is interesting to note that the mannose-binding protein of hepatocytes requires calcium ions [1, 2]. We were not able to measure the release of surface-bound invertase from hepatocytes by EGTA at 37° C by determining the amount of cell-associated radioactivity before and immediately after the addition of the chelator, presumably because the

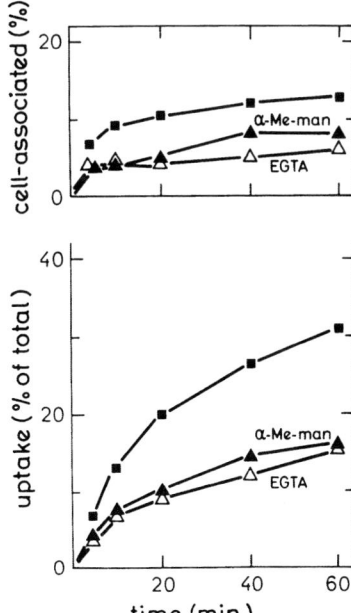

Fig. 2. Effects of α-methyl mannoside and EGTA on endocytosis of invertase. The cells were incubated with EGTA (3 mM) or α-methyl-mannoside (100 mM) for 10 min at 37° C. At time zero, 0.06 nM ^{125}I-invertase was added. Measurements and calculations are as in Fig. 1

amount of surfacebound ligand is very small compared to the total amount of cell-associated invertase.

These experiments show that the asialo-glycoprotein receptor is not involved in the uptake of yeast invertase by hepatocytes; the endocytosis may be mediated by a mannose/N-acetylglucosamine-binding protein with similar characteristics to that described previously [1, 2].

Intracellular distribution of invertase

Following endocytosis of asialo-fetuin (iodine-labelled) by hepatocytes and fractionation of the cells by isopycnic centrifuging in a sucrose gradient [8, 9], most of the ligand molecules are usually recovered in a single peak at a density close to 1.14 g/ml (Fig. 3). This peak contains only small amounts of lysosomal enzymes. The asialo-fetuin molecules in this part of the gradient are contained in a type of endosomes which deliver their contents to the lysosomes [8]. The lysosomes are found at 1.19-1.20 g/ml, and they usually contain very little labelled material because the degradation products cross the lysosomal membrane very quickly [9].

The intracellular distribution of invertase was different from that of asialo-fetuin. About 1/4 of the label from the invertase molecules was recovered in the lysosomal region of the gradient after a short incubation of the cells with ^{131}I-invertase (Fig. 3). In this experiment, extracellular invertase was removed after 10 min so that intracellular transport of the ligand could be studied without blurring of the picture by continuous influx of ligand into new endosomes. After 30

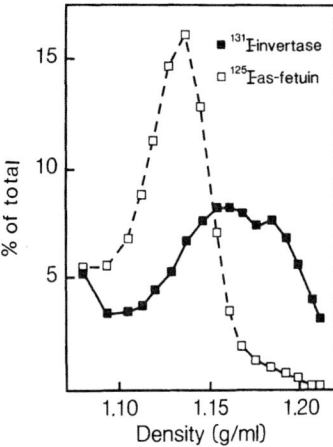

Fig. 3. Comparison of the intracellular distributions of invertase and asialo-fetuin. A hepatocyte suspension was incubated at 37° C in the presence of 0.2 nM ^{131}I-invertase and 0.04 nM ^{125}I-asialo-fetuin. After 10 min, the cells were chilled, washed twice in ice-cold medium in order to remove extracellular ligands, and reincubated for 10 min at 37° C. The cells were homogenized and fractionated by isopycnic centrifuging in a sucrose gradient [8, 9]

min of incubation in the absence of extracellular invertase, all of the ligand molecules had been transported into the lysosomes [5]. Thus, the rate of transport of invertase into the lysosomes is much higher than the corresponding rate for asialo-fetuin [9].

Even though invertase enters the lysosomes faster than asialo-fetuin does, invertase is degraded much more slowly. The reason is probably that the large carbohydrate chains shield the peptide from proteolytic attack [10].

General remarks

In the present study, we used a ligand of comparatively high molecular weight containing a very large number of terminal mannose residues. This ligand is probably able to compete efficiently with mannose-terminated glycoproteins which may contaminate the culture media. It may also be able to compete with mannose-terminated membrane proteins, which could be "natural" ligands of the hepatocyte mannose receptor on the cell surface.

"Leakage" of the intracellular receptor on to the cell surface may vary according to small variations in the conditions used during isolation and purification of hepatocytes: this has been shown to be a significant cause of variability in the surface binding capacity for asialo-glycoproteins [11]. For these and other reasons, we are not surprised that previous attempts to measure the uptake of mannose-terminated glycoproteins in hepatocytes have given divergent results [5, 12].

We were able to show that specific uptake of yeast invertase in hepatocytes occurs *in vivo* as well as *in vitro*. We also found that ß-galactosidase, a lysosomal enzyme which contains terminal mannose residues, is taken up into hepatocytes (Fig. 4) in analogy with previous work by Ullrich et al. [3]. It is an attractive possibility that the mannose receptor of hepatocytes serves to clear the circulation of

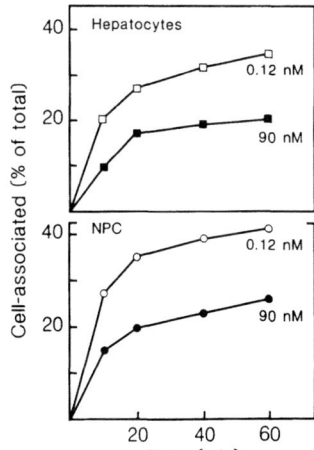

Fig. 4. Endocytosis of β-galactosidase by hepatocytes and nonparenchymal cells. Purified hepatocytes and a mixture of nonparenchymal cells (NPC) [5] were incubated with ^{125}I-β-galactosidase (from bovine testes) at two different concentrations

lysosomal enzymes possessing terminal mannose. This hypothesis would explain why hepatocytes are not seriously affected in I-cell disease [13], a condition in which newly synthesized lysosomal enzymes lack the Man-6-phosphate recognition marker. These enzymes are secreted into the circulation instead of being routed into the lysosomes. However, the defective enzymes could be taken up by hepatocytes (and also by macrophages, endothelial cells and other cell types possessing mannose-specific receptors)

References

1. Maynard Y, Baenziger JU (1982) J Biol Chem 257: 3788-3794
2. Mori K, Kawasaki T, Yamashina I (1983) Arch Biochem Biophys 222: 542-552
3. Ullrich K, Basner R, Gieselmann V, von Figura K (1979) Biochem J 180: 413-419
4. Prieels JP, Deschuyteneer M, May C, Wanson JC (1979) in Glycoconjugates (Schauer R, et al eds), pp 502-503 Georg Thieme Publishers Stuttgart
5. Tolleshaug H, Berg T, Blomhoff R (1984) Biochem J 223: 151-160
6. Trimble RB, Maley F (1977) J Biol Chem 252: 4409-4412
7. Lehle L (1980) Eur J Biochem 109: 589-601
8. Tolleshaug H (1984) Biochem Biophys Acta 803: 182-190
9. Tolleshaug H, Berg T (1981) Exp Cell Res 134: 207-217
10. Winkler JR, Segal H (1984) J Biol Chem 259: 1958-1962
11. Weigel PH (1980) J Biol Chem 255: 6111-6120
12. Madnick HM, Winkler JR, Segal HL (1978) Arch Biochem Biophys 191: 385-392
13. Neufeld EF, McKusick V (1983) in The metabolic Basis of Inherited Disease, 5th ed (Stanbury JB et al eds), pp 778-787 McGraw-Hill New York

Rapid Clearance of Lipoproteins and Liposomes by Hepatic Parenchymal or Kupffer Cells by Incorporation of a Tris-Galactoside-Terminated Cholesterol Derivative

H.J.M. Kempen[1], H.H. Spanjer[2], and T.J.C. van Berkel[3]

[1] Gaubius Institute TNO, Herenstraat 5d, 2313 AD Leiden
[2] Lab. Physiological Chemistry, Bloemsingel 10, 9712 KZ Groningen
[3] Dept. Biochemistry I, Erasmus University, P.O. Box 1738, 3000 DR Rotterdam

Introduction

A high plasma level of LDL increases the risk for atherosclerotic diseases [1, 2]. Any treatment to lower the plasma LDL level must either decrase the rate of LDL formation or speed up the rate of its clearance from the plasma. The latter can be effected by increasing the number or activity of the specific LDL-(or apo-B,E-) receptor in the liver, as is actually brought about by administration of bile acid sequestrants [3] and/or compactin or mevinolin [4].

Another strategy to enhance LDL clearance consists in modification of its surface leading to recognition of the particles by other receptors, not normally involved in LDL catabolism. This route became accessible by the synthesis of the triantennary galactosyl-terminated cholesterol derivative, N-(tris(β-galactosyloxymethyl) methyl)-N$^\alpha$-(cholesteryloxysuccinyl) glycinamide (tris-gal-chol).

This compound was found to dissolve easily in water and to attach itself with high affinity onto lipid particles like liposomes and lipoproteins [5]. These particles thereby are provided with galactosyl-moieties, able to be recognized by the hepatic lectin for asialoglycoproteins [6]. Previously, other workers have shown that lactosylated LDL is taken up effectively via this receptor by rat hepatocytes in culture [7].

In this chapter we describe the effect of incorporation of tris-gal-chol in radiolabeled liposomes and lipoproteins (LDL and HDL) on their clearance from the blood after intravenous injection in rats. Part of these data has been [5, 8] or shall be [9] published elsewhere.

Results and Discussion

Tris-gal-chol and liposomes

Small unilamellar vesicles composed of sphingomyelin and cholesterol (equimolar) and containing ^{14}C-inulin as marker for the internal space, were pretreated with tris-gal-chol (10 mole% of total lipid). This led to quantitative incorporation of tris-gal-chol in these particles, without causing leakage of the inulin [5]. Vesicles without tris-gal-chol are cleared very slowly from the plasma after intravenous injection, but after loading them with tris-gal-chol a portion of the liposomes is very rapidly cleared and taken up in the liver [5, 9]. After 10 min of circulation, the remaining tris-gal-chol liposomes disappear at the same slow rate as the unloaded vesicles, probably because they lose tris-gal-chol to plasma lipoproteins or blood cells. When the liver was taken out 10 min after injection of the loaded vesicles and perfused with collagenase at low temperature in order to isolate the different hepatic cell types, it was found that most of the label could be recovered in the Kupffer cells [9].

Expressed in another way, pretreatment of the vesicles with tris-gal-chol enhanced the uptake in the Kupffer cells about 10-fold, and that in the parenchymal cells by only 30-50%. This enhanced uptake was dependent on a galactose-Gal-NAc-receptor, since pre-injection of Gal-NAc (but not of Glc-NAc) could prevent the increased uptake nearly completely. There was no significant uptake in the liver endothelial cells [9].

Tris-gal-chol and LDL

Human LDL, isolated by density gradient centrifugation and radio-iodinated, was treated with tris-gal-chol in proportions between 0.05 and 10 μg per μg LDL-protein. As shown previously [10], human LDL is slowly cleared from the blood after intravenous injection in rats, and taken up mainly by the liver Kupffer cells. Incorporation of 0.2 μg or more tris-gal-chol per μg protein results in a dramatic increase of plasma clearance and liver uptake. As seen with the liposomes, there was a much greater stimulation of the uptake in the Kupffer cells than of that in the parenchymal cells [8]. Again, the stimulated uptake was mediated by a galactose-specific receptor, as deduced from the block exerted by Gal-NAc but not by Glc-NAc [8].

The uptake in both parenchymal and Kupffer cells is followed by transport of the LDL to and degradation in the lysosomes, as indicated by the appearance of trichloracid soluble radioactivity upon further incubation of the isolated cells at 37° C, and the inhibition of this appearance by ammonia and chloroquine [8].

Tris-gal-chol and HDL

The same kind of experiments were also done with radio-iodinated human HDL (apo-E free). Incorporation of tris-gal-chol in amounts of 0.2 μg or more per μg HDL-protein resulted in a dramatic increase of its plasma clearance and liver uptake, after intravenous injection in rats (Fig. 1). Now, however, by far the greatest part of label was recovered in the parenchymal cells, after isolation of the various cells by the cold collagenase technique. Pretreatment of HDL with 0.65 μg tris-gal-chol per μg protein led to 100-fold increase in uptake by parenchymal cells, and only 5-fold increase in the Kupffer cell uptake (Fig. 2). The enhanced liver association could be prevented by pre-injection of Gal-NAc (Fig. 3), attesting to the involvement of a galactose-specific uptake mechanism. As shown in Figure 1 the

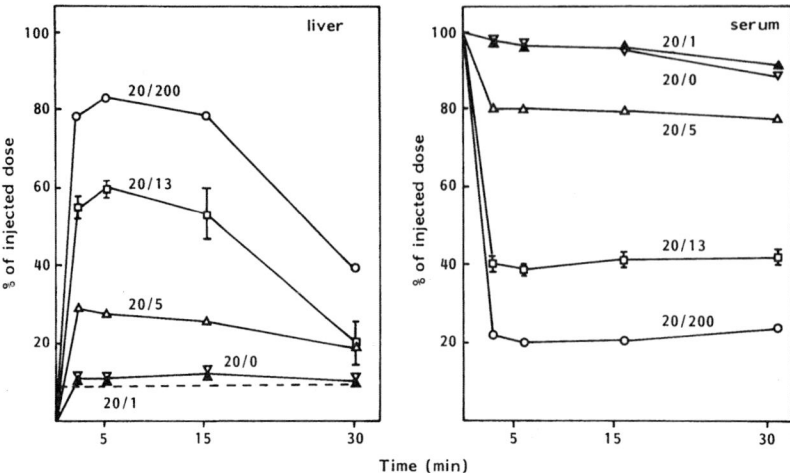

Fig. 1. Effect of Tris-Gal-Chol on the liver-association and serum decay of HDL. ^{125}I-HDL (20 μg of apolipoprotein) was mixed with 0 ( ); 1 (▲); 5 (Δ); 13 (□); or 200 μg of Tris-Gal-Chol (0). The mixture was injected into anesthesized rats and the liver-association and serum decay was determined. When indicated, bars represent S.E. for 3 animals. The livers were not perfused and the dotted line represents the maximal contribution of the serum value to the liver uptake (determined with ^{3}H-albumin)

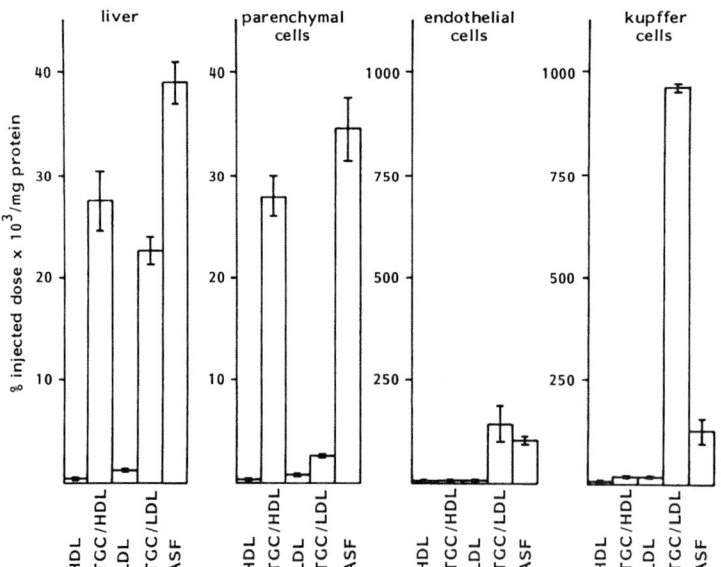

Fig. 2. The effect of Tris-Gal-Chol on the association of HDL and LDL to parenchymal, endothelial and Kupffer cells in comparison to the association of asialofetuin. ^{125}I-HDL or ^{125}I-LDL (20 μg of apolipoprotein) were mixed with 13 μg of Tris-Gal-Chol (TGC/HDL or TGC/LDL) or the equivalent amount of PBS (HDL or LDL). Ten minutes after injection of the apolipoproteins or ^{125}I-asialofetuin (9 μg), a liver perfusion was started and the total liver association (after an 8-min perfusion at 8° C) and the association to the subsequently isolated (at 8° C) parenchymal, endothelial and Kupffer cells was determined. The bars represent values ± S.E. (n = 3)

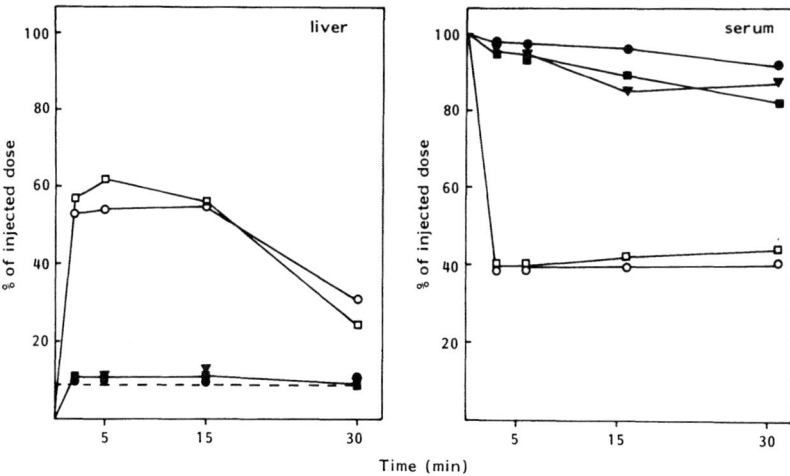

Fig. 3. Effect of asialofetuin, GalNAc and GlcNAc on the liver-association and serum-decay of Tris-Gal-Chol HDL. ^{125}I-HDL (20 µg of apolipoprotein) was mixed with 13 µg of Tris-Gal-Chol. One min prior to injection of Tris-Gal-Chol HDL, either solvent (□) 5 mg (▼) or 25 mg asialofetuin (■), 0.5 mmol GalNAc (●) or 0.5 mmol GlcNAc (○) was preinjected. Further conditions as in Fig. 1

amount of a label in the liver reaches its maximum after 5 min. The subsequent loss of label is probably due to breakdown of the HDL-apoproteins and discharge of the products. Evidence for the involvement of lysosomes was obtained in this case by pre-treatment of the rats with chloroquine or leupeptin prior to the injection of tris-gal-chol HDL. As can be seen in Fig. 4, this caused a marked decrease of label disappearance from the liver.

Fig. 4. The effect of leupeptin and chloroquine on the liver association of Tris-Gal-Chol HDL. ^{125}I-HDL (20 µg of apolipoprotein) was mixed with 13 µg of Tris-Gal-Chol. The mixtures were injected into rats who were preinjected with 5 mg leupeptin (60 min prior to the lipoproteins), or with chloroquine (120 and 60 min prior to injection of the lipoproteins). The control was preinjected at 60 min prior to the lipoproteins with PBS. The bars represent values ± S.E. (n = 3). Further conditions are as described in the legend to Fig. 1

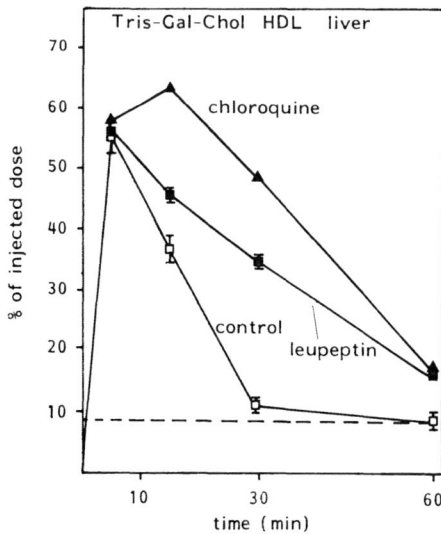

Table 1. Relative contribution of the different liver cell types to the total liver uptake of asialofetuin, tris-gal-chol HDL and tris-gal-chol LDL

Cell type	Asialofetuin	Tris-Gal-Chol HDL	Tris-Gal-Chol LDL
Parenchymal cells (%)	82.5	98.0	7.7
Endothelial cells (%)	9.3	0.5	15.5
Kupffer cells (%)	8.2	1.5	76.8

The amount of radioactivity per mg cell protein in the isolated cell fractions was multiplied with the amount of protein that each cell type contributes to total liver protein. Lipoproteins (20 μg apolipoproteins) were mixed with 13 μg tris-gal-chol. The values are calculated from the mean of 3 independent experiments for each substrate

Asialofetuin, clearance and effect as blocker of tris-gal-chol mediated uptake

In separate experiments we studied the fate of radio-iodinated asialofetuin in the rats. This protein was rapidly cleared from the blood and taken up by the liver, as expected from the published observations of many other workers. Upon isolation of the various liver cells by the cold collagenase procedure, the label was found mostly in parenchymal cells, and only for a small part (about 17%) in Kupffer and endothelial cells (Table 1). This is in good agreement with the autoradiographic findings of Hubbard et al. [11]. Uptake of labeled asialofetuin was greatly decreased by pre-injection of Gal-NAc or of 25 mg unlabeled asialofetuin.

Interestingly, pre-injection of 25 mg asialofetuin inhibited the effect of tris-gal-chol on the uptake of LDL in parenchymal cells, while it had no effect on the uptake of these particles in the Kupffer cells [8]. On the other hand, the plasma clearance and liver uptake of tris-gal-chol HDL was strongly depressed by pre-injection of only 5 mg asialofetuin (Fig. 3).

These effects confirm the findings described above on the difference in cell type involved in the uptake of tris-gal-chol LDL (Kupffer cells) or that of tris-gal-chol HDL (parenchymal cells), respectively.

The marked contrast in cellular destination between loaded LDL and HDL (see Table 1 for a comparison) might be due to the difference in size of these two lipoproteins. Roos et al. have shown previously [12] that the distribution of colloidal gold particles loaded with asialofetuin among parenchymal and nonparenchymal cells strongly depends on the size of the gold particle. Particles with a diameter of less than 10 nm could readily enter into both parenchymal and Kupffer cells, while those with diameters of 17 nm and larger ended up solely in the Kupffer cells. As yet, it is uncertain whether the same or different receptors is/are present in the two cell types.

These studies are the first phase in evaluation of tris-gal-chol as a potential hypocholesterolemic pharmacon. In this respect, the finding of enhanced removal of LDL via stimulation of Kupffer cell uptake is not ideal. It remains to be seen, if the LDL-cholesterol introduced in these cells can be transported to parenchymal cells and bile. Studies exploring this possibility are presently carried out. Concerning the increased removal of HDL by the parenchymal cells, this can be considered as a means to speed up the rate of centripetal cholesterol transport.

References

1. Wilson PW, Garrison RJ, Castelli WP, Feinleib M, McNamara PM, Kannel WB (1980) Am J Cardiol 46: 649-654
2. Goldstein JL, Brown MS (1977) Metab Clin Exp 26: 1257-1275
3. Slater HR, Packard CJ, Bicker S, Shepherd J (1980) J Biol Chem 255: 10210-10213
4. Kovanen PT, Bilheimer DW, Goldstein JL, Jamarillo JJ, Brown MS (1981) Proc Natl Acad Sci USA 78: 1194-1198
5. Kempen HJM, Hoes C, Van Boom JH, Spanjer HH, De Lange J, Langendoen A, Van Berkel TJC (1984) J Med Chem 27: 1306-1312
6. Ashwell G, Morell AG (1974) Adv Enzymol 41: 99-128
7. Attie AR, Pittman RC, Steinberg D (1980) Proc Natl Acad Sci USA 77: 5923-5927
8. Van Berkel TJC, Kruyt JK, Spanjer HH, Nagelkerke JF, Harkes L, Kempen HJM (1985) J Biol Chem 260: 2694-2699
9. Spanjer HH, Van Berkel TJC, Scherphof G, Kempen HJM (1985) Biochim Biophys Acta (in press)
10. Harkes L, Van Berkel TJC (1984) Biochem J 224: 21-27
11. Hubbard A, Wilson G, Ashwell G, Stukenbrok H (1979) J Cell Biol 83: 47-64
12. Roos PH, Kolb-Bachofen V, Schlepper-Schaefer J et al (1983) FEBS Letters 157: 253-256

Intracellular Degradation of Asialoglycoproteins in Rat Hepatocytes Studied by Fractionation in Nycodenz Gradients

T. Berg, G. Kindberg, T. Ford, and R. Blomhoff

Institute for Nutrition Research, University of Oslo, P.O. Box 1046 Blindern, 0316 Oslo 3, Norway

Introduction

Information about the intracellular transport of endocytosed ligands may be obtained by subcellular fractionation studies. We have used this approach to follow the intracellular path of asialoglycoproteins in isolated rat liver parenchymal cells (PC). In these studies asialoorosomucoid labeled with ^{125}I-tyramine cellobiose (^{125}I-TC-AOM) was used. When ligands labeled in this way are degraded, the labeled degradation products are trapped in the lysosomes as they do not penetrate the lysosomal membrane. Therefore, in subcellular fractionation studies the labeled degradation products may serve as markers for the organelles in which they are formed.

Experimental Design

Male Wistar rats (200 g) were used. Isolated rat liver parenchymal cells were prepared by collagenase perfusion of the liver [1]. ^{125}I-TC-AOM was prepared according to Pittman et al. [2]. Nycodenz gradients were prepared by mixing 0.25 M sucrose and 45% (w/v) Nycodenz [3, 4]. The uptake of ^{125}I-TC-AOM into the cells was synchronized by allowing the ligand first to bind to the surface receptors of the cells at 4° C. Then after removing the extracellular ligand the cells were transferred to 37° C, and at various times postnuclear fractions were prepared and centrifuged in Nycodenz gradients. Centrifugations were carried out in the Beckman SW 27 rotor at 85,000 x g. When the centrifugation time was kept short (45 min) it was found that small endocytic vesicles did not reach equilibrium density and could therefore be separated from larger endocytic vesicles and lysosomes [3]. Therefore, in most experiments the gradients were centrifuged for 45 min at 85,000 x g. The distribution of β-acetylglucosaminidase (β-AGA) was used as a marker for the lysosomes. All experiments were done with suspensions of PC. The cells were kept in a simple salt medium containing 1% albumin [5]. The cell concentration was about 5 x 10^6 cells/ml

Receptor-Mediated Uptake
in the Liver
Edited by H. Greten, E. Windler, U. Beisiegel
© Springer-Verlag Berlin Heidelberg 1986

Results and Discussion

Subcellular distribution of degraded and undegraded ^{125}I-TC-AOM in control cells

Fig. 1 shows the distribution of degraded (acid soluble) and undegraded (acid precipitable) ^{125}I-TC-AOM in Nycodenz gradients after centrifuging postnuclear fractions from cells that were incubated at 37° C for 1, 15, 30, 60 and 90 min. Prior to the incubation at 37° C the cells were allowed to bind ligand at 4° C for 1 hour. The result presented show that the ligand early (< 1 min) after uptake into the cells was in an organelle which banded at a relatively low density in the gradient (about 1.05 g/ml). At longer time intervals the ligand was transferred to more rapidly sedimenting structures (about 1.10 g/ml). The different distribution of "early" and "late" vesicles was due to differences in size and not in density. When the centrifugation time at 85,000 x g was extended from 45 min to 2 hours, the distribution of "early" and "late" vesicles nearly coincided [3]. The early small vesicles may be coated vesicles as the transit time for the ligand in these structures corresponds closely to that observed by electron microscopic techniques [6].

Analysis of acid soluble radioactivity in the cell suspensions revealed that degradation of the ligand started about 15 min after the start of its internalization. The first degradation products appeared in the Nycodenz gradient at a density of about 1.10 g/ml and coincided with the distribution of undegraded ligand (Fig. 1b). Fractionation of cells that had been incubated for longer time intervals revealed an additional peak of degradation products at about 1.13 g/ml. More and more acid soluble radioactivity became associated with the denser peak with time of incubation at 37° C. The present data indicate that degradation is initiated in a relatively light lysosome and completed in a denser lysosome. The distribution of a lysosomal marker enzyme (β-AGA) in the gradient showed a main peak at 1.14 g/ml. However, a "shoulder" could be seen coinciding with the "early" degradation products (Fig. 1f).

To get additional information about the relationship between the structures containing ligand we studied the effects of various inhibitors on the subcellular distribution of degraded and undegraded ^{125}I-TC-AOM.

Colchicine, an inhibitor of microtubuli formation, reduced the formation of acid soluble radioactivity in both the light and the dense lysosome (Fig. 2). It probably did not inhibit degradation as such, since no undegraded ligand accumulated in the dense lysosome. The drug probably prevented the uptake of ligand into the lysosomes by interfering with fusion between endosomes and lysosomes or with the directed movement of the organelles.

Leupeptin also strongly inhibited the formation of acid soluble radioactivity both in the light and the dense lysosomes (Fig. 3). Interestingly, leupeptin, in contrast to colchicine, did not prevent transfer of ligand to the dense lysosomes, and acid precipitable radioactivity accumulated in these organelles. This result suggests that the light lysosomes does not change gradually into a dense lysosome in parallel with ongoing degradation of ligand; rather, the light lysosome empties its contents into the dense lysosome. The dense lysosome containing labeled ligand could conceivably arise by fusion between the light-lysosome and a dense body. In accordan-

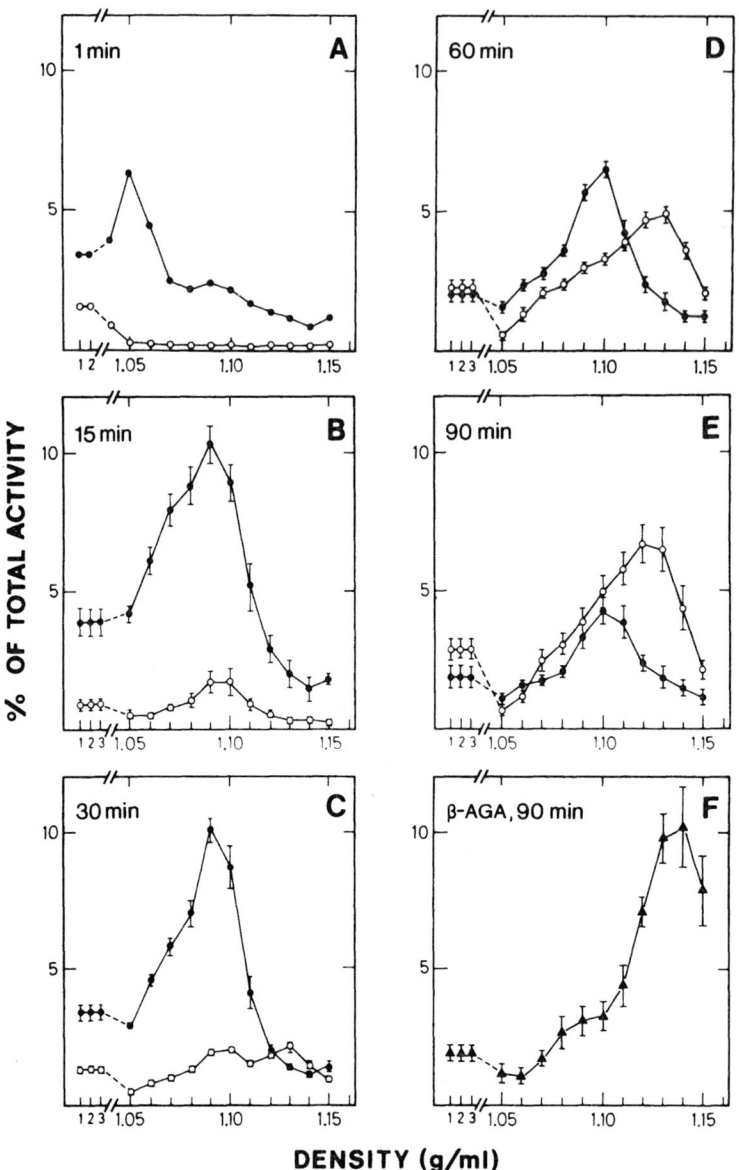

Fig. 1. Subcellular fractionation of hepatocytes containing degraded (○) or undegraded (●) ^{125}I-TC-AOM. The cells were first incubated at 4° C for 1 h in the presence of 50 nM ^{125}I-TC-AOM, and after removing extracellular ligand incubated at 37° C. At the indicated times cell aliquots were removed and fractionated in linear Nycodenz gradients. Panels A-E show distribution of acid soluble (○) and acid precipitable (●) radioactivity, and panel F shows the distribution of β-acetylglucosaminidase for cells incubated for 90 min. Radioactivities are presented as % of total cell-associated radioactivity at the start of the incubation at 37° C. Total cell-associated radioactivity changed insignificantly during the incubation at 37° C. β-acetylglucosaminidase is presented as % of total recovered activity in the gradient. Panel A (cells incubated 1 min at 37° C) shows the results from one typical experiment. The other results are means ± S.E. for 6 experiments

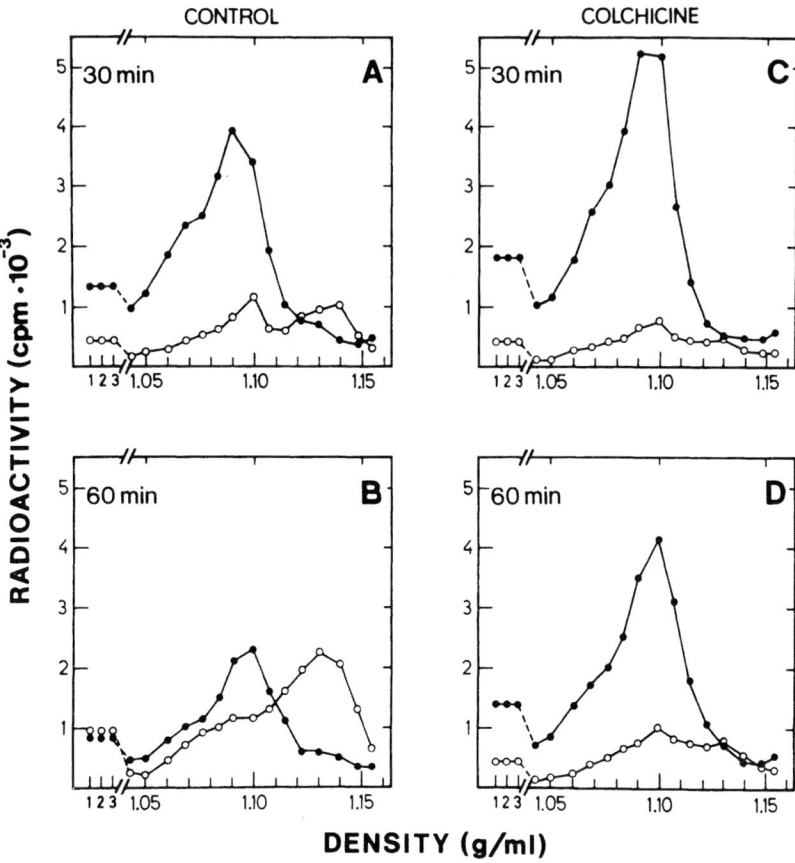

Fig. 2. Effect of colchicine on the distribution of degraded (○) and undegraded (●) ^{125}I-TC-AOM after centrifugation in Nycodenz gradients. Cells containing surface-bound ^{125}I-TC-AOM were incubated at 37° C in the presence or absence (control) of 100 μM colchicine. After 30 (A, C) and 60 (B, D) min samples of cells were removed and fractionated in Nycodenz gradients

ce with this notion the dense ligand containing lysosome was at a slightly lower density than the main peak of lysosomal enzymes. It is likely that the fusion between a light lysosome and a dense body results in a lysosome with an intermediary density.

Monensin disrupts proton gradients and would be expected to elevate pH in endosomes and lysosomes. Monensin practically abolished degradation (Fig. 4). However, no undegraded ligand seemed to accumulate at the position of the lysosomal enzyme β-AGA in the gradient. Therefore, monensin like colchicine prevented the uptake of ^{125}I-TC-AOM in the lysosomes. This is in accordance with earlier reports [7]. When monensin was added to cells that internalized surface bound ligand, it consistently led to two peaks in the distribution of ligand in the gradient

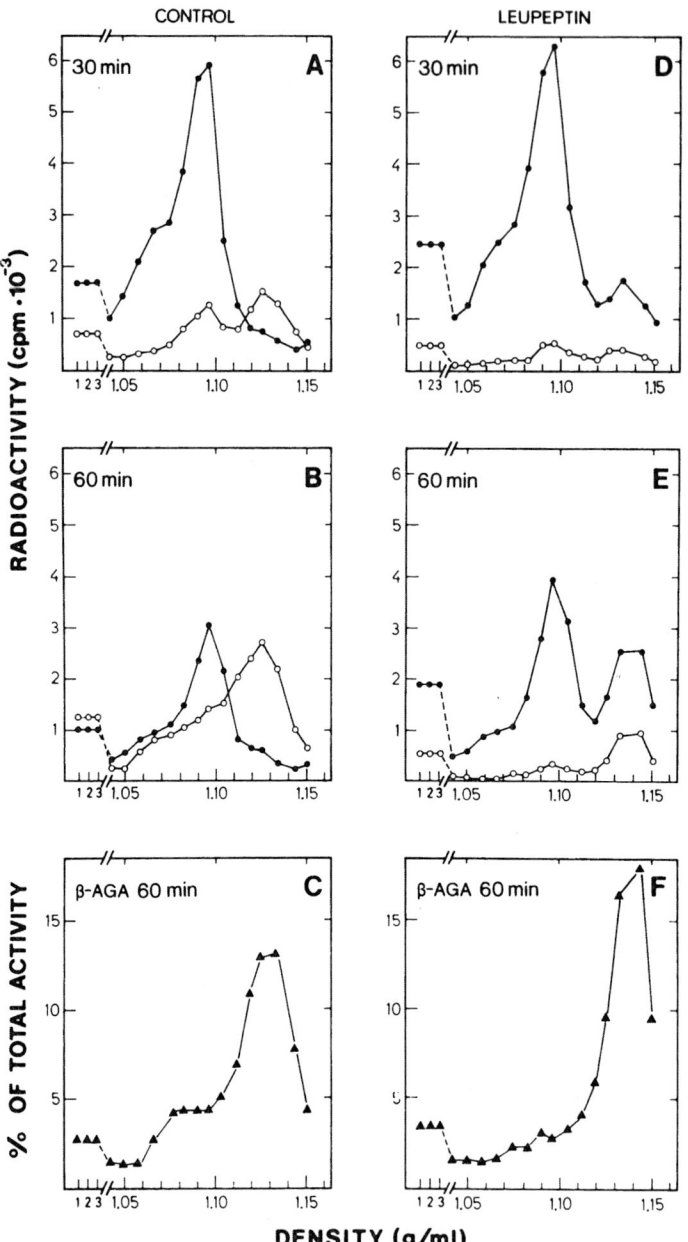

Fig. 3. Effect of leupeptin (0.05 mg/ml) on the distribution of degraded (○) and undegraded (●) ^{125}I-TC-AOM after centrifugation in Nycodenz gradients. Cells with surface-bound ligand were incubated at 37° C in presence (right panels) and absence (left panels) of leupeptin. Cell samples were fractionated in Nycodenz gradients after 30 and 60 min of incubation. Acid soluble and acid precipitable radioactivities as well as β-acetylglucosaminidase were measured in the gradient fractions. The two lower panels show the distribution of ß-acetylglucosaminidase for cells which had been incubated for 1 h in the absence (C) or the presence (F) of leupeptin

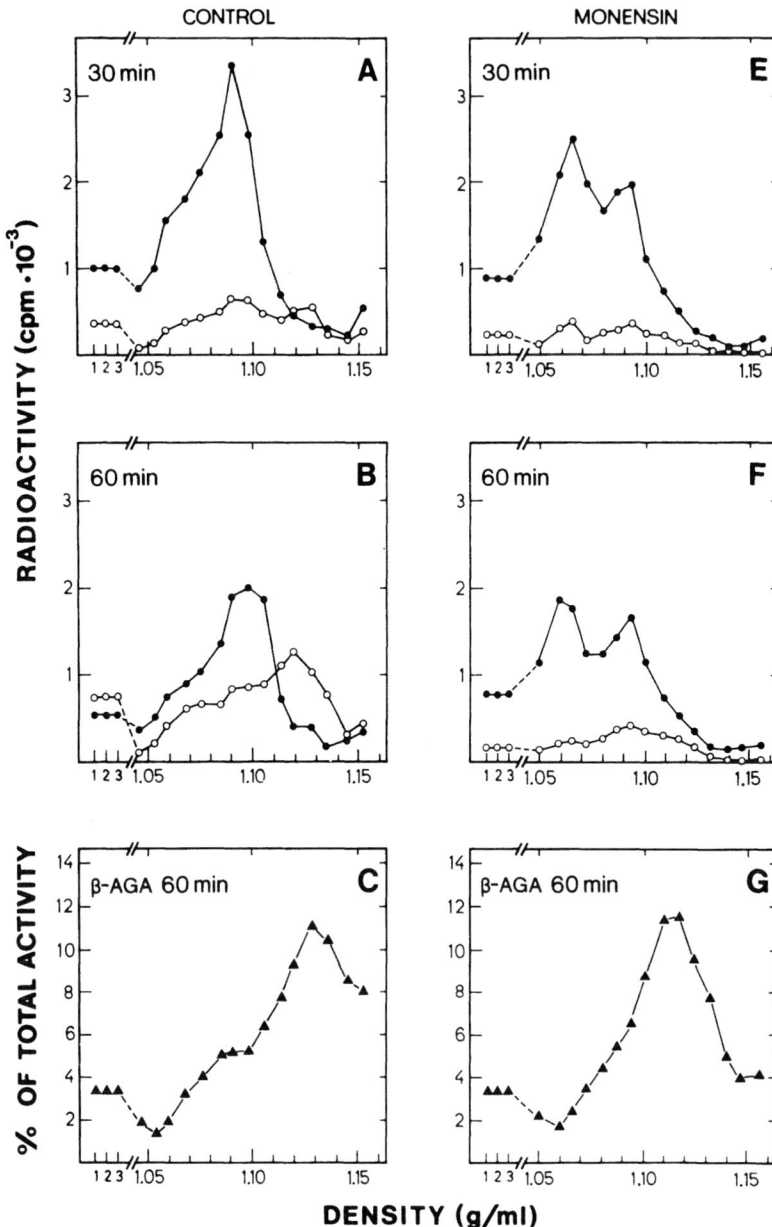

Fig. 4. Effect of monensin on the distribution of degraded (○) and undegraded (●) ^{125}I-TC-AOM after centrifugation in Nycodenz gradients. The cells were incubated for 1 h at 4° C in presence of 50 nM ^{125}I-TC-AOM and then, after washing to remove extracellular ligand incubated at 37° C in the presence (E, F, G) or absence (A, B, C) of 25 μM monensin. Aliquots of cells, removed after 30 and 60 min, were fractionated by centrifugation in Nycodenz gradients (as detailed in the method section). The two lower panels show the distributions of β-acetylglucosaminidase for control (C) and monensin-treated (G) cells incubated for 1 h at 37° C

(Fig. 4). The peak at lower density could be identical to the "early" vesicles, formed during the first minute after internalization of the ligand (Fig. 1a), and the effect of monensin could be to retard the transfer of ligand to the larger endosome. However, if monensin were added to cells that had first internalized ligand for 15 min or more, it again induced the formation of a peak at lower density, in addition of the peak at 1.10 g/ml (Fig. 5). Fig. 5 shows that the effect of monensin was established gradually during 15 min. However, even after 60 min two peaks were still discernible in the gradient. Thus, monensin did not direct all the ligand into a light vesicle; some of the ligand seemed to be in an organelle that was insensitive to monensin. Possibly, the ligand may be in an acid and a neutral compartment, and only the acid compartment is influenced by monensin. Monensin leads to rebinding of ligand to the receptor, if both the receptor and the ligand are in the same compartment [8]. The most likely explanation of the monensin induced light peak is that ligand remains associated with the receptor when the receptor is segregated into a vesicle destined for recycling to the plasma membrane.

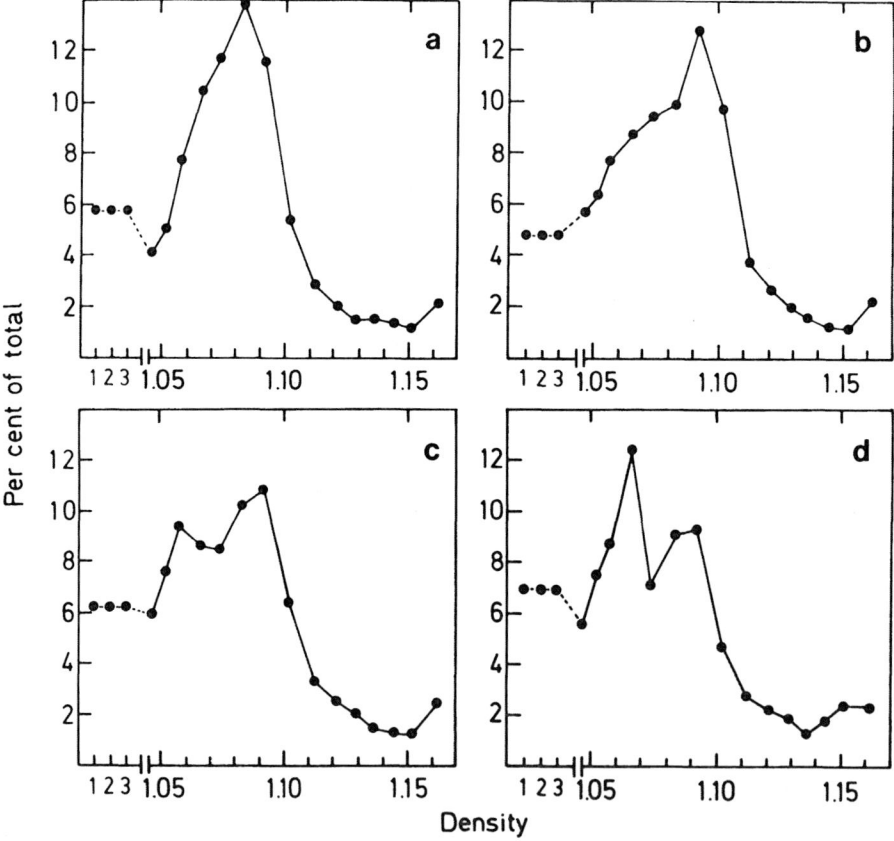

Fig. 5. The effect of adding monensin to cells which had internalized ^{125}I-TC-AOM for 15 min at 37° C. Cells with surface bound ligand were incubated at 37° C for 15 min (**a**). Monensin (25 μM) was then added and the incubation was continued for 1 min (**b**), 5 min (**c**), and 15 min (**d**)

Such a vesicle is probably small, and the progressive accumulation of ligand into this vesicle is also compatible with the notion that it is involved in recycling. If monensin "forces" ligand into a small recycling vesicle because it elevates intravesicular pH, then one would expect a similar effect of lysosomotropic amines. This was indeed found to be the case. The addition of ammonia (10 mM) to the cells led to two peaks in the distribution curve for ^{125}I-TC-AOM (not shown). It is tempting to relate the "monensin-insensitive" ligand-containing vesicle to the observation that substantial fractions of asialoglycoprotein ligands endocytosed by PC can subsequently be returned to the cell surface still bound to the receptor [9]. By adding EGTA to the cells 25-50% of the intracellular ligand may be released to the medium [9]. Since the ligand dissociated from the receptor at low pH it is conceivable that the recycling ligand is passed through a non-acidic intracellular compartment. This compartment could be the "monensin-insensitive" endosome. Interestingly, monensin and ammonia have been found not to influence the EGTA-induced release of asialoorosomucoid from rat PC [10]. We have also found that EGTA-induced ligand release from the cells reduces the peak of labeled ligand at 1.10 g/ml (the monensin-insensitive peak).

Summary

The present fractionation studies suggest that asialoglycoprotein ligands during their metabolism in PC are sequentially associated with at least 6 compartments (see Fig. 6):

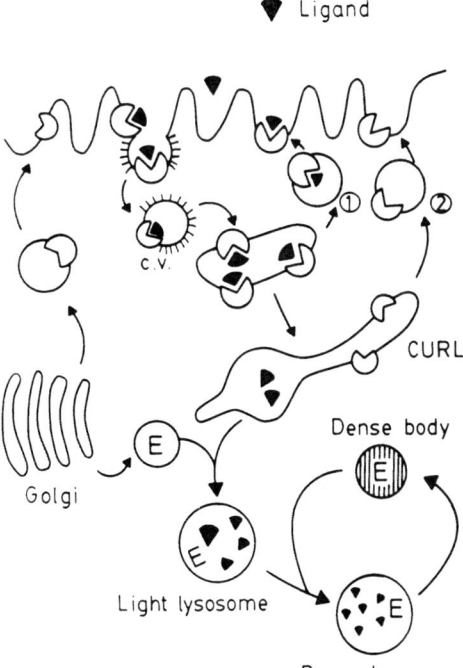

Fig. 6. Steps in the uptake and intracellular transport of asialoglycoproteins. Following binding in coated pits the receptor-ligand complex is internalized into coated vesicles (c.v.). These form an endosome from which the receptor-ligand complex may be recycled to the plasma membrane [1]. Larger endosomes (CURL) are formed in which ligand dissociates from the receptor due to drop in pH. A light lysosome is formed by uptake of primary lysosomes. By fusion with a dense body a dense lysosome is formed

1. The plasma membrane,
2. coated vesicles,
3. larger endosomes,
4. light lysosomes,
5. dense lysosomes.

Recycling of ligand may in addition be associated with a neutral vesicle.

In the presence of monensin all internalized ligand is bound to the receptors, and may, as suggested above, also follow the receptor in the enigmatic recycling vesicle.

Acknowledgements. The authors are grateful to Mrs. Ba Gørbitz for preparing the manuscript. The work was financially supported by the Norwegian Council for Science and the Humanities, the Nansen Foundation, and the Norwegian Council on Cardiovascular Diseases.

References

1. Seglen PO (1976) Methods in cell biology (ed DM Prescott) Adacemic Press New York vol 13: 29
2. Pittman RC, Carew TE, Glass CK, Green SR, Taylor CA, Attie AD (1983) Biochem J 212: 791
3. Kindberg GM, Ford T, Blomhoff R, Rickwood D, Berg T (1984) Anal Biochem 142: 455
4. Berg T, Ford T, Kindberg GM, Blomhoff R, Drevon CA (1985) Exp Cell Res 156: 319
5. Nilsson M, Berg T (1977) Biochem Biophys Acta 497: 171
6. Wall DA, Wilson G, Hubbard AL (1980) Cell 21: 79
7. Berg T, Blomhoff R, Naess L, Tolleshaug H, Drevon CA (1983) Exp Cell Res 148: 319
8. Harford J, Wolkoff AW, Ashwell G, Klausner RD (1983) J Cell Biol 96: 1824
9. Weigel P, Oka JA (1984) J Biol Chem 259: 1150
10. Chang TM, Kullberg DW (1984) Biochem Biophys Acta 805: 268

The Effect of Monensin on Receptor-Mediated Endocytosis of Asialofetuin and Secretion of Very Low Density Lipoproteins (VLDL) by Cultured Rat Hepatocytes

C.A. DREVON[1], A.C. RUSTAN[2], J.Ø. NOSSEN[2], and T. BERG[3]

[1] National Institute of Forensic Toxicology, Oslo, and
[2] Department of Pharmacology, Institute of Pharmacy and
[3] Institute for Nutrition Research, University of Oslo, Norway

Monensin is a carboxylic ionophore which is able to abolish ionic gradients across membranes (Pressman, 1976). There are indications that monensin inhibits fluid-phase endocytosis (Wilcox et al., 1982), entry of virus particles into fibroblasts and receptor-mediated endocytosis of LDL (Basu et al., 1981) and asialoglycoproteins (Berg et al., 1983). Monensin may cause swelling of the Golgi cisternae and decrease secretion of procollagen, fibronectin (Uchida et al., 1979) and immunoglobulins (Tartakoff and Vasalli, 1977). Certain experiments on endocytosis of epidermal growth factor, β-galactosidase, α_2-macroglobulin (Pastan and Willingham, 1981), insulin (Posner et al., 1982) and asialofetuin (Debanne et al., 1982) suggest that endosomes are directed to the Golgi complex. Conceivably, endo- and exocytosis might have a common pathway through this membrane system.

To test this possibility we studied endocytosis of asialoglycoproteins and exocytosis of VLDL under similar conditions in cultured rat hepatocytes. We also studied the effect of another proton gradient disrupting agent, DCCD, on VLDL secretion. Primary cultures of rat hepatocytes have maintained the selective ability to secrete VLDL (Davis et al., 1979, Drevon et al., 1980) and to bind, internalize and degrade asialoglycoproteins (Drevon et al., 1983), making these cells a good model for simulatenous studies of endo- and exocytosis.

Methods

Rat hepatocytes were isolated and plated in DME medium containing newborn calf serum (20%), glucose (20 mM), bovine insulin (10 ug/ml) and gentamicin (50 ug/ml). After overnight incubation, the cells were transferred to serum-free DME medium and monensin was added as fresh ethanolic solution (Rustan et al., 1985).

Asialofetuin was prepared and labeled with 125-I. Binding of labeled asialofetuin was measured after incubation at 4° C as EGTA-releaseable radioactivity (Drevon et al., 1983).

Secretion of VLDL triacylglycerol (TG) was measured as (3H)glycerol incorporated into medium TG. More than 95% of the secreted tritiated TG was recovered in the VLDL fraction as evaluated by ultracentrifugation (Nossen et al., 1984). Electron microscopy of the cells and measurement of protein synthesis were performed as described elsewhere (Nossen et al., 1984).

Receptor-Mediated Uptake
in the Liver
Edited by H. Greten, E. Windler, U. Beisiegel
© Springer-Verlag Berlin Heidelberg 1986

Results

Maximum inhibition of asialofetuin binding was about 60% of the control at 25 μM-monensin (Fig. 1). Scatchard plot analysis showed that the number of receptors decreased to half that was found in control cells, whereas the affinity was unaffected. Maximum inhibition of degradation of asialofetuin was 85% of the control at 25 μM-monensin. At 1 μM-monensin binding and degradation was hardly affected.

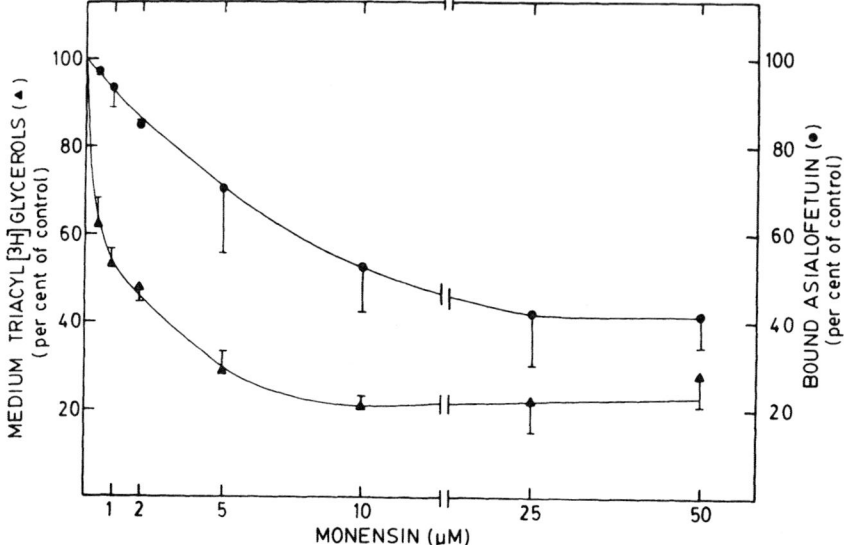

Fig. 1. Effect of monensin on binding of asialofetuin (●) and secretion of VLDL (▲). Asialofetuin binding: Hepatocytes were incubated in DME medium with increasing amounts of monensin at 37° C for 2 h, and then chilled on ice before (125I) asialofetuin (1 μ/ml) was added. After incubation at 4° C for 2 h, the amounts of EGTA- releasable (125I) asialofetuin was measured. Control value was equal to 17.4 ± 8.8 ng/mg of cell protein.
VLDL secretion: Hepatocytes were incubated in DME medium containing (3H)glycerol (5 μCi/ml). After 30 min preincubation, monensin was added and the cells were reincubated for 2 h before medium triacyl (3H)glycerols were measured. Control value was equal to 7000 cpm/mg of cell protein

Table 1. Effect of monensin on secretion of VLDL apolipoproteins and albumin

Monensin in media (μM)	Secreted proteins (% of controls)			
	Apo Bl	Apo Bs	Apo E	Albumin
0	100	100	100	100
5	4	17	25	25
25	13	0	4	16

Hepatocytes were incubated in DME medium containing 40 uCi/ml (3H)valine. After 60 min preincubation, the media were added monensin (0, 5 and 25 μM) and further incubated for 2 h. The amount of secreted, labeled VLDL apoproteins was determined after ultracentrifugation, SDS polyacrylamide gel electrophoresis (gradient (4/20%) and liquid scintillation. The data represent the means of two different experiments.
The apolipoprotein correspondend approximately for apo Bl (large) to MW 400,000, apo Bs (small) 250,000, apo E 33,000 and albumin 62,000, respectively

At 5 μM-monensin the secretion of (3H)TG was 25% of the control and even at 1 μM the secretion was decreased by about 50% (Fig. 1). The decreased secretion of VLDL-TG was also verified by mass measurement and was not due to a decrease in TG synthesis, as no change in cell-associated TG was found. The cellular content of α-glycerophosphate was not significantly affected by monensin. There was a marked inhibition of VLDL-apoprotein secretion at μM-monensin (Table 1).

It lasted 10-15 min before 10-25 μM-monensin decreased binding of asialofetuin (Fig. 2) and VLDL secretion (Fig. 3). The decreased binding of asialofetuin and secretion of VLDL caused by monensin was reversible 40-80 min after wash-out of the drug. Monensin did not affect the synthesis of TCA-precipitable (3H)labeled proteins as compared with controls at concentrations up to 50 μM, whereas secretion of these proteins decreased by 90%. By electron microscopy it was obvious that 5 μM-monensin caused a marked swelling of Golgi cisternae with VLDL particles trapped inside (Fig. 4).

We have also shown that other agents affecting proton gradients across membranes (chloroquine, propylamine, ammonia) can decrease asialofetuin binding as well as VLDL secretion (Drevon et al., 1983, Nossen et al., 1984). The addition of a proton ATP-ase inhibitor dicyclohexylcarbodiimide (DCCD) (Pedersen, 1982) also decreased secretion of VLDL-TG as shown in Fig. 5.

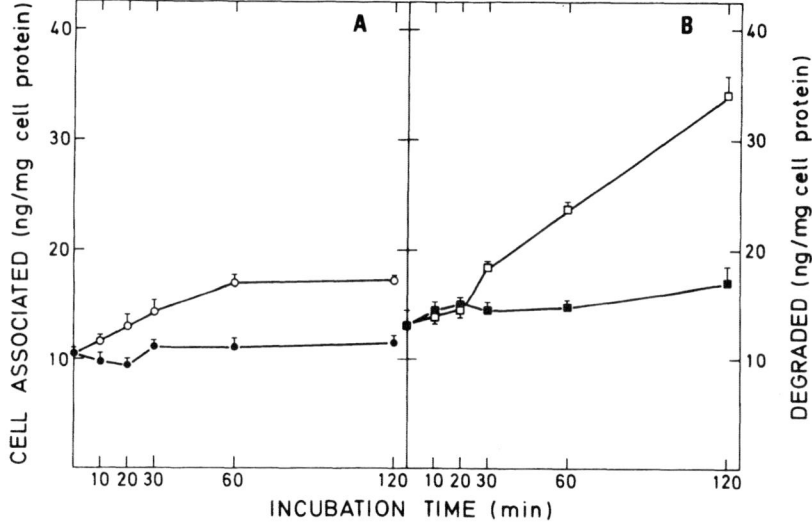

Fig. 2. Time course for the effect of monensin on cell-association (A) and degradation (B) of (125I) asialofetuin. Hepatocytes were incubated at 37° C in DME medium containing (^{125}I) asialofetuin (1 μg/ml). After 30 min preincubation, the cells were reincubated with (●, ■) or without (○, □) 25 μM monensin for the time periods indicated before cell-associated and degraded asialofetuin were measured.

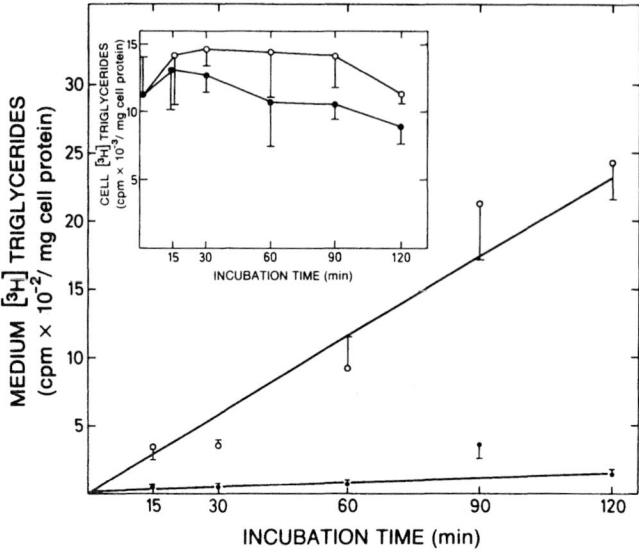

Fig. 3. Time course for the effect of monensin on secretion (main figure) and synthesis (inserted) of triacyl(3H)glycerols. Hepatocytes were incubated in DME medium containing (3H)glycerol. After 30 min preincubation, the cells were reincubated for the indicated periods with (●) or without (○) 10 μM monensin before triacyl(3H)glycerols in media and cells were determined

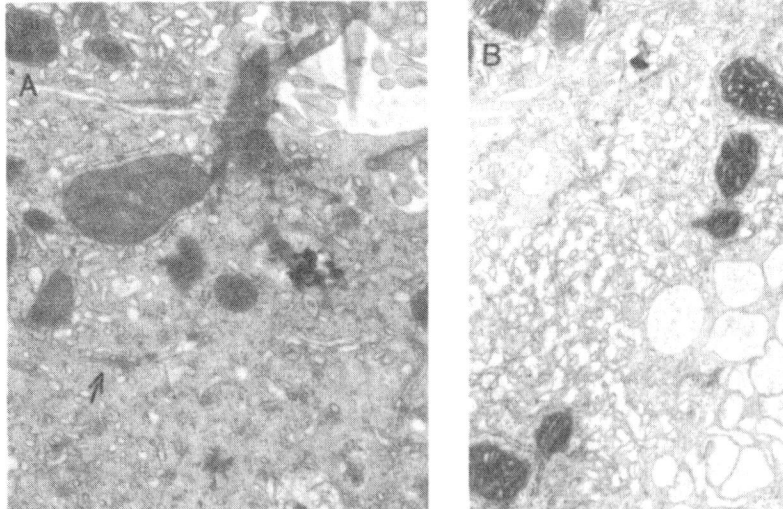

Fig. 4. Electron micrographs of control (A) and monensin-exposed hepatocytes (B). Hepatocytes were incubated in DME medium in the presence or absence of 5 μM monensin for 2 h, before the medium was removed and the cells prepared for electron microscopy. 6600x. Arrows indicate Golgi complex ($\rightarrow$)

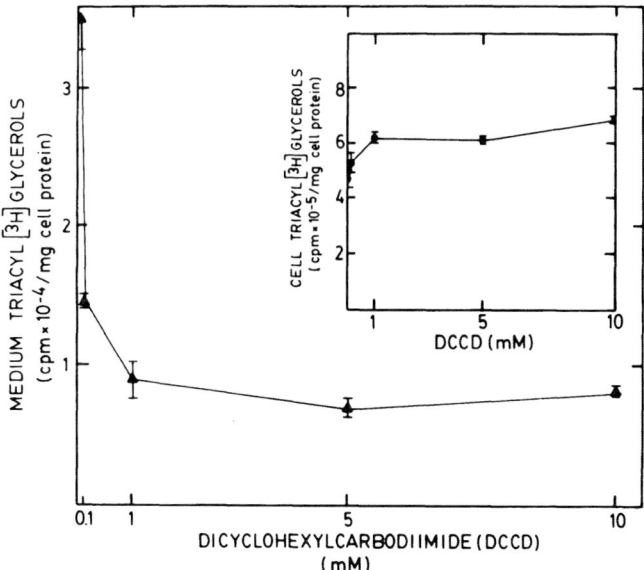

Fig. 5. Effect of dicyclohexylcarbodiimide (DCCD) on secretion (main figure) and synthesis (inserted) of triacyl(3H)glycerols. Hepatocytes were incubated in DME medium containing (3H)glycerol. After 30 min preincubation, the cells were added DCCD and reincubated for 2 h, before triacyl(3H)glycerols in media and cells were determined

Discussion

Our data demonstrate that monensin reversibly decreases receptor-mediated endocytosis of asialofetuin and secretion of VLDL in hepatocytes under similar conditions. The number of functional receptors goes down probably because monensin increases endosomal pH and this causes trapping of undissociated receptor-ligand complexes inside the cell (Harford et al., 1983).

The inhibitory effect of monensin VLDL secretion may be explained by its interference with the Golgi function, but the mechanism by which monensin works is unclear. It has been demonstrated that weak bases and DCCD promote a marked inhibition of VLDL secretion from cultured hepatocytes. In addition to our present data, those findings suggests that disruption of proton gradients might be crucial for cellular release of VLDL. In accordance with this, it has been shown that rat liver Golgi vesicles contain an ATP-dependent proton pump (Glickman et al., 1983, Zhang and Schneider, 1983). This suggests that certain compartments of the Golgi apparatus may contain acidic vesicles. The function of these compartments may be to release newly synthesized proteins from their postulated binding sites in vesicles responsible for transfer from endosplasmic reticulum to the Golgi compartment (Lodish et al., 1983).

Secretion of VLDL was more sensitive to low concentrations of monensin than was metabolism of asialofetuin. There was a marked decrease in VLDL secretion (at 1 μM-monensin), whereas binding and degradation of asialofetuin were almost unaffected.

One way to interpret these data is that monensin inhibits endo-and exocytosis via disturbance of proton gradients. It is most likely that monensin influences endosomes and Golgi apparatus separately, since the sensitivity to monensin of VLDL secretion is larger than that of endocytosis of asialofetuin. Another way to interpret our findings is that the asialofetuin receptor is recycled through a different compartment in the Golgi complex from that responsible for VLDL secretion. Although this explanation is possible, because of the well-recognized heterogeneity of the Golgi complex (Rothmann, 1981), most data support the idea that endocytosis of several ligands is independent of the Golgi function (Helenius et al., 1983).

Summary

1. Endo- and exo-cytosis were studied in cultured hepatocytes under similar conditions.
2. Monensin reversibly inhibits endocytosis of asialoglycoproteins and secretion of VLDL.
3. Disturbance of pH gradients may be the mechanism by which monensin exhibits its inhibitory effect on endo- and exocytosis. Other protein gradient disrupting agents e. g. weak bases (chloroquine, propylamine and ammonia) and dicyclohexylcarbodiimide (DCCD), a proton pump ATP-ase inhibitor, decrease secretion of VLDL.
4. The secretory process is more sensitive to low concentrations of monensin than receptor mediated endocytosis. Along with most other recent data this suggests that endo- and exocytosis are independent processes.

References

1. Basu SK, Goldstein JL, Anderson RGW, Brown MS (1981) Cell 24: 493-502
2. Berg T, Blomhoff R, Naess L, Tolleshaug H, Drevon CA (1983) Exp Cell Res 148: 319-330
3. Davis RA, Engelhorn SC, Pangburn SH, Weinstein DB (1979) J Biol Chem 254: 2010-2016
4. Debanne MT, Evans WH, Flint N, Regoeczi GE (1982) Nature (London) 298: 398-400
5. Drevon CA, Engelhorn SC, Steinberg D (1980) J Lipid Res 21: 1065-1071
6. Drevon CA, Tolleshaug H, Carlander B, Berg T (1983) Int J Biochem 15: 827-833
7. Glickman J, Croen K, Kelly S, Al-Awqati Q (1983) J Cell Biol 97: 1303-1308
8. Harford J, Wolkoff AW, Ashwell G, Klausner RD (1983) J Cell Biol 96: 1824-1828
9. Helenius A, Mellman I, Wall D, Hubbard A (1983) Trends Biochem Sci 8: 245-249
10. Lodish HF, Kong N, Snider M, Strous GJAM (1983) Nature (London) 304: 11-20
11. Nossen JØ, Rustan AC, Barnard T, Drevon CA (1984) Biochim Biophys Acta 803: 11-20
12. Pastan IH, Willingham MC (1981) Science 214: 504-509
13. Pedersen PL (1982) in Annals of the New York Academy of Sciences (Carafoli E, Scarpa A, ed) New York Academy of Science New York Vol 402: 1-20
14. Posner BI, Patel BA, Khan MN, Bergeron JJM (1982) J Biol Chem 257: 5789-5799
15. Pressmann BC (1976) Annu Rev Biochem 45: 501-530
16. Rothman JE (1981) Science 213: 1212-1219
17. Rustan AC, Nossen JØ, Berg T, Drevon CA (1985) J Biochem 227: 529-536
18. Tartakoff AM, Vassalli P (1977) J Exp Med 146: 1332-1345
19. Uchida N, Smilowitz H, Tanzer ML (1979) Proc Natl Acad Sci (USA) 76: 1868-1872
20. Wilcox DK, Kitson RP, Widnell CC (1982) J Cell Biol 92: 859-864
21. Zhang F, Schneider DL (1983) Biochem Biophys Res Commun 114: 620-625

Membrane Transport of Amphiphilic Compounds by Hepatocytes

H.-P. Buscher[1], G. Fricker[2], W. Gerok[1], W. Kramer[2], G. Kurz[2],
M. Müller[2], and S. Schneider[2]

[1] Medizinische Klinik der Universität, Freiburg, F.R.G.
[2] Institut für Organische Chemie und Biochemie, Freiburg, F.R.G.

Liver, being the central organ for degradation of compounds differing greatly in chemical and physical properties, must have the appropriate transport systems for vectorial membrane transport. Of outstanding interest are the transport systems for the great many of amphiphilic compounds, metabolites and xenobiotics, which are excreted hepatobiliarily, either unmetabolized or metabolized. In order to evaluate the number, the specificity, and the function of hepatic membrane transport

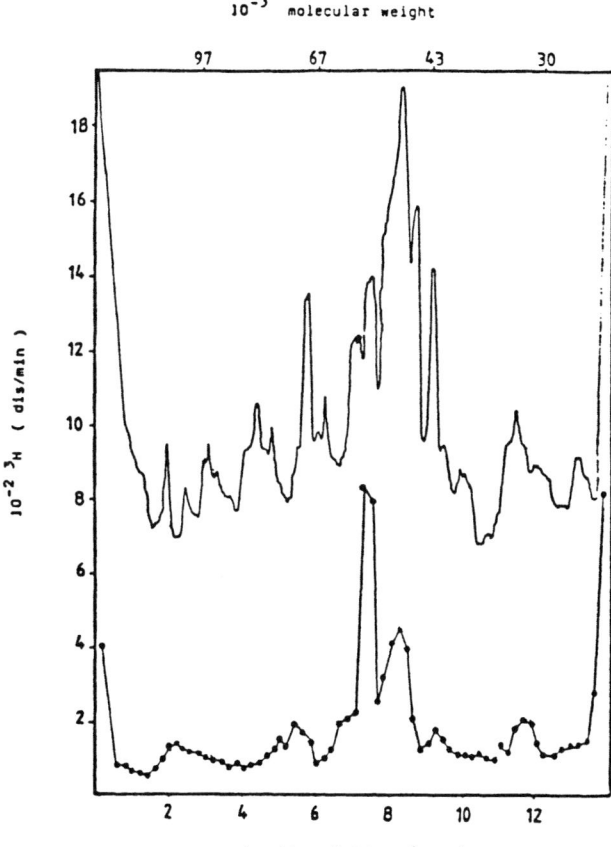

Fig. 1. Distribution of radioactivity after SDS-polyacrylamide gelelectrophoresis of the membrane fraction obtained after photoaffinity labelling of isolated hepatocytes with the sodium salt of (7,7-azo-3α, 12α-dihydroxy-5β-[3β, 12β-^{3}H]cholan-24-oyl)-2-aminoethanesulfonic acid (3.85 μM, 44 μCi). 5 ml suspension (5·10^6 cells per ml)

Receptor-Mediated Uptake
in the Liver
Edited by H. Greten, E. Windler, U. Beisiegel
© Springer-Verlag Berlin Heidelberg 1986

systems for amphiphilic substances representative compounds of characteristic substance classes and their appropriate photolabile derivatives were used for:

1. Kinetic studies   (K)
2. Photoaffinity labelling   (P)
3. Differential photoaffinity labelling   (D)

Because results obtained with membrane subfractions are of limited significance for the demonstration of an identified polypeptides function, and because hepatobiliary transport processes require the structural polarity of hepatocytes, photoaffinity labelling and differential photoaffinity labelling studies were not only performed with appropriate membrane subfractions but also with isolated hepatocytes and intact liver snips. Hepatocytes in such tiny liver snips (1-4 mm² cross-section, 2-5 mm height) have preserved their original structural integrity and their metabolic functions. Decisive for their suitability in transport studies is that they exhibit an intact hepatobiliary transport of bile salts, as demonstrated with the aid of the fluorescent derivative N-[7-(4-Nitrobenzo-2-oxa-1,3-diazol)]-3β-amino-7α, 12α-dihydroxy-5β-cholan-24-oate and its taurine conjugate [1].

Photoaffinity labelling studies with isolated hepatocytes using different photolabile bile salt derivatives, either unconjugated or taurine conjugated [2] result in

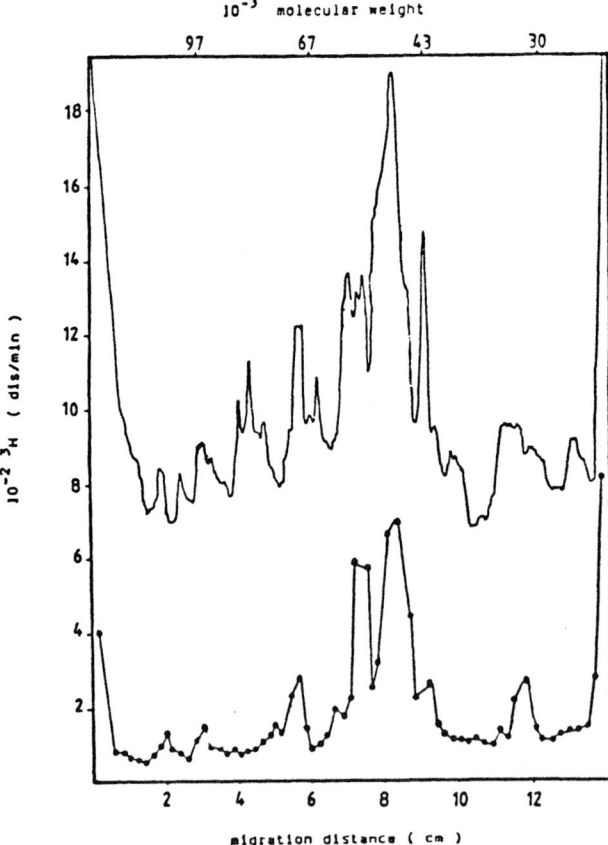

Fig. 2. Distribution of radioactivity after SDS-polyacrylamide gelelectrophoresis of the membrane fraction obtained after photoaffinity labelling of isolated hepatocytes with the sodium salt of (11-azido-12-oxo-3α, 7α-dihydroxy-5β-cholan-24-oyl)-2-amino [2-³H(N)] ethanesulfonic acid (3.56 μM, 26 μCi). 5 ml suspension (5·10⁶ cells per ml)

the labelling of two membrane polypeptides with apparent molecular weights of 54,000 and 48,000 (Fig. 1 and Fig. 2). The labelling of a polypeptide with the apparent molecular weight of 33,000 originates from a mitochondrial polypeptide [3], the isolation of which has been performed recently (U. Giese and G. Kurz, unpublished). The same two membrane polypeptides have been identified by photoaffinity labelling of a membrane subfraction enriched with sinusoidal surfaces [4].

The separability of membrane subfractions enriched with either of the two polypeptides by discontinuous density gradient centrifugation after photoaffinity labelling of sinusoidal membranes or of isolated hepatocytes (Fig. 3) suggests the existence of two different transport systems for bile salts in the membrane of hepato-

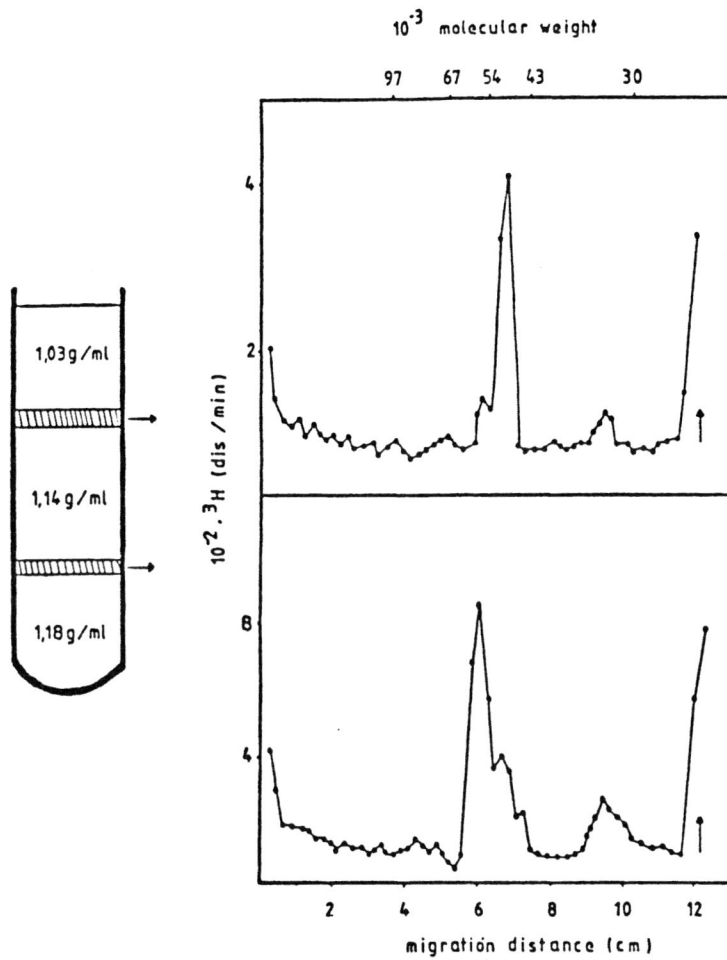

Fig. 3. Incorporation of radioactivity into polypeptides of plasma membrane subfractions of isolated hepatocytes by photoaffinity labelling with the sodium salt of (7,7-azo-3α, 12α-dihydroxy-5β-[3β, 12β-³H]cholan-24-oyl)-2-aminoethansulfonic acid. Photoaffinity labelling of a 5 ml suspension (5 x 10^6 cells per ml) with 0,22 μM (44 μCi) of the photo labile bile salt derivative. Subsequent to photoaffinity labelling plasma membrane subfractions were isolated by discontinuous sucrose density gradient centrifugation and subjected to SDS-polyacrylamide gelelectrophoresis

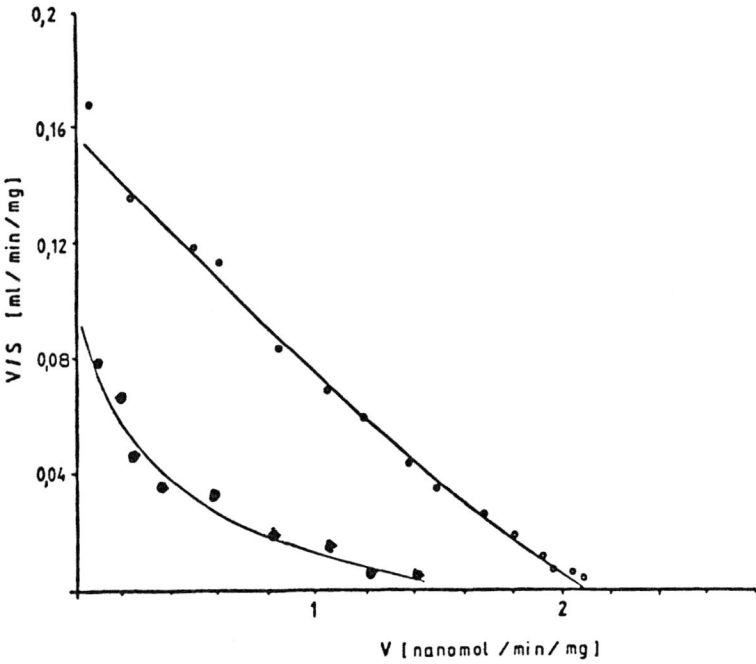

Fig. 4. Uptake of [³H]-taurocholate into isolated hepatocytes. The uptake was measured at 15, 30, 45, ..., 105 and 120 sec. The initial rate of uptake was calculated from the slope of uptake curves within the first 90 sec. (○) Uptake into hepatocytes prior to photoaffinity labelling. (●) Uptake into hepatocytes after photoaffinity labelling with sodium salt of (7,7-azo-3α, 12α-dihydroxy-5β-cholan-24-oyl)-2-aminoethansulfonic acid (400 μM). The cells were washed three times to remove unbound bile salt derivatives

cytes. This is in excellent accordance with the results of kinetic uptake studies (Fig. 4) which also revealed that two different uptake systems for bile salts are operative, the first with an apparent K_M for taurocholate of 11 μM and a V_{max} of 1,6 nmole/min/mg of protein and the second with an apparent K_M of 60 μM and a V_{max} of 0,5 nmole/min/mg of protein. The irreversible inhibition of both systems by photoaffinity labelling with the appropriate bile salt derivatives (Fig. 4) demonstrates that both polypeptides have a function in bile salt uptake by hepatocytes.

Photoaffinity labelling of liver snips and subsequent isolation of the membrane subfraction enriched with sinusoidal surfaces the labelling pattern of the membrane polypeptides demonstrates a clear incorporation of radioactivity into the polypeptides with the apparent molecular weights of 54,000 and 48,000 (Fig. 5). These polypeptides are also labelled at 4° C, where both bile salt uptake by hepatocytes and bile secretion are greatly reduced. This is in accordance with the results obtained with the membrane subfractions and proves that both polypeptides are localized in the sinusoidal membrane.

In the search for a bile salt secreting transport system subsequent to photoaffinity labelling of liver snips the membrane subfraction predominantly composed of

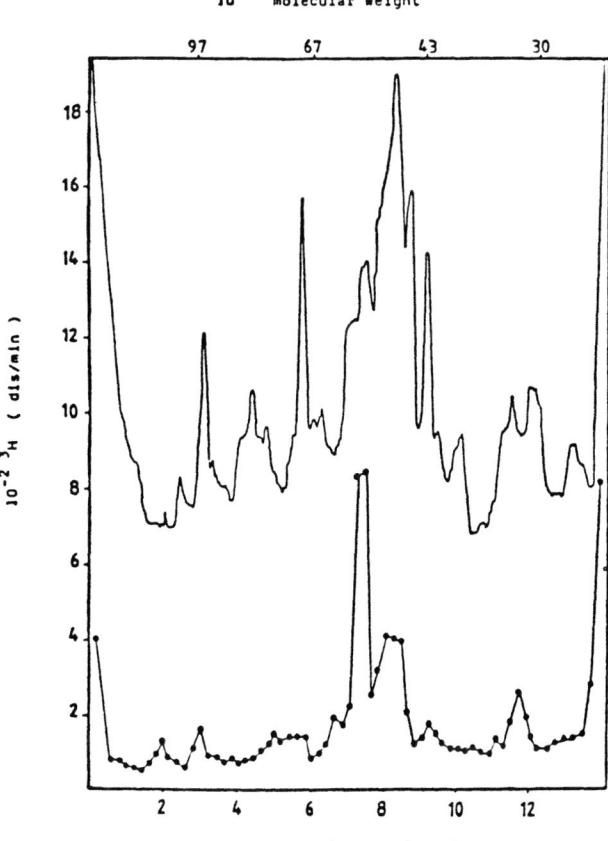

Fig. 5. Distribution of radioactivity after SDS-gelelectrophoresis of a sinusoidal plasma membrane fraction obtained after photoaffinity labelling of liver snips and subsequent removal of impaired cells with trypsin/DNAse. Photoaffinity labelling of liver snips with (7,7-azo-3α, 12α-dihydroxy-5β-[3β, 12β-³H]cholan-24-oyl)-2-aminoethanesulfonic acid. 20 snips were incubated with 1 μM (200 μCi) photolabile derivative

bile canalicular membranes was isolated and analyzed for labelled polypeptides (Fig. 6). The comparison of the resulting labelling pattern with that obtained after isolation of the membrane subfraction enriched with sinusoidal surfaces revealed that in addition to the polypeptides with the apparent molecular weights of 54,000 and 48,000 only one further polypeptide with the apparent molecular weight of 100,000 is labelled (Fig. 6). The labelling of this polypeptide is, compared with that of the other two membrane polypeptides, significantly lower at 4° C and does not occur in presence of Ca^{++} chelating agents. This polypeptide seems to be involved in the secretion process of bile salts, provided that the polarity of hepatocytes is preserved.

Kinetic studies suggest that the uptake of many other amphiphilic anions and even of phalloidin, a bicyclic toxic heptapeptide from the poisonous mushroom *Amanita phalloides* interferes with bile salt transport. In order to determine whether the same sinusoidal transport systems are involved in the uptake of these compounds differential photoaffinity labelling studies as well as direct photoaffinity labelling studies were performed with a photolabile derivative of phalloidin and

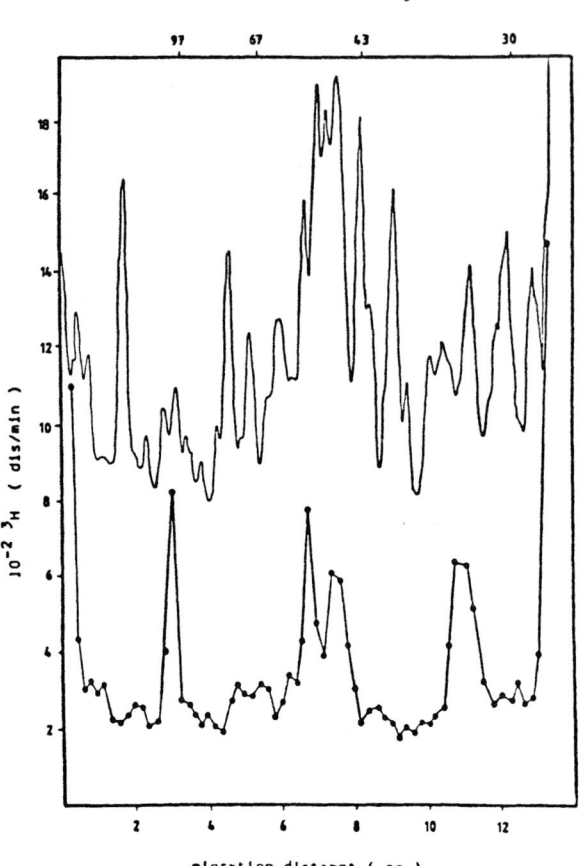

Fig. 6. Distribution of radioactivity after SDS-gelelectrophoresis of a bile canalicular membrane fraction obtained after photoaffinity labelling of liver snips and subsequent removal of impaired cells with trypsin/DNAse. Photoaffinity labelling of liver snips with (7,7-azo-3α, 12α-dihydroxy-5β-[3β, 12β-³H]cholan-24-oyl)-2-aminoethanesulfonic acid. 20 snips were incubated with 1 μM (200 μCi) photolabile derivative

of antamanide, a monocyclic decapeptide from the same toadstool, which inhibits the uptake of phalloidin into hepatocytes [5-7]. With both the photolabile derivative of phalloidin and of antamanide the same membrane polypeptides with apparent molecular weights of 54,000 and 48,000 were labelled as with the photolabile derivatives of unconjugated and conjugated bile salts (Fig. 7). The presence of bile salts and of antamanide decreased markedly the extent of labelling of the phalloidin-binding polypeptides (Fig. 8), just as bile salts and phalloidin decreased the incorporation of radioactivity into the antamanide-binding polypeptides.

Photoaffinity labelling of sinusoidal membrane subfraction as well as of isolated hepatocytes with bilirubin, a compound photolabile by itself, resulted in the labelling of the same two polypeptides (Fig. 7). By differential photoaffinity labelling studies and kinetic studies with a variety of anionic and uncharged compounds (Table 1) it becomes evident that the two sinusoidal transport systems are common for a multiplicity of amphiphilic anions and neutral compounds.

Amphiphilic monoquaternary and bisquaternary cations are readily taken up into liver. In order to see whether different transport systems are involved in the up-

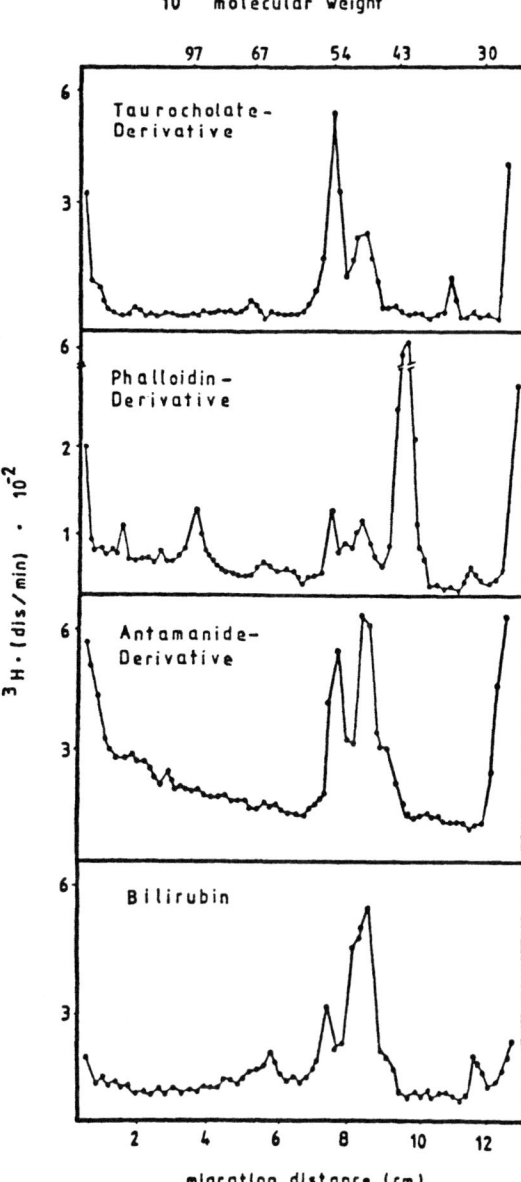

Fig. 7. Distribution of radioactivity after SDS-polyacrylamide gelelectrophoresis of the membrane fraction obtained after photoaffinity labelling of isolated hepatocytes. Photoaffinity labelling of a 5 ml suspension (5 x 10^6 cells per ml) with: **a)** Sodium salt of (7,7-azo-3α, 12α-dihydroxy-5β-[3β, 12β-^{3}H]-cholan-24-oyl)-2-aminoethanesulfonic acid (0,22 μM, 44 μCi). **b)** N^δ-4-[(1-azi-2,2,2-trifluoroethyl)benzoyl]-β-[2,3-^{3}]-alanyl-δ-aminophalloin (0,29 μM, 37 μCi). **c)** N^ϵ-[4-(1-azi-2,2,2-trifluoroethyl)-benzoyl]-[4,5-^{3}H]lys^6]-antamanide (0,32 μM, 40 μCi). **d)** Bilirubin (21 μM, 20 μCi). Subsequent to photoaffinity labelling the plasma membranes were isolated and the polypeptides were separated by SDS-polyacrylamide gelelectrophoresis

take of amphiphilic cations, anions and neutral compounds or the same, kinetic investigations were performed in combination with photoaffinity labelling studies using N-alkyl-21-deoxyajmalinium salts and appropriate photolabile derivatives. These amphiphilic compounds are monoquaternary cations under physiological conditions. Kinetic studies of uptake of N-(n-propyl)-21-deoxyajmalinium salts

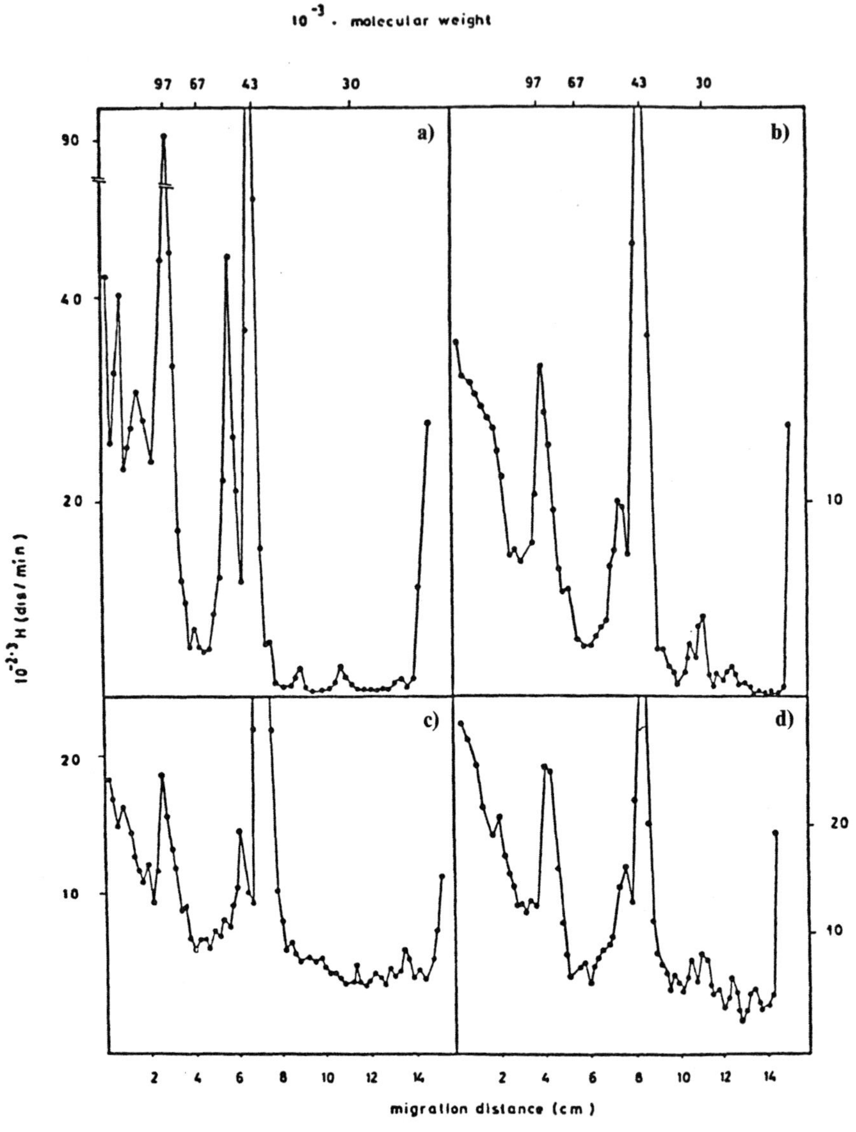

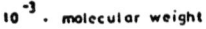

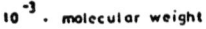

Fig. 8. Distribution of radioactivity after SDS-polyacrylamide gelelectrophoresis of the membrane fraction obtained after photoaffinity labelling of isolated hepatocytes. Photoaffinity labelling of a 5 ml suspension (5 x 10^6 cells per ml) with N^δ-4-[(1-azi-2,2,2-trifluoroethyl)benzoyl]-β-[2, 3-^{3}H]alanyl-δ-aminophalloin (0,39 μM, 50 μM), **a)** no additions, **b)** Presence of taurocholate (250 μM), **c)** Presence of antamanide (250 μM), **d)** Presence of cholate (250 μM). Subsequent to photoaffinity labelling the plasma membranes were isolated and subjected to SDS-polyacrylamide gelelectrophoresis

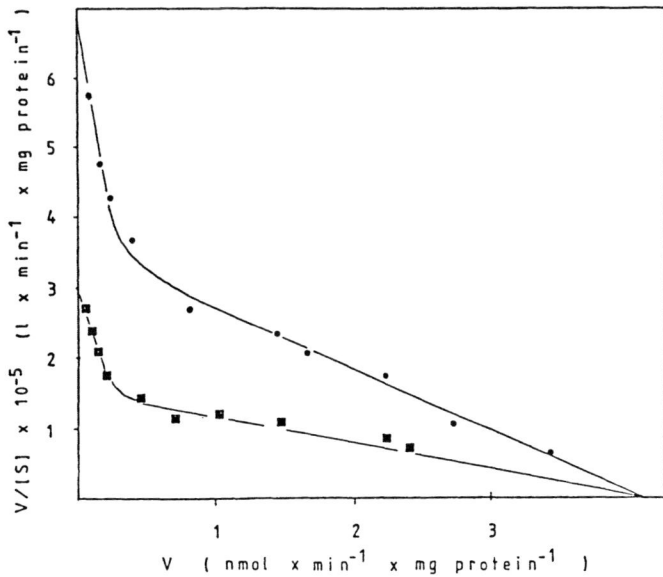

Fig. 9. Uptake of N-(n-propyl)-21-deoxy[21-³H]ajmalinium into isolated hepatocytes. The uptake was measured at 15, 30, 45,... 105 sec. The initial rate of uptake was calculated from the slope of the uptake curves within the first 90 sec. ○ no addditions, ■ presence of taurocholate (80 μM)

Table 1. Amphiphilic compounds competing for hepatic uptake Anions (acidic compounds)

bile acids	P.D.K.
bilirubin	P.D.K.
bromosulfophthalein	D.K.
indocyanine green	D.K.
iopodate	D.K.

neutral compounds	
phalloidin	P.D.K.
antamanide	P.D.K.
cholestanetriol	P.D.K.
hydrocortisone	D.K.
progesterone	D.K.
silybin	D.K.

cations (basic compounds)	
N-alkyl-deoxyajmalinium salts	P.D.K.
quinidine	D.K.
d-tubocurarine	D.K.
reserpine	D.K.
rifampicin	D.K.
procainamide	D.K.

P = photoaffinity labelling
D = differential photoaffinity labelling
K = kinetic studies

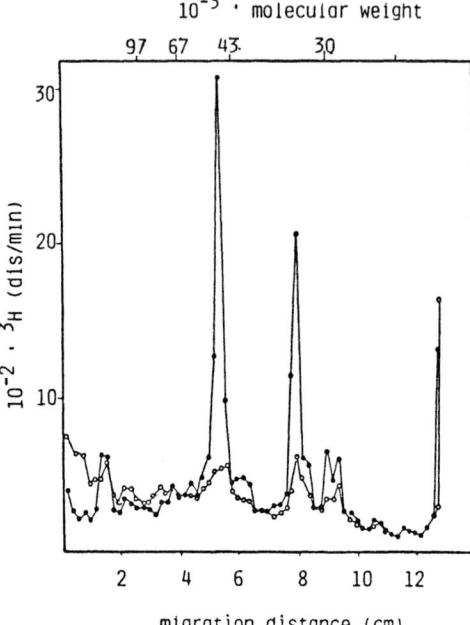

Fig. 10. Distribution of radioactivity after SDS-polyacrylamide gelelectrophoresis of the membrane fraction obtained after photoaffinity labelling of isolated hepatocytes. Photoaffinity labelling of a 1 ml suspension ($5 \cdot 10^6$ cells per ml) with N-(4,4-azo-n-pentyl)-21-deoxy [21-^{3}H]ajmalinium (3 μM, 7 μCi). ● no additions, ○ presence of quinidine (200 μM). Subsequent to photoaffinity labelling the plasma membranes were isolated and subjected to SDS-polyacrylamide gelelectrophoresis

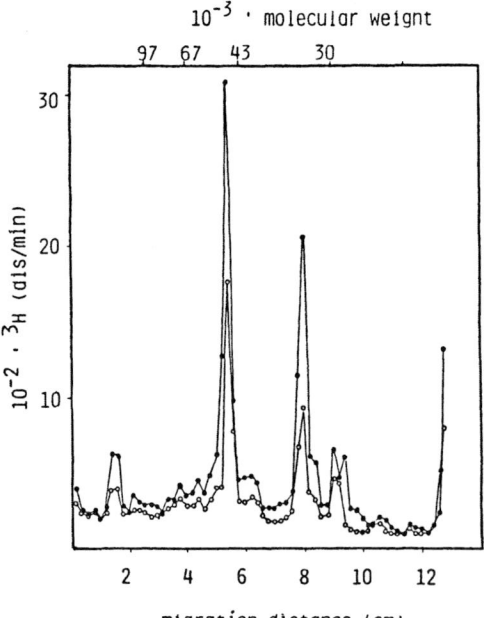

Fig. 11. Distribution of radioactivity after SDS-polyacrylamide gel-electrophoresis of the membrane fraction obtained after photoaffinity labelling of isolated hepatocytes. Photoaffinity labelling of a 1 ml suspension ($5 \cdot 10^6$ cells per ml) with N-(4,4-azo-n-pentyl)-21-deoxy [21-^{3}H]ajmalinium (3 μM, 7 μCi). ● no additions, ○ presence of taurocholate (200 μM). Subsequent to photoaffinity labelling the plasma membranes were isolated and subjected to SDS-polyacrylamide gelelectrophoresis

into hepatocytes showed that two different transport systems are involved, the first with an apparent K_M of about 1 μM and a V_{max} of 0.15 nmole/min/mg of protein and the second with an apparent K_M of 80 μM and a V_{max} of 4.0 nmole/min/mg of protein (Fig. 9).

Uptake of the N-(n-propyl)-21-deoxyajmalinium salts is not only competitively inhibited by amphiphilic cations as quinidine, d-tubocurarine, and by neutral compounds (Table 1) but also by taurocholate (Fig. 9). Photoaffinity labelling of the plasma membrane subfraction enriched with sinusoidal surfaces and of isolated hepatocytes with N-(4,4-azo-n-pentyl)-21-deoxy-[21-^{3}H]ajmalinium salt resulted once more in the labelling of membrane polypeptides with the apparent molecular weights of 54,000 and 48,000 (Fig. 10 and Fig. 11). It is evident that the extent of labelling of the polypeptid with the apparent molecular weight of 48,000 exceeds that of the polypeptid with the apparent molecular weight of 54,000, which appears only as slight shoulder in the peak caused by the other polypeptid. The appearance of a labelled polypeptie with the apparent molecular weight of 33,000 is caused by the mitochondrial polypeptia mentioned above.

Differential photoaffinity labelling with the monoquaternary cation quinidine (Fig. 10) and the anion taurocholate (Fig. 11) demonstrates that the same sinusoidal membrane polypeptides interact with amphiphilic anions and cations.

Summary

In accordance with the important function of liver in detoxification amphiphilic organic anions, neutral compounds, and cations are taken up into hepatocytes by two different uptake systems with a relative broad specificity.

References

1. Buscher HP, Gerok W, Kurz G, Schneider S (1985) in: Enterohepatic Circulation of Bile Acids and Sterol Metabolism, eds Paumgartner G, Stiehl A, Gerok W (MTP Press, Lancaster, England) in press
2. Kramer W, Kurz G (1983) J Lipid Res 24: 910-923
3. Abberger H, Buscher HP, Fuchte K, Gerok W, Giese U, Kramer W, Kurz G, Zanger U (1983) in: Bile Acids and Cholesterol in Health and Disease, eds Paumgartner G, Stiehl A, Gerok W (MTP Press, Lancaster, England) pp 77-87
4. Kramer W, Bickel U, Buscher HP, Gerok W, Kurz G (1982) Eur J Biochem 129: 13-24
5. Nassal M (1983) Liebigs Ann Chem 1510-1523
6. Nassal M, Buc P, Wieland T (1983) Liebigs Ann Chem 1524-1532
7. Wieland T, Nassal M, Kramer W, Fricker G, Bickel U, Kurz G (1984) Proc Natl Acad Sci USA 81: 5232-5236

Studies on Hepatocellular Uptake of Fatty Acids

W. STREMMEL, R. HÖDTKE, P. D. BERK, and G. STROHMEYER

Medizinische Klinik D der Universität Düsseldorf, FRG, and Mount Sinai School of Medicine, New York, USA

Supported by the Grant STR 216/2-1/2 from the Deutsche Forschungsgemeinschaft, Bonn, West-Germany

Introduction

Long-chain fatty acids are quantitatively the most important substrates for energy production. Their uptake by the liver is rapid, but little is known about the mechanism by which they permeate the plasma membrane. Investigation of fatty acid permeation, however, is potentially important since the influx of other major energy-yielding substrates, such as glucose and amino acids, has been shown to be a site of metabolic and hormonal control. The lipophilic character of fatty acids suggests that they might diffuse directly through the phospholipid bilayer of the membrane [1-3]. However, several recent observations suggest that at least a portion of fatty acid uptake might be mediated by a specific transport system [4, 5]. Studies with cardiac cells and adipocytes showed fatty acid uptake to be a saturable phenomenon [6, 7]; furthermore fatty acid oxidation in hepatocytes was inhibited by trypsin pretreatment of the cells [8]. Some investigators have argued that the apparent saturation of uptake observed in those studies, as well as the effect on uptake produced by sex hormones [9], fasting [10] and clofibrate [11] reflected saturation of an intracellular metabolic step rather than of membrane transport [12, 13].

For further evaluation of the uptake process determination of the driving forces and of the specific membrane transport machinery at the molecular level was essential. Therefore the aims of the present studies are:
1. To determine the interaction of free fatty acids with isolated liver plasma membranes;
2. To examine the nature of the hepatocellular uptake kinetics for free fatty acids in an isolated hepatocyte preparation.

Methods

Rat liver plasma membranes enriched in sinusoidal components were prepared from livers of male Sprague-Dawley rats by differential centrifugation [14] and characterized by electron microscopy and analysis of enzymatic markers [15]. Binding of a representative free fatty acid, ^{14}C-oleate, to rat liver plasma membranes was assessed by a centrifugation assay as described earlier in detail [16]. A specific

Receptor-Mediated Uptake
in the Liver
Edited by H. Greten, E. Windler, U. Beisiegel
© Springer-Verlag Berlin Heidelberg 1986

fatty acid binding protein was isolated from Triton X-100 extracts of total sinusoidal liver plasma membrane protein by affinity chromatography over oleate agarose [17]. After its physicochemical characterization [17] a monospecific antibody to the fatty acid binding membrane protein (FABMP) was prepared by intradermal immunization of rabbits. The distribution of the FABMP in various rat tissues was dermined by indirect immunofluorescence [17].

Rat hepatocyte suspensions were prepared by the collagenase perfusion technique of Berry and Friend [18]. Hepatocytes were incubated with 173 μM ^{14}C-oleate in the presence of various concentrations of bovine serum albumin, which served to modulate the free oleate concentration. After 10 sec to 7 min incubation, cell aliquots were transferred to 1 ml 200 μM phloretin/0.1% albumin to stop influx and efflux and remove surface-bound ligand, prior to determination of uptake by vacuum filtration [4]. For antibody inhibition studies hepatocytes were pretreated with the IgG-fraction of a rabbit antiserum to FABMP or with the pre immune serum as controls. Isolated hepatocytes (2 x 10[6]/ml) were incubated for 1 hour at 4° C with 100-800 μg of the appropriate IgG-fractions in a total volume of 3 ml. Antibody pretreated cells (2 x 10[6] cells/ml) were incubated with ^{14}C-oleate and for comparison with ^{35}S-BSP, ^{3}H-cholate and ^{14}C-taurocholate bound to albumin in various molar ratios.

Results

Since binding to plasma membranes represents the first step in any cellular uptake mechanism, binding of a representative fatty acid, ^{14}C-oleate, to rat liver plasma membranes was studied. Binding was shown to be saturable exhibiting a binding constant (K_{av}) of 2 x 10[8]M[-1], to be reduced by 50% following incubation of the membranes with trypsin and inhibited by heat denaturation of the membranes. The suggestion, that high affinity binding is due to an intrinsic membrane protein was confirmed by isolation of a single specific fatty acid binding membrane protein (FABMP) by affinity chromatography of the solubilized membrane protein mixture over oleate agarose (Fig. 1). This protein with a high binding affinity for variouslong-chain fatty acids but not for phospholipids, cholesterolesters, bile acids, sulfobromophthalein (BSP), or bilirubin, consists of a 40 kDa polypeptide chain with a pI of 9.0 lacking either lipid or carbohydrate components. The protein does not share immunologic determinants with either ligandin or the cytosolic fatty acid binding protein (Z-protein). A rabbit antibody to this membrane FABMP selectively inhibited specific binding of ^{14}C-oleate but not of other organic anions to rat liver plasma membranes. Immunofluorescence studies localized the antigen in liver cell plasma membranes (Fig. 2) as well as in plasma membranes of other major sites of fatty acid utilization (myocardium, small intestine, macrophages).

In studies with isolated hepatocytes initial rates of fatty acid uptake (v_O) were determined under conditions where membrane permeation is rate limiting [4]. Influx of ^{14}C-oleate was shown to be saturable (K_m = 9.7 x 10[-8] M; V_{max} = 210 pmol x min[-1]/10[4] hepatocytes), reversible, pH- and temperature dependent with optima at 37° C and pH 7.4, reduced in trypsin treated cells, and therefore, pre-

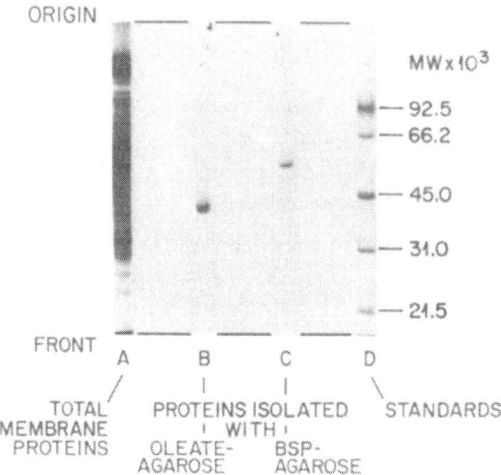

Fig. 1. Affinity chromatography of Triton X-100 solubilized proteins from rat liver plasma membrane proteins. Shown are Coomassie blue-stained cyclindrical gels after NaDod SO$_4$/PAGE of total solubilized membrane proteins (gel A), 40 kDa protein eluted from oleate agarose with 8M urea (gel B), 55 kDa protein eluted from BSP-agarose with BSP (20) (gel C), and standards (gel D; molecular masses in kDa, to right)

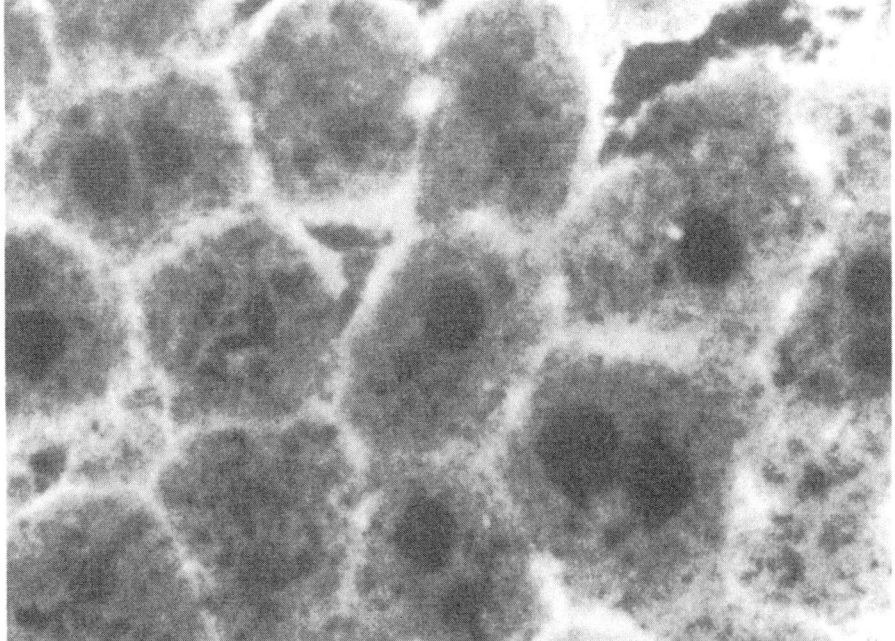

Fig. 2. Indirect immunofluorescence staining of the plasma membranes of hepatocytes in normal rat liver sections after incubation with an antibody to the fatty acid binding membrane protein

sumtively, carrier mediated. To evaluate the physiologic significance of the previously isolated rat liver plasma membrane FABMP as putative carrier protein in the hepatocellular uptake of fatty acids, the effect of the antibody to this protein on hepatocellular ^{14}C-oleate uptake was examined. When oleate uptake by hepatocytes pretreated with varying concentrations of the IgG-fraction of this antibody was compared with that of a control cell preparation pretreated with pre immune

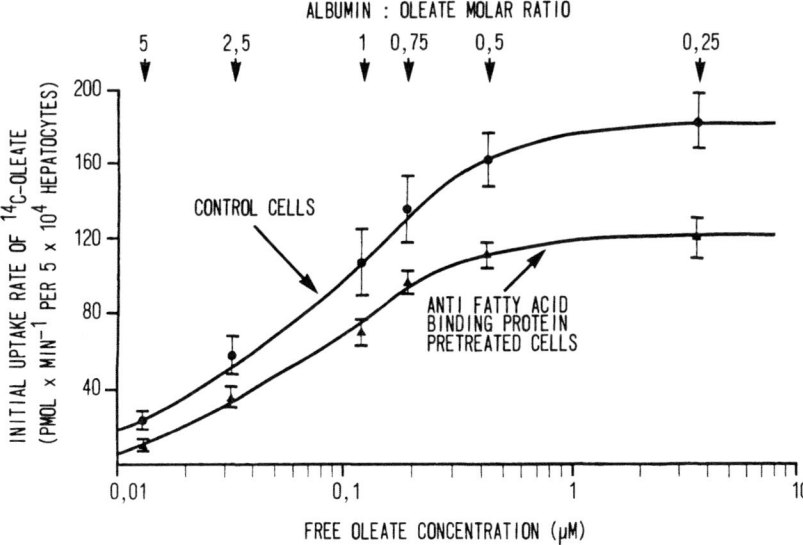

Fig. 3. Inhibition of ^{14}C-oleate uptake into isolated hepatocytes by the anti-fatty acid binding membrane protein. Cells pretreated with 400 μg of the IgG-fraction of the immune serum were compared to a control preparation pretreated with the pre immune serum. 250 μl of the cell suspensions (2 x 10^6 cells/ml) were incubated with 173 μM ^{14}C-oleate bound to albumin in various molar ratios at 37° C in 1 ml PBS. Illustrated are the initial uptake rates as a function of the calculated free oleate concentrations in the incubation media. ^{14}C-oleate influx is significantly reduced by the anti-fatty acid binding membrane protein

serum, a statistical significant inhibition of initial uptake velocity by the anti-membrane FABMP was clearly demonstrated (Fig. 3). In contrast, this antibody had no effect on the hepatocellular uptake of either taurocholate, BSP or cholic acid.

Since the anti-membrane FABMP inhibits the uptake of ^{14}C-oleate by isolated hepatocytes, these studies indicate that the liver plasma membrane FABMP must have a significant role in the hepatocellular uptake of free fatty acids. Furthermore, driving forces mediating the hepatocellular uptake of free fatty acids were determined. Hepatocellular uptake of ^{14}C-oleate by isolated rat hepatocytes is significantly decreased when 143 mM NaCl in the incubation medium is isoosmotically replaced by other inorganic salts (LiCl, KCl) or sucrose (Table 1). Quabain, which inhibits Na$^+$, K$^+$-ATPase, reduced the initial rate of oleate uptake by an average of 39%, suggesting that uptake might be linked to the activity of this enzyme. Phloretin, a potent inhibitor of a variety of cellular transport processes, inhibited uptake by a mean of 81%. Uncouplers of oxidative phosphorylation (2.4-DNP, CCCP) as well as the respiratory inhibitors (antimycin, KCN) also significantly inhibited oleate uptake. The effects of Na$^+$ substitution, ouabain and metabolic inhibitors are compatible with the hypothesis, that a component of fatty acid uptake is energy requiring, sodium linked and dependent on membrane Na$^+$, K$^+$-ATPase.

Table 1. Influence of external Na$^+$ on ^{14}C-oleate uptake by isolated rat hepatocytes

Buffer containing	initial uptake rate
143 mM NaCl	116 ± 11*
110 mM KCl/25 mM NaCl	75 ± 9
143 mM LiCl	57 ± 8
246 mM Sucrose	47 ± 7

* pmol x min^{-1} per 5 x 10^4 hepatocytes

Conclusion

Accumulating evidence thus suggests that the entry of free fatty acids into hepatocytes involves at least a component of membrane-associated carrier mediated transport. Since the membrane binding protein responsible for this process in hepatocytes also has been isolated from the principal site of fatty acid absorption, the jejunum [19], and identified in other sites of fatty acid utilization such as cardiac muscle and the macrophage [17], this transport system may prove to be an important aspect of the overall disposition of fatty acids throughout the mamalian organism.

References

1. Kuhl WE, Spector AA (1970) J Lipid Res 11: 458-465
2. Scow RD, Blanchette-Mackie, Smith LC (1980) Fed Proc 39: 2610-2617
3. Heimberg M, Goh EH, Lausner HJ, Soler-Argilaga C, Weinstein J, Wilcox HG (1978) In: JM Dietschy, AM Gotto, JA Onthro, Eds. Disturbances in Lipid and Lipoprotein Metabolism. Baltimore, Williams and Wilkins pp 251-267
4. Abumrad NA, Perkins RC, Park JH, Park CR (1981) J Biol Chem 256: 9183-9191
5. Abumrad NA, Park JH, Park CR (1984) J Biol Chem 259: 8945-8953
6. Samuel D, Paris S, Ailhaud GH (1976) Eur J Biochem 64: 583-595
7. Paris S, Samuel D, Romey G, Ailhaud G (1979) Biochemie 61: 361-367
8. Mahadevan S, Sauer F (1979) Arch Biochem Biophys 164: 185-193
9. Kushlan M, Gollan J, MA WL, Ockner R (1981) J Lipid Res 22: 431-436
10. Christiansen RZ (1977) Biochim Biophys Acta 448: 249-272
11. Renaud G, Foliot A, Infante R (1978) Biochim Res Commun 80: 327-334
12. DeGrella RF, Light RJ (1979) J Biol Chem 255: 9731-9738
13. DeGrella RF, Light RJ (1979) J Biol Chem 255: 9739-9745
14. Fisher MM, Bloxam DL, Oda M, Phillips MJ, Yousef YM (1975) Proc Soc Exp Biol Med 150: 177-184
15. Reichen J, Blitzer BL, Berk PD (1981) Biochem Biophys Acta 640: 298-312
16. Stremmel W, Kochwa S, Berk PD (1983) Biochem Biophys Acta 112: 88-95
17. Stremmel W, Strohmeyer G, Borchard F, Kochwa S, Berk PD (1985) Proc Natl Acad Sci USA 82: 4-8
18. Berry MN, Friend DS (1969) J Cell Biol 43: 506-520
19. Stremmel W, Lotz G, Strohmeyer G, Berk PD (1985) J Clin Invest 75: 1068-1076
20. Stremmel W, Gerber MA, Glezerov V, Thung SN, Kochwa S, Berk PD (1983) J Clin Invest 71: 1796-1805

Inter- and Intracellular Transport of Retinol in the Liver

Rune Blomhoff, Kaare R. Norum, and Trond Berg

Institute for Nutrition Research, University of Oslo, Norway

Introduction

Following absorption and esterification by enterocytes in the small intestine, retinol is transported in lymph in chylomicrons [1]. In rats, the retinyl esters are relatively nonexchangeable components of the chylomicrons and their remnants [2]. Accordingly, nearly all the retinyl esters follow the chylomicron remnants when they are taken up by the liver [3]. Several studies have shown that chylomicron remnants are removed from the circulation by hepatic parenchymal cells [4-5], and that these cells express high affinity receptors that recognize the apo E of the chylomicron remnant particles [6-7]. We have studied the hepatic handling of chylomicron remnant retinyl esters. These results indicate that retinol taken up by parenchymal cells as part of chylomicron remnants may have two destinations.

Transfer of retinol from parenchymal cells to perisinusoidal stellate cells

First, some retinol taken up by the parenchymal cells may be transferred to stellate cells in liver for storage. This conclusion is based on a series of experiments in which chylomicrons labeled with radioactive retinyl esters were injected into rats [5, 8]. After 30 min, about 80% of the radioactivity injected was recovered in isolated parenchymal liver cells (Fig. 1). However, during the next 2-4 hours, a redistribution of radioactivity occured in liver. The amount of radioactive retinol decreased in parenchymal cells and reappeared partly in the perisinusoidal liver stellate cells [8]. After 4 hours, these stellate cells contained 60-80% of the total radioactivity recovered in liver [5,8] (Fig. 1).

Mass analysis of retinoids (retinol metabolites) in the various types of liver cells isolated from rats fed a normal pelleted diet, revealed that about 80-90% of the total amount of retinoids in liver was located in the perisinusoidal stellate cells as retinyl esters, with the rest located in parenchymal liver cells [9] (Table 1). Negligible amounts of retinoids were recovered in isolated liver endothelial cells or Kupffer cells. This massive storage of retinyl esters in stellate cells may be due to the observed transfer of newly absorbed retinol from parenchymal to stellate cells.

The transfer of newly absorbed retinoids from parenchymal to stellate cells in liver seems to be specific. Neither cholesterol [5] nor vitamin D_3 [10] which is taken up in parenchymal liver cells together with retinoids as part of the chylomicron

Receptor-Mediated Uptake
in the Liver
Edited by H. Greten, E. Windler, U. Beisiegel
© Springer-Verlag Berlin Heidelberg 1986

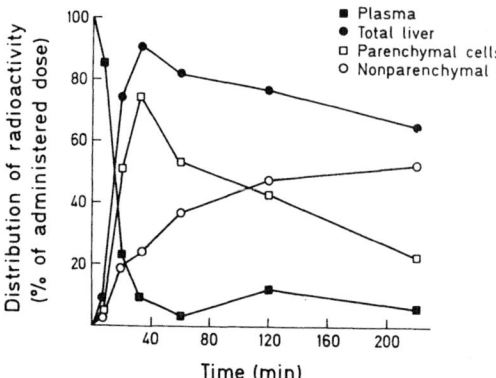

Intravenous injection of chylomicron
retinyl ester (4 I.U. [³H]-retinol)

Fig. 1. Intravenous injection of chylomicron retinyl ester (4 I.U. [³H]-retinol). The distribution of radioactivity in various liver cells was determined after intravenous injection of chylomicron (³H)reti-nyl ester into rats [5[. Radioactivi-ty in the nonparenchymal liver cells is almost exclusively due to radioactivity in perisinusoidal stel-late cells [8].

Table 1. Distribution of retinoids in liver cells

	nmol/10⁶ cells	nmol/g liver	% of total
Parenchymal cells	0.6	74	10-20
Endothelial cells	< 0.1	< 1	-
Kupffer cells	< 0.1	< 1	-
Stellate cells	31.0	354	80-90

The various liver cells were isolated from three-month-old male Wistar rats and the total retinoid content was determined. When converting values per 10⁶ cells to gram liver, it was assumed that the liver contain 190 x 10⁶ cells/gram wet weight, and that parenchymal, endothelial, Kupffer and stellate cells constitute 65%, 19%, 10% and 6% of the hepatic cells, respectively. The values are derived from Blomhoff *et al.* [9]

remnants, are transferred to any of the nonparenchymal liver cells. Furthermore, the transfer to stellate cells is strictly regulated by the vitamin A status of the ani-mal [5].

In addition to retinoids, some other molecules and particles are also known to be transferred between individual liver cells. One of these are hepatic lipase which is synthesized in the parenchymal cells and is then transferred to liver endothelial cells [11]. Other examples are carcinoembryonic antigen [12] and malaria parasite [13] which are cleared rapidly from the circulation by Kupffer cells. After modifi-cation in Kupffer cells, they are subsequently transferred to the parenchymal cells where degradations is completed. In addition, we have in a parallel study [14] shown that cholesteryl ester labeled acetyl-LDL is removed rapidly from the circu-lation by liver endothelial cells. About 1 hour after injection into rats, radioactive cholesterol was transferred to the parenchymal cells, and after a lag phase of 4 hours, significant amounts of radioactivity were recovered in the bile [14]. Little is at present known about the mechanisms of transfer for these various molecules between the different types of liver cells.

Transfer of retinoids from parenchymal cells to extrahepatic target cells

The second destination for retinol taken up by parenchymal liver cells as part of the chylomicron remnant particles, may be secretion from the parenchymal cells and transport to extrahepatic target cells. We have studied the intracellular transport of chylomicron remnant retinyl esters in parenchymal liver cells by means of subcellular fractionation in Nycodenz gradients [15]. Initially, radioactive retinyl esters are located in low density endosomes (d = 1.08-1.09 g/ml) (Fig. 2). Retinol is subsequently transferred to a denser vesicle (d = 1.14-1.16 g/ml) which comigrates with marker enzymes for lysosomes and endoplasmic reticulum [15] (Fig. 2).

Rate zonal centrifugation of Nycodenz gradients as well as equilibrium centrifugation of sucrose gradients indicated that this denser vesicle which contain radioactive retinol is not a lysosome since various lysosomal markers may be well separated from the vesicle containing radioactive retinol [15]. However, in all of these experiments, the dense retinol-containing vesicle comigrates completely with marker enzymes for endoplasmic reticulum.

We have also compared the intracellular transport of chylomicron remnant retinyl ester with the receptor mediated endocytosis of asialofetuin, which is a thoroughly studied system [15] (Fig. 3). Our results suggest that the (³H)retinoid and ^{125}I-asialofetuin follow the same path initially to the endosomes. After transit in endosomes, the intracellular transport differs. While asialofetuin is transported to

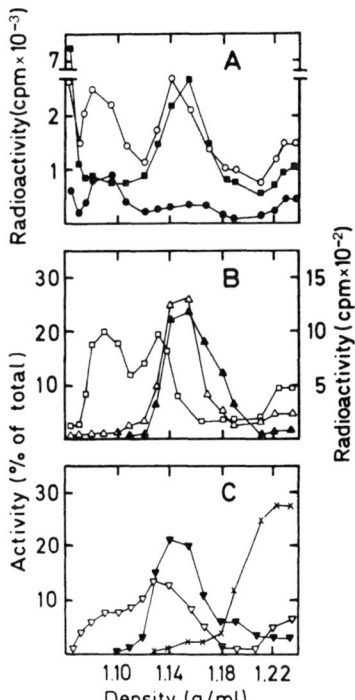

Fig. 2. Subcellular distribution in parenchymal liver cells of (³H)retinyl ester-labeled chylomicrons endocytosed in vivo. Cytoplasmic extracts from parenchymal liver cells prepared from rats which had received labeled lymph 15 min, 30 min, and 70 min prior to liver perfusion were analyzed in Nycodenz-gradients centrifuged to equilibrium. a) ³H-radioactivity was determined in the fractions (●, 15 min; ○, 30 min; ■, 70 min). b) ^{125}I-asialofetuin (□), glucose-b-phospastase (△) and rotenon insensitive NADPH cytochrom c reductase (▲) were determined in the fractions. ^{125}I-asialofetuin was injected 5 min before the start of the liver perfusion. c) 5' nucleotidase (▽), β-acetylglucosaminidase (▼) and catalase (x) were determined in the fractions (ref. 15)

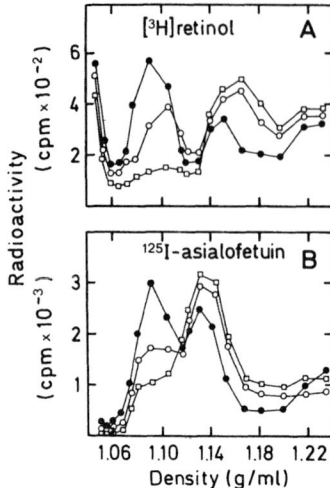

Fig. 3. Comparison of the subcellular distribution of endocytosed asialofetuin and retinyl ester-labeled chylomicrons. Parenchymal liver cells were loaded with **a)** (^{3}H)retinyl ester labeled chylomicrons (loaded 12 min *in vivo*) or **b)** ^{125}I-asialofetuin (loaded 5 min *in vivo*). Following incubation at 37°C for 0 min (●), 15 min (○) and 45 min (□) the cells were fractionated on Nycodenz gradients (85,000 x g for 5 hours) (ref 15)

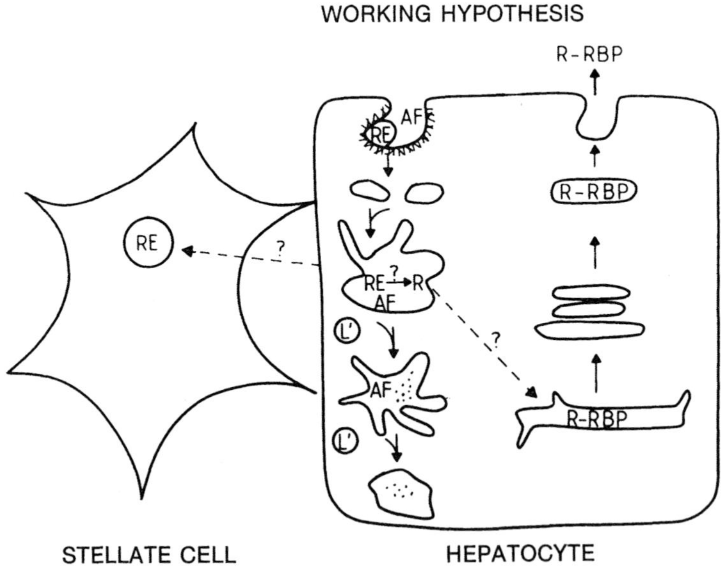

WORKING HYPOTHESIS

STELLATE CELL   HEPATOCYTE

Fig. 4. Working hypothesis for the intracellular transport of chylomicron remnant retinyl esters in liver parenchymal cells. The results suggest that chylomicron remnant retinyl ester and asialofetuin follow the same path initially to the endosomes. After transit in endosomes (or CURL) the intracellular transport differs. While asialofetuin is transported to a subgroup of lysosomes where the protein is degraded, the retinoid is probably transferred to endoplasmatic reticulum. Binding of retinol to RBP in endoplasmic reticulum results in a translocation of the retinol-RBP complex to the Golgi apparatus and then secretion from the cells. (RE, retinyl ester; R, retinol; RBP, retinol binding protein; AF, asialofetuin)

a subgroup of lysosomes where the protein is degraded, the retinoid is probably transferred to endoplasmic reticulum (Fig. 4).

It is known from other studies that retinol binding protein (RBP), the plasma transport vehicle for retinol, is found in high concentrations in rough and smooth endoplasmic reticulum [16]. Furthermore, binding of retinol to RBP located in endoplasmic reticulum seems to be a necessity for translocation of RBP from endoplasmic reticulum to Golgi and then secretion from the cells [17]. Hence, our suggestion that retinol is transferred from endosomes to endoplasmic reticulum fits well with the present hypothesis for retinol mobilization from the liver.

References

1. Goodman DS, Blaner WS (1984) In The Retinoids (MB Sporn, AB Roberts, DS Goodman eds) Academic Press Inc. Vol 2, pp 1-39
2. Blomhoff R, Helgerud P, Dueland S, Berg T, Pedersen JI, Norum KR, Drevon CA (1984) Biochem Biophys Acta 772: 109-116
3. Goodman DS, Huang HS, Shiratori T (1965) J Lipid Res 6: 390-396
4. Lippiello PM, Dijkstra J, van Galen M, Scherphof G, Waite M (1981) J Biol Chem 256: 7454-7460
5. Blomhoff R, Helgerud P, Rasmussen M, Berg T, Norum KR (1982) Proc Natl Acad Sci USA 79: 7326-7330
6. Windler E, Chao Y, Havel R (1980) J Biol Chem 255: 5475-5480
7. Hui DY, Innerarity TL, Mahley R (1981) J Biol Chem 256: 5646-5655
8. Blomhoff R, Holte K, Naess L, Berg T (1984) Exp Cell Res 150: 194-204
9. Blomhoff R, Rasmussen M, Nilsson A, Norum KR, Berg T, Blaner WS, Kato M, Mertz JR, Goodman DS, Eriksson U, Peterson PA (1985) J Biol Chem 260 (in press)
10. Dueland S, Helgerud P, Pedersen JI, Berg T, Drevon CA (1983) Am J Physiol 245: E326-E331
11. Jansen H, Hulsman WC (1980) Trends Biochem Sci 5: 265-268
12. Toth CA, Thomas P, Broitman SA, Zamcheck N (1985) Cancer Res 45: 392-397
13. Danforth HD, Aikawa M, Cochrane AH, Nussenzweig RS (1980) J Protozool 27: 193-202
14. Blomhoff R, Drevon CA, Eskild W, Helgerud P, Norum KR, Berg T (1984) J Biol Chem 259: 8898-8903
15. Blomhoff R, Eskild W, Kindberg GM, Prydz K, Berg T (1985) J Biol Chem 260 (in press)
16. Rask L, Valtersson C, Anundi H, Kvist S, Eriksson U, Dallner G, Peterson PA (1983) Exp Cell Res 143: 91-102
17. Ronne H, Ocklind D, Wiman K, Rask L, Øbrink B, Peterson PA (1983) J Cell Biol 96: 907-910

The Dynamics of Clathrin and the Coated Vesicle Pathway

CLIFFORD J. STEER and G. GARY SAHAGIAN*

Laboratory of Biochemistry and Metabolism, National Institutes of Arthritis, Diabetes, and Digestive and Kidney Diseases, National Institutes of Health, Bethesda, Maryland 20892

* Department of Physiology, Tufts University School of Medicine, 136 Harrison Avenue, Boston, Massachusetts 02111

Introduction

Eukaryotic cells display specialized regions of the plasma membrane which are involved in the endocytosis of macromolecules. These so-called "coated pits" were initially described in oocytes as 140 nm surface membrane diameter depressions exhibiting a 20 nm bristle-like coat on the convex cytoplasmic side [1]. Invagination of the coated pits gave rise to distinct subcellular organelles referred to as coated vesicles. Although coated vesicles have been implicated in a variety of cellular processes such as membrane transfer, membrane recycling, and intracellular shuttling of macromolecules, their major impact has been in the area of receptor-mediated endocytosis [2, 3]. Internalization of receptor-bound molecules at the surface membrane is achieved by clustering of complexes into coated pit regions which ultimately invaginate and pinch off to form coated vesicles. In most cell types, coated pits comprise about 2% of the surface area, turn over approximately every 3 minutes and number between 1000-2000. Under conditions of random diffusion, it has been determined that certain receptors encounter coated pits as frequently as every 3-4 seconds. The mechanism by which receptor-ligand complexes cluster in coated pits is, however, unknown [4, 5].

Electron Microscopy of Coated Structures

Coated pit regions of the hepatocyte surface membrane as seen by thin-section electron microscopy (Fig. 1 and 2) reveal that the structures are abundant along the base of microvilli and can be distinguished by their fuzzy or bristle-like appearance on the cytoplasmic surface. The clathrin coat, as it is now generally referred, is composed almost entirely of a 180,000 molecular weight protein (clathrin) which is capable of assembling into defined geometric arrays exhibiting five and six-sided faces. Kanaseki and Kadota were first to describe the geometric make-up of the coat material [6]. They were able, with the use of high magnification electron microscopy, to detail the clathrin coat as an array of hexagons and pentagons capable of transforming the underlying membrane into a coated pit and subsequently a coated vesicle. The mechanism by which clathrin initially assembles onto the surface membrane is unknown. However, Heuser using a technique of freeze-etching has beautifully illustrated that the coat does not form by coalescence of patches, but

Receptor-Mediated Uptake
in the Liver
Edited by H. Greten, E. Windler, U. Beisiegel
© Springer-Verlag Berlin Heidelberg 1986

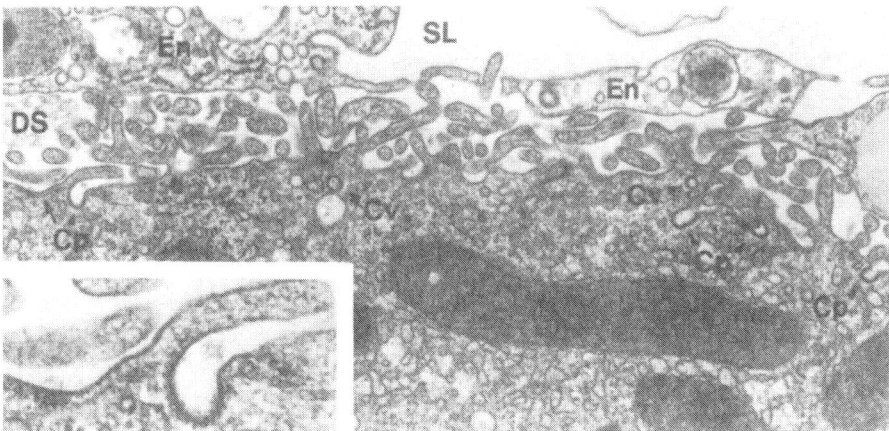

Fig. 1. Thin section electron micrograph of the sinusoidal region of an hepatocyte. Microvilli can be seen extending into the space of Disse (DS) which is separated from the sinusoidal lumen (SL) by an endothelial cell (En). Several coated pits (Cp) are seen at the base of microvilli. Coated vesicles (Cv) and numerous smooth-surfaced membrane vesicles are found within the cytoplasm. The inset shows a portion of the cell surface at high magnification to illustrate the coating on the cytoplasmic surface of a coated pit. (Reprinted with permission from Wall et al, *Cell* 1980; 21: 79-93.)

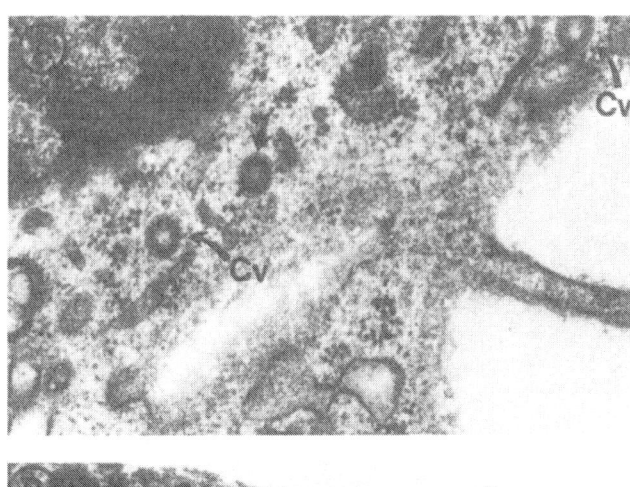

Fig. 2. Thin section electron micrograph of the plasma membrane region of liver cells stained with tannic acid to accentuate the clathrin coat of coated vesicles in an (**a**) hepatocyte and an (**b**) endothelial cell

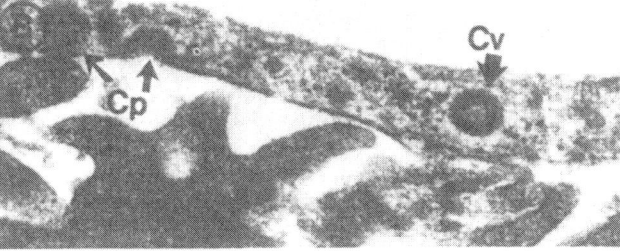

rather by piecemeal assembly [7]. The flat membrane is initially coated on its cyto-plasmic side by an array of hexagons afterwhich pentagons are introduced in order to curve the structure. Using a combination of freeze-fracture, deep-etching and rotary replication, Heuser has provided a superlative view of the dynamics of the coated membrane at the hepatocyte cell surface (Fig. 3).

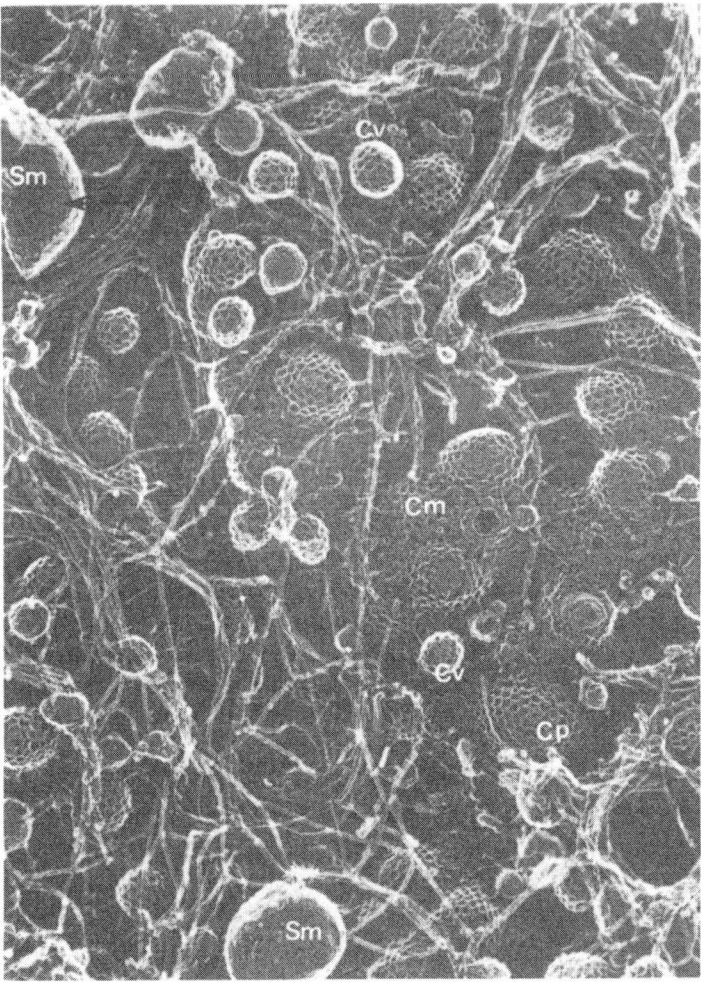

Fig. 3. Survey view of the cytoplasmic surface of a liver cell plasma membrane in a non-junction area. Prominent are numerous clathrin basketworks forming coated membranes (Cm), coated pits (Cp) and coated vesicles (Cv) as well as many smooth-surfaced membranes (Sm) and interme-diate filaments (thick arrow). Intramembranous particles are particularly prominent in the smooth-surfaced vesicles (thin arrow). (Reprinted with permission from Hirokawa and Heuser, *Cell* 1982; 30: 395-406.)

Dynamics of Coated Vesicle Formation

In an attempt to explain the unique properties of the coated pit region, early studies focused not only on the protein content but also the lipid make-up of that domain of cell membrane. The original reports that isolated coated vesicles were devoid of membrane cholesterol were corroborated by subsequent studies employing Filipin, a polyene antibiotic, as a cholesterol probe [8, 9]. Absence of Filipin binding in the coated pit regions suggested that in some way these coated membranes represented specialized domains which acted as molecular filters for removing cholesterol and perhaps other lipids. The absence of sterol was considered important in increasing the lipid disorder and allowing the membrane to adopt the appropriate curvature necessary for coated vesicle formation. Subsequent biochemical studies, however, revealed that coated vesicles were not devoid of cholesterol. Also, the negative response of a coated membrane to Filipin was a result of the stabilizing influence of the clathrin coat inhibiting the characteristic structural perturbation of the Filipin-cholesterol complex [10]. The results, taken together, revealed that the lipid environment of both coated vesicles and coated pits was not significantly different from uncoated membrane domains. It has, however, been shown that the presence of the clathrin lattice on the membrane surface of intact coated vesicles increases the lipid disorder and therefore, the so-called, "membrane fluidity". Using infrared spectroscopy and comparing the lipid acyl chain symmetric methylene stretching modes at the range of 2850 cm^{-1}, it was recently shown that the clathrin coat significantly increases the number of *gauche* chain conformers in the bilayer matrix of the coated membrane assembly [11]. This membrane perturbation was felt to represent a fundamental requirement for the structural rearrangement asociated with membrane invagination and coated vesicle formation This marked membrane disorder was furthermore, present in the absence of a deep penetration by the clathrin lattice into the lipid bilayer.

Cellular Distribution of Clathrin

A number of studies have examined the cellular distribution of clathrin using immunocytochemical techniques (Fig. 4). The staining pattern of the anticlathrin antibody has revealed two distinct distributions of fluorescence in all cell types examined: a random perinuclear distribution as well as an orderly linear arrangement, which upon close examination was noted to be on or near the cell surface membrane [12, 13]. Staining patterns were unlike those of structural proteins including tubulin, tropomyosin and fibronectin. However, the linear dotted clathrin pattern followed closely the orientation of stress fibers as seen by phase contrast and anti-actin antibody immunocytochemistry. The results are interesting in light of a recent report that during axonal transport within the neuron, clathrin travels not with the fast moving membrane elements but rather with the slow moving cytoskeletal elements [14]. In particular, kinetic analysis revealed a preferential movement with actin in contrast to tubulin and neurofilament protein. Studies using sophisticated and improved staining techniques together with thin section electron micros-

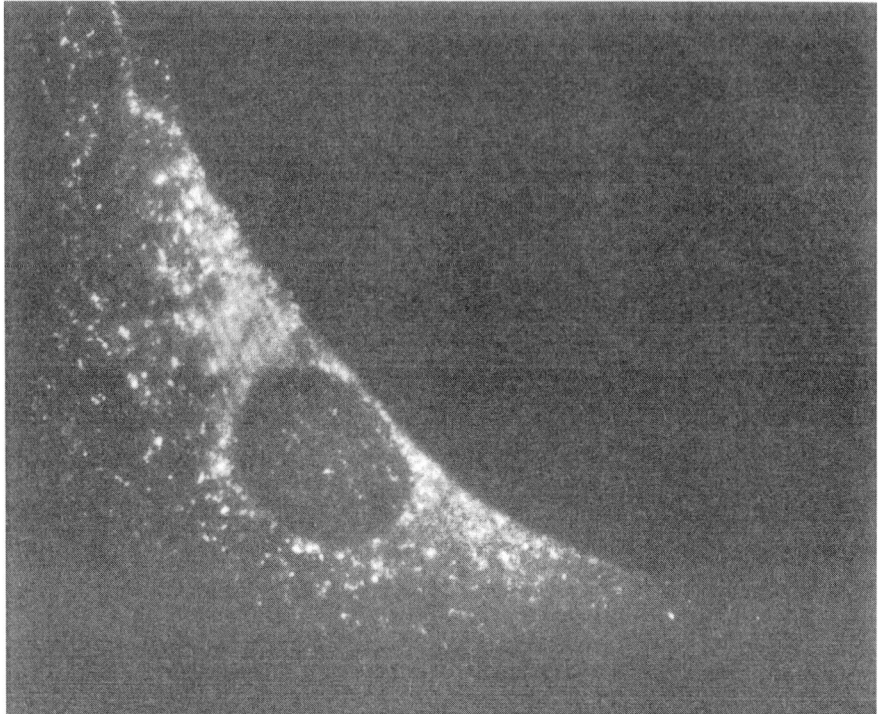

Fig. 4. Immunofluorescent localization of clathrin in a Swiss-3T3 fibroblast cell microinjected with antibody to clathrin. Aside from the punctate distribution over the entire cell, clathrin is concentrated in the perinuclear Golgi-GERL region. The lack of fluorescence in the cell located upper right indicates that only previously injected cells showed labeling with fluorescent antiglobulin. (Reprinted with permission from Wehland et al, *Cold Spring Harbor Symposium* 1982; 46: 743-753.)

copy revealed a similar distribution of coated vesicles, ie those involved in endocytosis at the plasma membrane and those involved in intracellular shuttling of macromolecules in the Golgi and peri-nuclear regions.

Although early studies argued against the presence of a soluble form of clathrin, more recent immunocytochemical studies using polyclonal antibodies argue in favor of its existence [15]. Furthermore, Louvard et al. have recently produced a monoclonal antibody that recognizes an epitope present on the clathrin heavy chain [16]. The monoclonal antibody gives a diffuse staining throughout the cytoplasm of cells suggesting the presence of a soluble, or non-membrane bound pool of clathrin. Further proof of the existence of an unassembled form of clathrin has been provided by Goud and co-workers who, by using polyclonal antibodies raised against clathrin, developed an enzyme-linked immunoassay that could specifically measure the quantity of clathrin in crude cell extracts [17]. Their results indicated that with the exception of brain cortex (0.7%), the amount of detectable clathrin is relatively constant among the various cell types (0.1-0.2% of total cellular protein). However, the fraction of assembled clathrin appeared significantly higher in those cells more active in endocytosis than exocytosis.

Coated Vesicles as Secretory Structures

There is increasing evidence that coated vesicles are intimately involved in secretory processes as well as intracellular shuttling of newly synthesized molecules. Early descriptions of identifiable secretory products in coated vesicles included prolactin, in cells of the anterior pituitary, glycoprotein components in seminal vesicle epithelium, as well as lipoprotein granules in isolated rat hepatocytes [18]. Friend and Farquhar studied the role of coated vesicles in the epithelium of the rat vas deferens and concluded that large coated vesicles (greater than 1000 Å in diameter) were derived from plasma membrane and served as vehicles to transport absorbed protein to lysosomes. In contrast, smaller coated vesicles (less than 750 Å) derived from the Golgi and peri-nuclear regions were felt to be involved in transport of hydrolytic enzymes from the Golgi complex to lysosomes [19]. More recently, several reports have appeared in which isolated coated vesicles were shown to contain newly synthesized lysosomal enzymes as well as certain precursor forms [20, 21]. Coated vesicles have been implicated in the transport of newly synthesized G protein of vesicular stomatitis virus as well as membrane proteins of the Semliki Forest virus to the surface of infected cells [22]. Bursztajn and Fischbach, using cultured embryonic chick myotubes, detected a subpopulation of coated vesicles which appeared to be involved in the transport of newly synthesized acetylcholine receptors to the cell surface [23]. Numerous other reports are providing increasing evidence for the role of the coated vesicle pathway in secretory processes as well as in phagocytosis and certain cellular growth characteristics [24, 25].

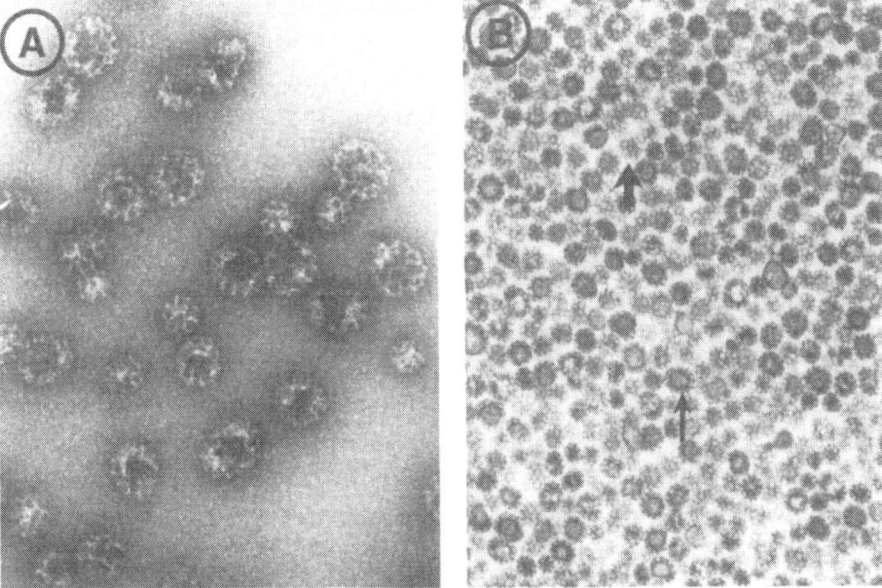

Fig. 5. Coated vesicles isolated from rat liver negatively stained with 1% uranyl acetate (**a**). Similarly prepared coated vesicles examined by thin section electron microscopy (**b**). The thin arrow points to a coated vesicle with an intact lipid bilayer in contrast to the thick arrow which identifies an empty coat structure.

Isolation of Coated Vesicles

A major breakthrough in the understanding of their molecular properties occurred in 1975 when Pearse purified coated vesicles from porcine brain to near homogeneity using sucrose density gradient centrifugation [26]. Coated vesicles have since been isolated from a number of tissues including human placenta, chicken oocytes, bovine adrenal medulla, bovine and porcine brain, rat liver and various established cell lines as well as bovine heart, liver, pancreas, spleen and thyroid. Since the original report, the Pearse procedure has been modified in several ways. Most important has been the use of deuterium oxide (D_2O) to replace the very high sucrose concentrations which were shown to have a dissociating effect on interaction of the coat protein with the lipid bilayer [27]. The modifications have resulted in not only elimination of very lengthy equilibrium runs, but have also resulted in greater yields of more homogeneous preparations of coated vesicles. The use of sizing columns such as Sephacryl S-1000, agarose gel electrophoresis and immunoadsorption of coated vesicles to polyclonal anti-clathrin antibody coated Staphylococcus aureus have provided the means of isolating extremely pure preparations of coated vesicles (Fig. 5). Furthermore, advances in electron microscopic techniques have provided more effective ways in which to examine the actual structural make-up of coated vesicles (Fig. 6).

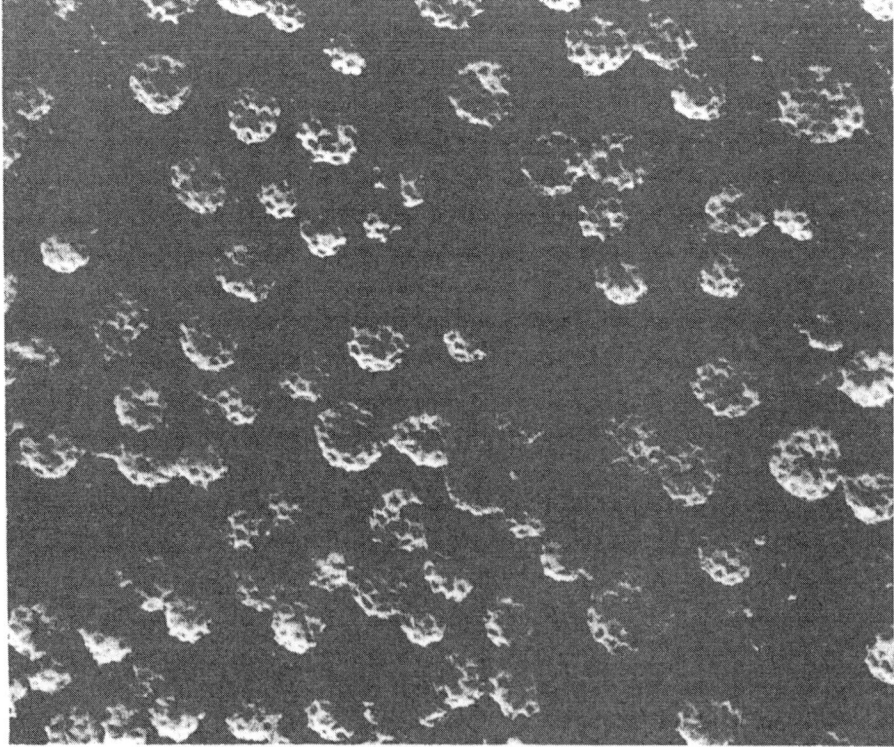

Fig. 6. Electron micrograph of coated vesicles isolated from rat liver and visualized by rotary shadowing. A contaminating smooth-membrane vesicle is identified by the arrow

Molecular and Biochemical Aspects of Coated Vesicles

Despite the common distinguishing feature of the surface lattice of protein molecules which form the coat, electron microscopic examination of coated vesicles isolated from various sources reveal marked heterogeneity in size [28]. Coated vesicles isolated from porcine brain range in diameter from 45-60 nm, in contrast to those isolated from human placenta which exhibit diameters of 70-120 nm. Recently, Steven and co-workers characterized rat liver and bovine brain coated vesicle size by computer analysis of scanning transmission electron micrographs of unstained specimens. They showed that brain coated vesicles ranged in diameter from 50 to 90 nm, whereas liver coated vesicles ranged from 50 to 150 nm [29]. The mass of brain coated vesicles ranged from 20 to 100 megadaltons with a weighted average of 35 megadaltons, while liver coated vesicles ranged in mass from 20 to 220 megadaltons with a weighted average of 66 megadaltons (Fig. 7 and 8). Examination of the mass to diameter distribution revealed that variation of mass to given diameter was a function of intravesicular content, in contrast to changes in the dimensions of the clathrin coat lattice.

Although an extensive size range is encountered among coated vesicles isolated from the various cell types, they appear amazingly similar on SDS-gel electrophoresis (Fig. 9). The 180,000 MW clathrin subunit accounts for 30 to 50% of the total coated vesicle protein, and appears to have been highly conserved across tis-

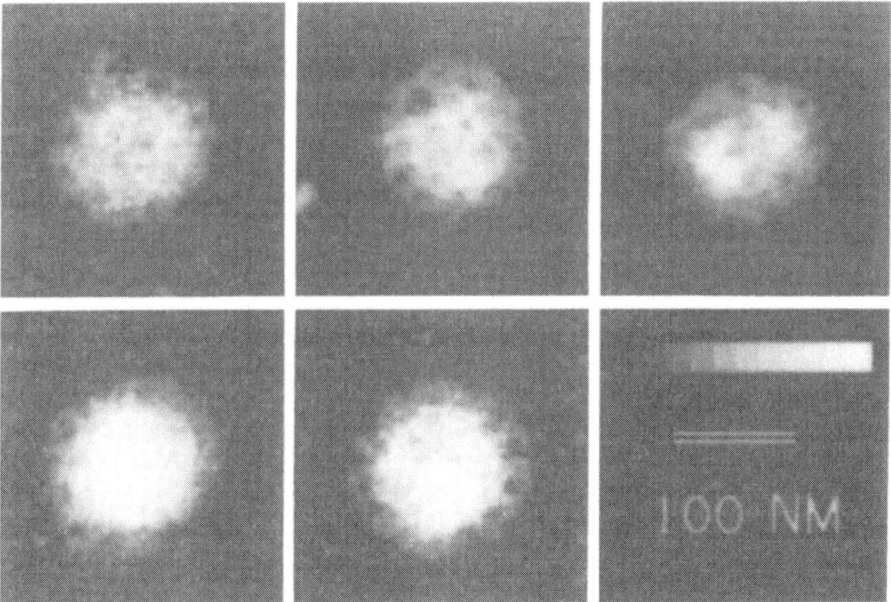

Fig. 7. STEM dark field images of unstained liver coated vesicles (LCV's). These particles were selected to illustrate the variation in mass among LCV's and, in particular, the variability in their vesicular internal contents. These particular LCV's have outer diameters of approximately 135 nm. (a) 104 Mdaltons (b) 95 Mdaltons (c) 85 Mdaltons (d) 186 Mdaltons and (e) 169 Mdaltons. (Reprinted with permission from Steven et al, *J Cell Biol.* 1983; 97: 1714-1723.)

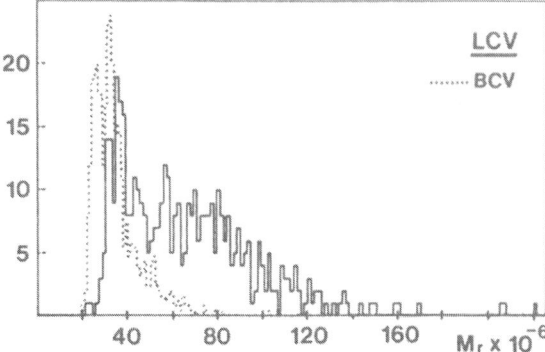

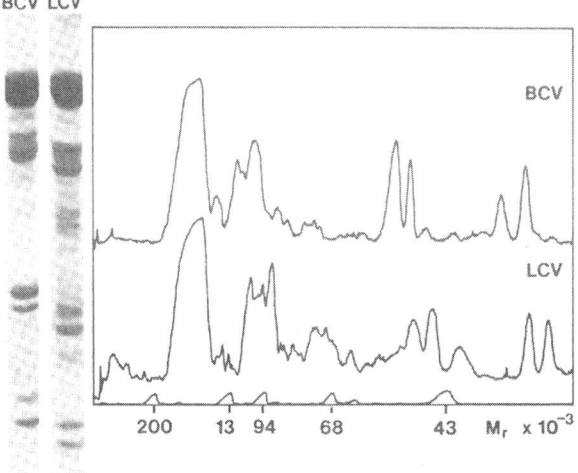

Fig. 8. Histogram illustrating the distribution of particle masses encountered in purified populations of liver (LCV) and brain (BCV) coated vesicles. (From Fig. 7 reference.)

Fig. 9. SDS-PAGE of purified coated vesicles from bovine brain (BCV) and rat liver (LCV). Densitometric scan compares the protein composition of the respective isolates. (From Fig. 7 reference.)

sue and species lines [30]. The patterns of secondary bands (ie 100,000 MW, 50,000 MW and 30,000 MW groupings) are also qualitatively similar to each other with perhaps some displacement in molecular weight. Several recent studies suggest that the 100,000 MW polypeptides are possibly involved in the assembly of the clathrin polyhedron as well as the putative binding of the lattice to the membrane surface [31, 32]. Antibodies against the 100 kd proteins, for example, have been shown to inhibit binding of radiolabeled clathrin to stripped coated vesicles. Similar results were noted after cleavage of the 100 kd peptides by gentle treatment of the intact coated vesicles with protease [33]. Aside from evidence to implicate the 50 kd proteins as an assembly factor to initiate lattice formation, attention has focused on the existence of protein kinase activity in this molecular weight range. Several groups have shown that at least one cyclic nucleotide-calcium independent protein kinase exists in the 50 kd range of proteins [34, 35]. Whether this protein kinase is involved in regulation of assembly factors is unknown. Pfeffer et al. has suggested that phosphorylation of the 51,000 MW polypeptide my play a role in the regulation of coated vesicle interaction with microtubules [36]. In this light, brain coated vesicles are particularly abundant with alpha and beta tubulin. Campbell and co-workers have recently described the existence of a phosphatidylinositol kinase in highly purified preparations of coated vesicles from bovine brain as well as rat liver and chick embryo skeletal muscle [37]. The production of phosphatidylinosital 4-phosphate by coated vesicles may play an important role in cellular phosphatidylinosital metabolism.

The Clathrin Triskelion

Coated vesicles are quite stable when isolated by procedures described above. They remain sedimentable and the coat remains intact, as determined morphologically and biochemically, for weeks at 4 ° C. Various reagents, however, have been found to promote the release of the coat lattice from the vesicle membrane, including various amines, low concentrations of urea, as well as slightly alkaline pH [38, 39]. Treatment of coated vesicles with such reagents results in release of the vast majority of the 180,000 dalton clathrin as well as other coat components, including two polypeptides in the molecular weight range of 30,000 to 36,000 (commonly referred to as "light chains"). Electron micrographs of the released coat material reveal pin-wheel-like structures exhibiting 3 extended arms of equal dimension (Fig. 10a). The three 445 Å legs bent at approximately 190 Å form a common vertex, were subsequently shown to interact with neighboring units to from the characteristic polyhedral coat surrounding the vesicle membrane (Fig. 10b). This legged trimer consisting of three 180,000 MW clathrin subunits together with three light chains of approximately 35,000 MW is referred to as a "triskelion" [40]. Under defined conditions, dissociated triskelions are capable of reassembly into cagelike structures resembling the surface lattice of coated vesicles (Fig. 10c). This ability to reas-

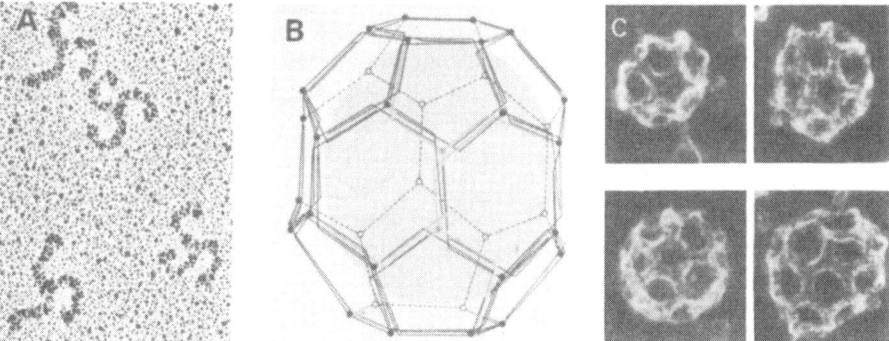

Fig. 10. (a) Electron micrograph of brain clathrin triskelions visualized by rotary shadowing. Magnification is 500,000 X (courtesy of Dr. Daniel Branton). (b) A schematic representation of the triskelions as they form the clathrin shell of a coated vesicle. 36 triskelions are organized to form a network of 12 pentagons and 8 hexagons. (Modified from *Molecular Biology of the Cell* 1983; pp. 255-318). (c) Clathrin shells reformed from brain triskelions. Each of the structures is composed of 12 pentagons and a variable number of hexagons depending on the size of the coat. Magnification is 230,000 X (courtesy of Dr. John Heuser)

semble appears to be based on an inherent flexibility of triskelions to not only remain compact but also to exhibit considerable overlapping properties.

Reassembly Properties of Triskelions

A number of studies have examined in detail the reassémbly properties of triskelions. Several groups have shown, for example, that disassembled triskelions exhibit 50% of the peptide backbone as α-helix [41, 42]. By examining infrared spectroscopic amide I and II vibrational frequency regions, Vincent and co-workers showed that as triskelions assemble into polyhedral structures they undergo a decrease in α-helical content, suggesting a significant change in secondary structure [43]. Based upon electron microscopic results of partially assembled cages, Crowther and Pearse postulated a system in which the clathrin arm represents a relatively stiff assembly unit exhibiting a variable joint at the vertex and a hinge approximately 160 Å from the common junction [44]. Protein assembly therefore, is the result of cross-over packing that permits each leg to interact with nearest neighbors and distant units. The model permits portions of the clathrin protein to form projecting knobs which may link the clathrin coat to the membrane vesicle. Using proteolytic dissection, Kirchhausen and Harrison have recently fragmented the clathrin arm and have generated a 52,000 MW subunit corresponding to the knob-like terminal domain at the tip of each arm [45]. It ist interesting to note that reassembly of triskelions into cages or onto vesicle membranes always results in polyhedral structures whose faces consist of 12 pentagons and a variable number of hexagons. Theoretical calculations show that such polyhedral structures can be constructed from a single species according to the principle of lowest strain energy [46].

Role of the Coated Vesicle Pathway in Receptor-Mediated Endocytosis

Aside from recent interest in the biochemical and biophysical characteristics of triskelions and the assembled clathrin coat, a major focus has continued as to the role of coated vesicles in receptor-mediated endocytosis. Binding of ligand to receptor at the cell surface is the first step in this endocytic process. The resulting ligand-receptor complexes diffuse within the plane of the membrane and cluster in coated pits. It has been suggested that ligand binding induces a change in the molecular shape of the receptor which in some way promotes clustering. Presently, there are a number of receptors which have been detected in coated vesicles from various sources, including those for LDL, transferrin, epidermal growth factor, α_2-macroglobulin, insulin, the asialoglycoproteins, the chicken hepatic lectin, as well as those for phosphomannosyl glycoproteins [47, 48]. Common to each of these receptors is the fact that the binding site is located within the vesicle lumen, ie outside the cell, and that in those cases studied exhibits a transmembrane orientation [49]. In the case of the mannose-6-phosphate receptor in brain coated vesicles (Fig. 11), a 12,000 MW portion of the polypeptide chain containing the COOH-terminal end was shown to be susceptible to proteolysis by both proteinase K and carboxypeptidase Y [50]. The orientation of this receptor with its C-terminal end exposed to the cytoplasm is similar to that of the LDL receptor. However, that

Fig. 11. Effect of protease treatment on the mannose-6-phosphate receptor of brain coated vesicles. (a) Intact vesicles or vesicles permeabilized with 0.1 % deoxycholate (DOC) were incubated at room temperature for 1 hr with or without proteinase K (PK) at a final concentration of 10 µg/ml. The vesicles were subjected to a 7 % polyacrylamide gel electrophoresis after which the mannose-6-phosphate receptor was detected by immunoblotting. (b) Intact vesicles or vesicles permeabilized with DOC were treated with carboxypeptidase Y (CPY) at the indicated concentration and/or 100 µg/ml of proteinase K and subjected to similar analysis as above. (Modified from Sahagian and Steer, *J Biol Chem.* 1985; 260: 9838-9842.)

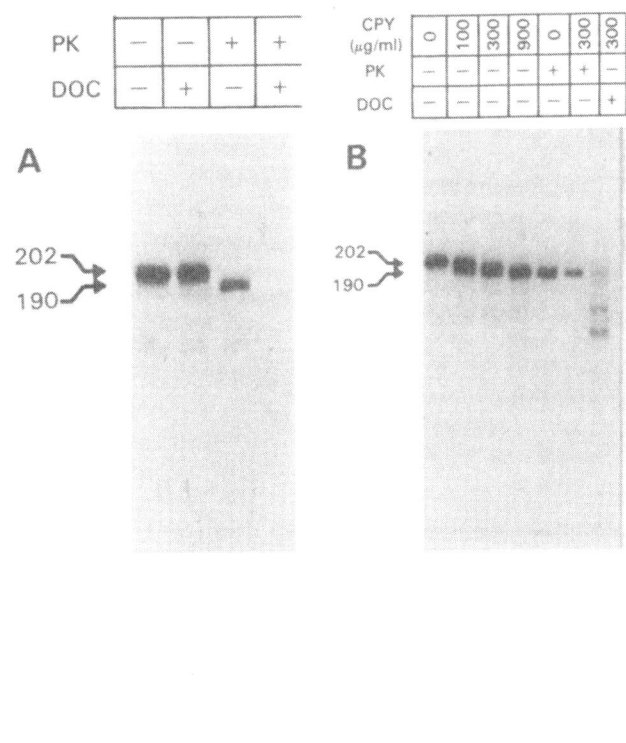

membrane topology differs from that of the transferrin receptor, the chicken hepatic lectin and the asialoglycoprotein receptor, all of which span the hepatocyte plasma membrane with the NH_2-terminus in the cytoplasm and their COOH-terminus exposed at the cell surface [51]. The significance of these divergent transmembrane orientations among the various receptors is speculative. However, it is not inconceivable that in either case, ligand binding promotes interaction between the receptors' cytoplasmic portion and a particular cytoplasmic factor, such as a component of the clathrin lattice.

The Uncoating ATPase

Many factors involved in coated pit/coated vesicle formation remain unknown. Even in the absence of ligands, electron microscopic studies have shown that membranes undergo the natural sequence of events to form coated vesicles. Under all conditions, however, once a coated vesicle is formed, it very rapidly loses its clathrin coat. Although coated vesicles have been shown to exhibit an ATP-dependent proton pump, which mediates intravesicular acidification and ligand-receptor dissociation, no correlation has been drawn between its activation and the spontaneous release of the clathrin coat [52]. Rather, Rothman and co-workers have recently isolated and characterized an ATP-dependent 70,000 MW uncoating ATPase which mediates the dissociation of clathrin from coated vesicles [53, 54]. The uncoating process was subsequently dissected into a two stage process [55, 56]. Initially, ATP hydrolysis drives the transient displacement of a portion of a triskelion from the polyhedron. In the second stage, the uncoating ATPase then captures the displaced triskelion by binding to a newly exposed site on the clathrin that had previously been hidden in the polyhedral lattice. The clathrin that is released consists of triskelions in a stoichiometric complex with the uncoating ATPase. Interestingly, there is evidence to suggest that the 30,000 MW light chains are required for the initial interaction with the clathrin coat by the uncoating ATPase [57].

Conclusion

A tremendous fountain of information has emerged since the initial discovery of coated vesicles in the late 1950's. They have shown themselves to be involved in a number of cellular functions including intracellular shuttling of molecules and membranes, as well as to play a major role in endocytosis. Numerous unanswered questions remain concerning their role in cellular homeostasis. Although the structural unit of the coat has been identified and characterized, many components of the polyhedron as well as their function(s) have yet to be discovered. Future studies will no doubt elucidate upon the "why's and how's" of coated vesicle formation and function.

References

1   Roth TF, Porter KR (1964) J Cell Biol 20: 313-332
2.   Goldstein JL, Anderson RGW, Brown MS (1979) Nature 279: 679-685
3.   Pearse BMF, Bretscher MS (1981) Annu Rev Biochem 50: 85-101
4.   Barak LS, Webb WW (1982) J Cell Biol 95: 846-852
5.   Goldstein B, Wofsy C, Bell G (1981) Proc Natl Acad Sci USA 78: 5695-5698
6.   Kanaseki T, Kadota K (1969) J Cell Biol 42: 202-220
7.   Heuser JE (1980) J Cell Biol 84: 560-583
8.   Severs NJ, Robenek H (1983) Biochim Biophys Acta 737: 373-408
9.   Montesano R, Perrelet A, Vassalli R, Orci L (1979) Proc Natl Acad Sci USA 76: 6391-6395
10. Steer CJ, Bisher M, Blumenthal R, Steven AC (1984) J Cell Biol 99: 315-319
11. Steer CJ, Vincent JS, Levin IW (1984) J Biol Chem 259: 8052-8055
12. Anderson RGW, Vasile E, Mello RJ, Brown MS, Goldstein JL (1978) Cell 15: 919-933
13. Willingham MC, Keen JH, Pastan IH (1981) Exp Cell Res 132: 329-338
14. Garner JA, Lasek RJ (1981) J Cell Biol 88: 172-178
15. Lin CT, Garbern J, Wu JY (1982) J Histochem Cytochem 30: 853-863
16. Louvard D, Morris C, Warren G, Stanley K, Winkler F, Reggio H (1983) The EMBO J 2: 1655-1664
17. Goud B, Huet C, Louvard D (1985) J Cell Biol 100: 521-527
18. Steer CJ, Klausner RD (1983) Hepatology 3: 437-454
19. Friend DS, Farquhar MG (1967) J Cell Biol 35: 357-376
20. Campbell CH, Rome LH (1983) J Biol Chem 258: 13347-13352
21. Schulze-Lohoff E, Hasilik A, von Figura K (1985) J Cell Biol 101: 824-829
22. Saraste J, Hedman K (1983) The EMBO J 2: 2001-2006
23. Bursztajn S, Fischbach GD (1984) J Cell Biol 98: 498-506
24. Aggeler J, Werb Z (1982) J Cell Biol 94: 613-623
25. Bastiani MJ, Goodman CS (1984) Proc Natl Acad Sci USA 81: 1849-1853

26. Pearse BMF (1975) J Mol Biol 97: 93-98
27. Nandi PK, Irace G, van Jaarsveld PP, Lippoldt RE, Edelhoch H (1982) Proc Natl Acad Sci USA 79: 5881-5885
28. Keen JH (1985) in: Endocytosis (MC Willingham, I Pastan eds), Plenum Press, 85-130
29. Steven AC, Hainfeld JF, Wall JS, Steer CJ (1983) J Cell Biol 97: 1714-1723
30. Pearse BMF (1978) J Mol Biol 126: 803-812
31. Zaremba S, Keen JH (1983) J Cell Biol 97: 1339-1347
32. Pearse BMF, Robinson MS (1984) The EMBO J 3: 1951-1957
33. Unanue ER, Ungewickell E, Branton D (1981) Cell 26: 439-446
34. Pauloin A, Bernier I, Jolles P (1982) Nature 298: 574-576
35. Campbell C, Squicciarini J, Shia M, Pilch PF, Fine RE (1984) Biochemistry 23: 4420-4426
36. Pfeffer SR, Drubin DG, Kelly RB (1983) J Cell Biol 97: 40-47
37. Campbell CR, Fishman JB, Fine RE (1985) J Biol Chem 260: 10948-10951
38. Keen JH, Willingham MC, Pastan IH (1979) Cell 16: 303-312
39. Woodward MP, Roth TF (1979) J. Supramolec Struct 11: 237-250
40. Ungewickell E, Branton D (1981) Nature 289: 420-422
41. Pretorius HT, Nandi PK, Lippoldt RE, Johnson ML, Keen JH, Pastan I, Edelhoch H (1981) Biochemistry 20: 2777-2782
42. Steer CJ, Klausner RD, Blumenthal R (1982) J Biol Chem 257: 8533-8540
43. Vincent JS, Steer CJ, Levin IW (1984) Biochemistry 23: 625-631
44. Crowther RA, Pearse BMF (1981) J Cell Biol 91: 790-797
45. Kirchhausen T, Harrison SC (1984) J Cell Biol 99: 1725-1734
46. Katsura I (1983) J Theor Biol 103: 63-75
47. Mello RJ, Brown MS, Goldstein JL, Anderson RGW (1980) Cell 20: 829-837
48. Steer CJ, Wall DA, Ashwell G (1983) Hepatology 3: 667-672
49. Holland EC, Leung JO, Drickamer K (1984) Proc Natl Acad Sci USA 81: 7338-7342
50. Sahagian GG, Steer CJ (1985) J Biol Chem 260: 9838-9842
51. Chiacchia KB, Drickamer K (1984) J Biol Chem 259: 15440-15446
52. Van Dyke RW, Steer CJ, Scharschmidt BF (1984) Proc Natl Acad Sci USA 81: 3108-3112
53. Patzer EJ, Schlossman DM, Rothman JE (1982) J Cell Biol 93: 230-236
54. Schlossman DM, Schmid SL, Braell WA, Rothman JE (1984) J Cell Biol 99: 723-733
55. Schmid SL, Rothman JE (1985) J Biol Chem 260: 10044-10049
56. Schmid SL, Rothman JE (1985) J Biol Chem 260: 10050-10056
57. Schmid SL, Braell WA, Schlossman DM, Rothman JE (1984) Nature 311: 228-231